HANDBOOK FOR HEALTH CARE ETHICS COMMITTEES

handbook

FOR HEALTH CARE ETHICS COMMITTEES

Linda Farber Post

Jeffrey Blustein

Nancy Neveloff Dubler

the johns hopkins university press baltimore

The views expressed herein by Kenneth A. Berkowitz are his and do not necessarily reflect the views of the VHA National Center for Ethics in Health Care, the Veterans Health Administration, or the Department of Veterans Affairs.

The views expressed herein by Jack Kilcullen do not necessarily reflect those of the Washington Hospital Center.

The views expressed herein by Tia Powell do not necessarily reflect those of the New York State Task Force on Life and the Law.

Nothing contained in this book is meant to imply or suggest any sponsorship, affiliation, or endorsement by Montefiore Medical Center of any of the opinions or positions taken in the book.

© 2007 The Johns Hopkins University Press
All rights reserved. Published 2007
Printed in the United States of America on acid-free paper
9 8 7 6 5 4 3 2

The Johns Hopkins University Press
2715 North Charles Street
Baltimore, Maryland 21218–4363
www.press.jhu.edu

LIBRARY OF CONGRESS CATALOGING-IN-PUBLICATION DATA
Post, Linda Farber.
Handbook for health care ethics committees / Linda Farber Post,
Jeffrey Blustein, and Nancy Neveloff Dubler.
p.   ; cm.
Includes bibliographical references and index.
ISBN 0-8018-8448-9 (pbk. : alk. paper)
1. Medical ethics committees—Handbooks, manuals, etc.
I. Blustein, Jeffrey. II. Dubler, Nancy N. III. Title.
[DNLM: 1. Ethics Committees, Clinical—ethics. 2. Bioethical Issues.
3. Ethics, Clinical. WB 60 P857h 2006]
R725.3.P67 2006
610—dc22   2006012324

A catalog record for this book is available from the British Library.

To all the health care ethics committees
whose work continually enhances
the quality of health care

CONTENTS

Anyone who has been paying attention to health care—patient, family member, professional care provider, policy maker, or interested observer—appreciates the profound changes during the past decades. Major advances in scientific knowledge, clinical skill, and technology have been paralleled by significant developments in how health care decisions are made and implemented. Decision making that used to be confined to the patient and family doctor now includes a whole cast of additional players, including consulting clinicians, relatives, health care proxy agents, risk managers, attorneys, judges, ethicists, organizational administrators, insurers, and other interested parties.

Among the most effective and valued resources in the health care decision-making process is you—the institutional ethics committee. As medicine becomes more complex, fiscal and bureaucratic pressures mount, and governmental regulations expand, clinicians and administrators increasingly look to you for analysis and guidance in resolving health care problems. Depending on the size and needs of the institution, the ethics committee typically serves as moral analyst, information clearing house, dispute mediator, educator, policy reviewer, and clinical consultant. The importance and scope of these responsibilities suggest that committees should be familiar and comfortable with bioethical theory and analysis, clinical consultation skills, institutional policies, legal precedents, organizational function, and resource allocation.

At this point, you have every right to say, "Are you kidding? Our committee is made up of clinicians and administrators who volunteer our time because we are interested in the ethical issues in health care. But it's all we can do to keep up with what we need to know to meet our clinical and administrative responsibilities. Don't ask us to take a course in bioethics."

Your very legitimate concern is what prompted this book—a handbook, not a textbook—that distills the important information and presents a basic foundation of bioethical theory and its practical application in clinical and organizational settings. Bioethics raises complex questions that require essays rather than short answers, and we have packed a great deal into this volume, including theory, vignettes, discussion questions, and suggested strategies. To make the material more accessible and useful, we have provided illustrative cases and ethical analyses to explain how the principles and concepts apply to what you do. The book is divided into the following sections, each of which addresses one or more ethics committee functions:

- an eight-chapter ethics curriculum, organized according to the issues that ethics committees typically address
- an introduction to clinical ethics consultation, including examples of clinical cases raising ethical issues that trigger requests for consultation by an ad hoc group and/or review by the full committee
- examples of memoranda, guidelines, and protocols that can be generated and discussed by ethics committees
- examples of institutional policies that would be drafted or reviewed by ethics committees
- an example of an institutional code of ethics
- summaries of key legal cases in bioethics
- a transcript demonstrating how an ethics committee would address a difficult issue referred for its consideration

This handbook grew out of the twenty-seven-year history of the Montefiore Medical Center Bioethics Committee and Consultation Service and the frequent requests from other committees to share what we have learned. While the examples are drawn largely from the Montefiore experience, our goal is to provide information and suggestions that can be adapted to the needs of a wide range of committees. In the pages that follow, we talk to the members of both well-established and newly formed ethics committees in large academic medical centers, small community hospitals, nursing homes, and other care-providing agencies. We hope that this resource will stimulate your committee, inform its deliberations, and enhance its contribution to the care delivered in your institution.

■

This handbook owes its existence and utility to numerous individuals and groups, whose invaluable contributions must be acknowledged. Because the book's inspiration is drawn from our collective experience at Montefiore Medical Center, most of those who were so helpful are part of that remarkable institution.

First and most important is the Montefiore Medical Center Bioethics Committee. Since its establishment in the mid-1980s, this multidisciplinary body has steadily increased the scope of both its membership and agenda, developing a considerable body of knowledge and skill in clinical and organizational ethics. The committee's eagerness to address new, sometimes controversial issues, its willingness to revisit previous recommendations in light of recent developments, and its determination to be actively involved in education, consultation, and policy review have made it a respected and routinely accessed institutional resource. This handbook reflects the considerable experience and insights of the Montefiore Bioethics Committee, which we hope your committee will find useful.

The effectiveness of an ethics committee depends in large part on whether it is marginalized or fully integrated into the functioning of the institution. The Montefiore administrative and clinical leadership has historically demonstrated support and respect for the Bioethics Committee, encouraging its robust role throughout the medical center. The collaborative relationship with the offices of the medical director, nursing, social work, legal affairs, and risk management has contributed significantly to the practical application of ethics described in this book. Medical Directors Dr. Brian Currie and Dr. Gary Kalkut, Director of Clinical Affairs Lynn Richmond, and Associate Legal Counsel Mary Scranton deserve special gratitude for their assistance in shaping the manuscript. Drs. David Hoenig, Martin Levy, Grace Minamoto, and Albert Sauberman provided important feedback on draft chapters that were piloted in their resident training programs. Dr. Kalmon D. Post read and reread the manuscript through its numerous incarnations and contributed valuable clinical insights. Maria denBoer provided meticulous manuscript review and editing, and Kim Johnson carefully guided the manuscript through production editing. Our extraordinary editor, Wendy Harris, shepherded the book from first draft to finished product with skill, support, tact, attention to detail, and surpassing patience.

Several people contributed their considerable expertise by writing selected portions of the handbook. Dr. Tia Powell, executive director of the New York State Task Force on Life and the Law, co-authored the introduction on the nature and functioning of ethics committees, which provides the context for the book. Dr. Kenneth Berkowitz, chief, Ethics Consultation Service, Veterans Administration National Center for Ethics in Health Care, co-authored chapter 9, "Approaches to Ethics Consultation," in part II. Dr. Jack Kilcullen, surgical critical care attending at Washington Hospital Center and former member of the Montefiore Bioethics Committee, wrote "Allocating Critical Care Resources: Keeping the Teeth in ICU Triage," which appears in part III. Research assistants Dr. Kiyoshi Kinjo, Katharine Michi Ettinger, and Margot Eves were enormously helpful in gathering and organizing material. Several institutions generously shared their policies for comparison in parts IV and VI, including The Cleveland Clinic, Hennepin County Medical Center, Lenox Hill Hospital, Long Island Jewish Medical Center, The Methodist Hospital, Montefiore Medical Center, Mount Sinai Medical Center, Oregon Health and Science University, University of California at San Diego Healthcare, and Wyckoff Heights Medical Center.

Finally, this book would not have been possible without the encouragement, critical commentary, and general forbearance of our families.

HANDBOOK FOR HEALTH CARE ETHICS COMMITTEES

Introduction:
The Nature and Functioning
of Ethics Committees

TIA POWELL, M.D., AND JEFFREY BLUSTEIN, PH.D.

Ethics committees vary from institution to institution along every significant dimension, including the number and qualifications of members, types of activities performed, the visibility of those activities, and perceived quality and usefulness. Across the country, some committees flourish while others fail to thrive. New committees, as well as those of long duration, can assess and change a variety of factors that may improve their chances of survival and add to their success in supporting the ethical practice of health care at their institutions.

FUNCTIONS

Traditionally, ethics committees have addressed some or all of three functions: education, policy development, and consultation. These functions are discussed in later chapters; here, we focus on the committee's obligation to define for itself which of these activities it will take on. In each of the three domains, the responsible committee members should clarify their goals and assess how they might attain them more effectively. For instance, if the ethics committee will provide ethics education, the committee should define its goals for education. A discussion aimed at improving educational efforts might focus on questions like the following: Toward whom should education be directed and in what format? Do committee members have sufficient expertise to teach ethics? Can they improve their knowledge base through continuing ethics education? If the hospital is affiliated with a medical school, are ethics committee members involved in teaching students? If not, can those who do teach students join the committee and lend their expertise to other groups within the institution? Are teaching activities geared to the needs of the institution? For instance, have members met with various groups, such as nursing, outpatient clinics, and the Emergency Department to see if they have a troubling case or other specific request for ethics teaching? Is there a set of basic topics in ethics for which the committee can offer instruction? Are there helpful articles and other prepared materials to distribute as part of the educational effort? Do teachers routinely provide evaluation forms so that they can learn which topics and instructors are well received and useful?

Similarly, the committee should assess its goals for policy development. If other groups also handle policy development, the ethics committee might collaborate in some cases or take over development of policies in others, depending on the policy in question. For instance, the ethics committee might serve as consultant to colleagues in palliative care for policies on pain control at the end of life, but might have primary responsibility for revising a policy on do-not-resuscitate orders. The ethics committee should not attempt to duplicate work that is already handled well elsewhere, particularly in the domain of policy development. Rather, designated committee members can reach out to other divisions within the institution so that ethics expertise may be incorporated into policies throughout all hospital departments.

ETHICS CONSULTATIONS AND COMMITTEES

Clinical ethics consultation is a particularly challenging function and is handled differently at different institutions. In some cases, consultation is handled by a subgroup of the ethics committee, while in other facilities an entirely separate group or individual provides consultation (Fox, 2002). If the ethics committee will take primary responsibility for ethics consultation, it needs to provide requisite training and support for consultants. This book provides a curriculum for such training; consultants may also wish to consider some of the training programs that are now emerging across the country.

MEMBERSHIP

The committee should examine whether its membership reflects sufficient diversity to represent the whole institution. While some early ethics committees were constituted entirely of physicians, a committee with such a limited range of members is unlikely to be an effective resource to the entire institution. For instance, a committee composed only of doctors is not best qualified to understand, support, and provide ethics expertise for nurses, social workers, and other health professionals. These distinct health professions adhere to specific codes of ethics and confront dilemmas that can differ from those that physicians face. Thus, allied health professionals will be represented on a well-designed ethics committee. Some committees, though by no means all, include community representatives as a way of bringing the patient's voice into the committee's deliberations. Community members who participate in clinical discussions regarding patient information must offer the same guarantee of confidentiality as health professionals.

Ethnic and cultural diversity is also important within the committee membership, because a significant number of consults stem from differences in religious practices and cultural expectations. For example, patients and family members from many cultures fear that full disclosure of a cancer diagnosis will rob patients of all hope (Powell, 2006). An ethics committee member from the same community serves as an educational resource to colleagues and as a helpful liaison to patients, professionals, and the committee.

As much as an effective committee requires diversity of representation, it also needs stability of membership. A frequently changing membership decreases the ease with which colleagues can identify those with ethics expertise. Moreover, the committee cannot build upon the experience and continued training of its membership if it is constantly changing. Committees with a high rate of turnover (or a significant proportion of no-show members) should view this as a sign of failure to thrive; busy professionals will not devote their time to a group that accomplishes little or whose work is of poor quality. In contrast, committees known for effective and skillful work enjoy a flow of volunteers seeking to join. Poor meeting attendance and a high drop-out rate signal the immediate need for intervention. The committee needs to address frankly every aspect of its functioning, from who chairs meetings and how effectively they are run, to whether the committee's goals are clear, realistic, useful, and adequately met.

The committee membership should be diverse in terms of whom it represents, but also must include a broad range of skills and knowledge. The American Society for Bioethics and Humanities produced a valuable report in 1998 entitled *Core Competencies for Health Care Ethics Consultation,* which is required reading for any ethics consultation service. Though specifically geared to the task of ethics consultation, these core competencies are also a useful benchmark for ethics committees that provide education and policy development. The skills and knowledge described need not all be present in the same individual. In fact, a great benefit of the committee structure is that collective expertise can surpass that of any one person. Some of the skills noted in *Core Competencies* are the abilities to identify and analyze values conflict, facilitate meetings, listen and communicate well, and elicit the moral views of others. Necessary knowledge areas are quite broad and include moral reasoning, bioethics issues, institutional policies, relevant health law, and beliefs and perspectives of staff and patients. Committees that function at a high level monitor their strengths and gaps in expertise and skill, and address those gaps by adding skilled members and/or encouraging continuing education for individual members and the group as a whole. In addition to ongoing educational efforts for members, a committee can also devise an orientation manual and a set of educational expectations for new members. Such a manual might include a list of useful reference works and journals in medical ethics, as well as copies of relevant institutional policies. Mentorship by a senior committee member to whom questions may be addressed, and information about continuing education opportunities would also be valuable. Providing a useful orientation for members new to the committee can be particularly helpful to those committees that have suffered from high turnover or low interest. Sitting through a series of meetings without having a clear role or understanding of the goals can lead new members to drift away instead of staying and contributing to the success of the committee.

EXPERTISE IN ETHICS

Ethics committees perform a unique function within a health care institution by virtue of the fact that they possess expertise in the area of ethics, an expertise that other bodies in the organization generally lack. Doubts may be raised, however, about whether there is such a thing as ethics "expertise" and, hence, whether any individual or group can possess it. The notion of expertise in ethics is not particularly fashionable these days in a culture like ours where relativism, or at least what passes for relativism, is in the ascendance and traditional views of legitimacy and authority are called into question. The notion of expertise in ethics also smacks of elitism, whereas it seems to be a hallmark of our democratic society that everyone is entitled to her own opinion about right and wrong. It is critical, therefore, to characterize accurately the sort of ethics expertise that ethics committees can offer.

As already noted, the expertise at issue here involves several components. Knowledge of general ethical concepts and principles and some understanding of ethical theory are important requirements, but not all committee members need have extensive philosophical training in ethics. Every committee, however, should have among its members an ethicist with at least some formal background in this area who is conversant with the relevant ethics literature and can educate other committee members in the fundamentals of ethics. In addition to familiarity with principles and concepts, committee members should be able to distinguish issues about which there is consensus in the literature from those that are controversial, to think about ethical problems in a critical and analytic fashion, and to be sensitive to and knowledgeable about cultural differences and power asymmetries in clinical practice. Clearly, there is much that committee members have to learn and, for this reason, committee self-education cannot be a one-time effort but must be an ongoing process.

Skills are also important ingredients of the ethics expertise that ethics committees possess, and they too require practice and continual honing. These include the following: the ability to communicate effectively and teach others; the ability to facilitate discussion and mediation of ethical conflicts; and, as a foundation for the rest, skill at discerning the existence and nature of particular ethical problems and dilemmas.

There are widely accepted ethical (to say nothing of legal) principles that limit the options available for solution of ethical problems, and there is a consensus within the medical and ethics literature on particular issues. Even when ethics committees have to work through cases involving patients and families from different cultures, cultural sensitivity, not a relativism of ethical view, seems to be the appropriate response. Finally, there is no basis for the charge of elitism if it is understood that everyone on the committee can make a valuable contribution to the identification, analysis, and resolution of ethical issues.

LEADERSHIP

Committee leadership is of crucial importance in shaping the nature and success of the committee. The tenure of the committee chair should be long enough for both hospital leadership and other colleagues to identify the leader with the ethics committee and its work. Though some committees have adopted a rotating chair, this strategy has the disadvantage of diffusing authority and decreasing visibility. On the other hand, some chairs do not provide effective leadership and an effort to support term limits may be a way to bring new energy to such a committee. The ethics committee chair should be a person respected within the institution, as well as someone with ethics expertise, yet not every facility contains a person who fits this description ideally. Committees whose chair has great institutional credibility but limited formal training should be especially conscientious in continual self-education and efforts to enlist ethics professionals with formal training. A committee whose chair offers formal ethics expertise but limited clinical experience or institutional recognition must build collegial relationships with clinicians. A strong, knowledgeable, and well-respected committee chair is critical to ethics committee survival. The ethics committee chair functions as liaison between the committee and the rest of the institution. When the committee finds that a difficult recommendation is nonetheless the right one, a chair with strong collegial ties to leadership can help present the committee's views effectively. A committee chair who antagonizes colleagues with judgmental or arrogant pronouncements about what is and is not ethical undermines the work of the committee and may even cause its demise. In contrast, a chair who mediates conflict and addresses ethical tensions effectively and respectfully is an invaluable asset to the committee and the institution.

SECURING A FOOTHOLD

The ethics committee should be situated within the overall structure of hospital governance. Whether the committee reports to the medical board or directly to the hospital leadership, a clear reporting structure creates accountability for the ethics committee, as is appropriate for any workgroup in the institution. At the same time, the reporting structure shows the committee where it may turn when it requires additional support. That support may be financial, for example, funding for a lecture series, or it may be political, as when the committee wants to address a controversial topic like questionable billing practices in one hospital division.

An ethics committee will not flourish and may not even survive in a useful way unless it has the support of the institution, from both leadership and staff. Hospitals in which senior leaders are committed to ethics reflect that commitment in large and small ways throughout the institution. On the other hand, if a key leader—for instance, the chair of a powerful department—doubts the value of ethics endeavors, the institution will follow that lead and ethics activities will be peripheral to the hospital's mission. New committees and those hoping to improve their efficacy need to examine their level of institutional support. Keeping in mind that hospital directors face extraordinary demands on their time, attention, and financial resources, the ethics committee may wish to consider ways in which support might be increased. Before approaching leadership to ask for support in terms of space, money, or other resources, the committee should define what it offers the institution in exchange for that support. An ethics committee that can show that its current or planned services are important and effective is far more likely to win initial or sustained support than a committee that can define neither its goals nor its accomplishments. The task of clearly defining goals and seeking more effective ways to attain them is a key aspect of earning and deserving support from hospital leadership. Ethics committees that assume that their name alone assures them of support are unlikely to flourish.

Support does not only come from above. A committee may enjoy strong backing from leadership but fail to win the respect of colleagues; such a committee will not thrive. Therefore, in addition to winning the confidence of the institution's leadership, the committee must gain a broad base of support from staff in different departments and roles. The best way to earn support, of course, is to provide a valuable service. A committee that actively seeks out ways in which it can be helpful and provides useful assistance in addressing ethical problems will enjoy the support of its lucky institution; an ethics committee that sits alone in the boardroom waiting for consults will fail. The delicate balance here is to avoid intruding while providing easy and broad access to ethics expertise. Some ethics committees and consultants make rounds with medical teams as a means of increasing visibility and offering real-time assistance. The benefit of this approach is that it brings ethics into the daily fabric of clinical care, which is where it should be. The liability is that many ethics dilemmas cannot be solved on the spot. Consultants must avoid the urge to please colleagues by providing quick answers that lack depth. For example, consultants who round with medical and surgical teams must have the confidence and experience to note when a situation requires a more lengthy and in-depth resolution process than can be provided during rounds.

In summary, ethics committees that flourish have several elements in common. Their goals are clearly defined, and continual efforts are made to improve the ways in which these goals are met. Membership is professionally and culturally diverse, and includes significant expertise in ethics. The committee seeks to build strong collegial relationships with both leadership and colleagues. Committees that provide effective ethics education, policy development, and consultation support the delivery of excellent health care at their institutions.

REFERENCES

American Society for Bioethics and Humanities, Task Force on Standards for Bioethics and Humanities. 1998. *Core Competencies for Health Care Ethics Consultation: The Report of the American Society of Bioethics and Humanities*. Glenview, IL: American Society for Bioethics and Humanities.

Fox E. 2002. Ethics consultations in U.S. hospitals: A national study and its implications. Paper presented at the Annual Meeting of the American Society of Bioethics and Humanities, October 24, 2002, Baltimore, MD.

Powell T. 2006. Culture and communication: Medical disclosure in Japan and the U.S. *The American Journal of Bioethics* 6(1):18–20.

Curriculum for Ethics Committees

Part I is an eight-chapter curriculum designed to introduce the fundamentals of bioethics, explain the key concepts, and provide a basic analytic framework for addressing and resolving ethical dilemmas. Each chapter highlights a set of ethical issues that commonly arise in the clinical setting and generate requests for ethics committee attention. It is beyond the scope of this handbook to provide a comprehensive treatment of these topics, and our discussion of the basic ethical principles and concepts draws on the work of expert theorists and practitioners who have contributed to the vast scholarly and clinical literature.

We encourage you to consult the selected but by no means exhaustive references listed at the end of each chapter. Classic texts, such as Beauchamp and Childress's *Principles of Biomedical Ethics,* anthologies, such as Arras, Steinbock, and London's *Ethical Issues in Modern Medicine,* newsletters, such as *Medical Ethics Advisor,* as well as journals, such as the *Hastings Center Report,* the *Journal of Law, Medicine & Ethics, The American Journal of Bioethics,* and the *Journal of Clinical Ethics,* should be part of any ethics committee's library. The American Society for Bioethics and Humanities' forthcoming publication *Improving Competence in Ethics Consultation: A Learner's Guide* will be a valuable resource for individuals and organizations providing clinical ethics consultation and education. Finally, Websites, such as www.asbh.org (American Society for Bioethics and Humanities) and www.ethicsweb.ca/resources/bioethics/institutes.html (a comprehensive list of resources with links to ethics institutes and organizations), are an important source of current information about what is happening in bioethics. These references are essential, providing ready access to the relevant research and in-depth analysis applicable to the cases and issues that committees consider.

1

Ethical Foundations
of Clinical Practice

||| As a member of your hospital's ethics committee, you have been called by Dr. Thomas, a second-year surgical resident who was paged for the following consult: Ms. Lawrence is a 23-year-old woman who was returning home from her bridal shower when her car skidded on the ice and hit an oncoming truck. Although her multiple injuries are serious, with immediate surgery and replacement of lost blood, her chances of full recovery are excellent.

Ms. Lawrence is in considerable pain, but she appears coherent and her answers to Dr. Thomas's questions reflect understanding of her condition, the treatment options, and their consequences. Because of her beliefs as a Jehovah's Witness, however, she will not accept blood or blood products and will not consider surgery unless she is promised that it will be done without transfusions.

Dr. Thomas knows that surgical and hemodynamic intervention can prevent this patient's almost certain death. He also knows that saving her life in this way will violate Ms. Lawrence's deeply held religious convictions. What are the conflicting medical, legal, and ethical obligations? What is the role of the ethics committee in resolving this dilemma? What resources are available to help you?

Perhaps the threshold question that should begin our discussion is, What is bioethics and why does it matter? The short answer is that bioethics is the discipline that addresses the ethical issues that arise in the health care setting. As will become clear in the following pages, however, bioethics does not lend itself to short answers, and further definition is necessary. The concerns of bioethics include the well-being and dignity of the patient; matters of choice and decision making; rights and responsibilities of the patient, family, and care team; access to care; and fairness and justice in health policy.

These matters are neither new nor exotic, but they have become more prominent. Health care has traditionally dealt with the profound moral issues of human existence, including life, self-determination, suffering, and mortality. What has changed are the complexity of medicine, the increased range of choices, and the way care is accessed and delivered. The ethical implications of these matters have attracted heightened attention, especially from those who make clinical and policy decisions. As applied ethics has become an integral part of the health care setting, institutional ethics committees have become increasingly visible and active in clinical and organizational decision making. The goal of this handbook is to help your committee be a knowledgeable, skillful, and effective ethics resource for your institution.

THE ROLE OF ETHICS IN CLINICAL MEDICINE

Ethics has a long and distinguished history grounding both the practice of medicine and the laws related to it. Society considers ethical principles so important that it gives them legal sanction in statutory and case law. Thus, ethical principles, such as respect for autonomy and privacy, are translated into laws about informed consent and confidentiality. It is important to note, however, that issues related to providing and forgoing medical treatment are governed almost exclusively by state law, creating wide variation in the way these matters are handled. For example, decisions about withholding or withdrawing life-sustaining measures might be very different if the patient were being treated in New York or New Jersey. For this reason, your ethics committee should have some familiarity with how your state laws and regulations address these issues.

Ironically, some of the most potentially beneficial developments have generated some of the most difficult ethical problems. In critical, acute, and long-term care settings, the very existence of new therapies often creates demand for their use, whether or not they are medically indicated or ethically appropriate. Clinical research raises issues of information disclosure, comparative levels of risks and benefits, and conflicts of interest. Budgetary pressures constrain the allocation of resources. Standing at the intersection of medicine, ethics, and law, bioethics provides a useful analytic framework for committees charged with helping to resolve these dilemmas.

ETHICS COMMITTEES IN THE HEALTH CARE SETTING

The development of bioethics as a powerful influence on the way health care is perceived and practiced was part of a larger social transformation. A hallmark of the latter half of the twentieth century was the heightened notion of individual rights. Virtually every social sphere was affected by the effort to promote equality and redress inequities in race, gender, class, and education. In the context of the various rights movements, the ethical principle of autonomy became the major support for individual empowerment and self-determination in health care, most prominently in the doctrine of informed consent and refusal. In the process, patients became both partners in health care decision making and informed health care consumers.

Ethical, legal, and scientific developments created an obligation to evaluate critically the process of gathering scientific information, translating it into therapeutic applications, and using it responsibly. Advances in medical knowledge and skills generated a new array of treatment options, as well as the concern that the *ability* to intervene could become the *obligation* to intervene. For the first time, questions were raised not only about *how* and *when,* but *whether* to treat. Under what circumstances should therapies be withheld or withdrawn? When does the burden of an intervention outweigh its benefit? How should decisions be made about the allocation of limited medical resources? At the same time, the law was becoming involved in life-and-death matters that used to be confined to the doctor-patient interaction.

Bioethics as a discipline is generally considered to have developed between the 1960s and the 1980s as it became apparent that emerging issues could benefit from thoughtful analysis by people with both clinical and nonclinical perspectives. Philosophers, social scientists, theologians, legal scholars, and biomedical scientists increasingly focused their attention on clinical research, allocation of limited resources, transplantation of organs, reproductive technologies, genetic testing and treatment, terminal illness and end-of-life care, and the obligations in the clinical interaction. Of particular relevance to ethics committee background, these deliberations revealed that ethical analysis had practical application in the research and clinical settings.

The hospital ethics committee was an early institutional effort to bring a formal ethical perspective to the clinical setting, otherwise described as "a politically attractive way for moral controversies to be procedurally accommodated" (Moreno, 1995, pp. 93–94). Hospitals began to establish ethics committees during the mid-twentieth century to answer questions and help make decisions about health care issues with ethical dimensions. These committees had their roots in several types of small decision-making groups, each intended to address specific ethical problems. Sterilization committees, composed mainly of physicians with expertise in psychiatry and psychology, functioned mainly during the 1920s and 1930s to determine which individuals with mental disabilities should be involuntarily sterilized. Abortion selection committees functioned in many hospitals before the 1973 U.S. Supreme Court decision in *Roe v. Wade* legalized abortion. Beginning in 1945, their purpose was to evaluate the requests of women who wished to terminate their pregnancies and determine whether therapeutic abortions were indicated to preserve the life or health of the prospective mother. Dialysis selection committees emerged during the early 1960s in response to the development of the dialysis machine, the first publicly recognized life-sustaining technology. Composed of lay members of the community, they were charged with choosing among the candidates with end-stage renal disease and determining who would receive chronic hemodialysis.

Beginning in the 1960s, institutional review boards (IRBs) responded to revelations of abuse in medical experimentation by reviewing all government-funded research using human subjects. The 1974 federal mandating of IRBs represented the first codified suggestion of institutional obligation to address ethical concerns. Prognosis committees were occasionally convened by the mid-1970s to assess the projected course of patients' illnesses. In its 1976 decision in *In re Quinlan,* the New Jersey Supreme Court referred to an article by Dr. Karen Teel and recommended that hospitals have an ethics committee to deal with termination of life-sustaining treatment for incapacitated patients. Although the court used the term *ethics committee,* it was actually suggesting a *prognosis committee* that would render opinions on the likely benefits of continued treatment for patients with grave and irreversible illness.

Infant care review committees began appearing in the wake of the 1982 "Baby Doe" ruling that permitted parents to approve withholding life-saving treatment from a neonate with Down's syndrome. These committees, which were intended to review care plans for severely disabled newborns, were also recommended by the President's Commission for the Study of Ethical Problems in Medicine and Behavioral Research in 1983 and endorsed by the U.S. Department of Health and Human Services and the American Academy of Pediatrics.

Medical-morals committees met in Catholic hospitals to address sensitive issues, including those related to reproduction, analgesia, and extraordinary interventions at the end of life, in terms of Church doctrine.

Against this backdrop, clinical and administrative staffs began to meet for interdisciplinary deliberations about issues of high-tech care, undertook self-education, and exhibited a growing professional awareness of ethical implications. During the 1970s and 1980s, hospitals began to establish ethics committees to provide guidance about health care issues with ethical dimensions. Over time, these committees have taken on the additional functions of staff education, clinical guideline development, institutional policy advisement, and case review. Some ethics committees also advise on resource allocation and express or reinforce the institution's commitment to certain values.

Since 1992, the Joint Commission on Accreditation of Healthcare Organizations (JCAHO) has required as a condition of accreditation that each health care institution have a standing mechanism to address ethical issues and resolve disputes. In addition, several states have passed statutes requiring hospitals to have ethics committees. The result is that almost all hospitals in the United States have ethics committees that meet on a regular basis.

As you read though this handbook, it is important to bear in mind that your committee does not own ethics in your institution. As discussed in the introduction, the committee should strive to develop ethics expertise, but it would be counterproductive to encourage the notion of ethics exclusivity and the perception that ethics resides only in a select group. Rather, one of your most valuable roles is that of a resource that, through education, policy development and consultation, helps clinical and administrative staff to integrate ethics knowledge and skills into their daily practice.

An important committee function is helping staff to identify ethical issues and conflicts, develop the skills to handle routine cases in ways that you have modeled in consultation on similar cases, and distinguish complex cases that require the attention of your consultation service. One mark of a successful ethics consultation is when you are stopped in the hall by someone who says, "Remember that case you consulted on two weeks ago? Well, we had another one just like it and we *didn't* have to call you. But now, we've got one that really has us stumped and we need your involvement again."

While your committee retains the responsibility to provide ethics expertise, education and guidance, it is important to reinforce the notion that the health care organization and all those who practice in it are moral agents with ethical obligations that cannot be delegated.

FUNDAMENTAL ETHICAL PRINCIPLES

As you no doubt expected, any discussion of applied bioethics must begin with a review of its theoretical underpinnings. Understanding the key concepts and how they relate to clinical practice is essential to the effective functioning of ethics committees.

The core ethical principles that support the therapeutic relationship and give rise to clinician obligations include

- respecting patient autonomy—supporting and facilitating the capable patient's exercise of self-determination in health care decision making
- beneficence—promoting the patient's best interest and protecting the patient from harm
- nonmaleficence—avoiding actions likely to cause the patient harm
- distributive justice—allocating fairly the benefits and burdens related to health care delivery

Respecting Patient Autonomy

Autonomy is the ethical principle widely considered most central to health care decision making because of its focus on self-governance and individual choice. Autonomy includes determination of health care goals, power over what is done to one's body, and control of personal information. Only when the individual cannot make decisions are others asked to choose. Autonomy gives priority to personal values and wishes, supporting choices that are informed and uncoerced, and confers the professional obligation to respect patient privacy and confidentiality.

The significance of autonomy to health care decision making is seen in the ethical concepts of decisional capacity, informed consent and refusal, and truth telling. Patients exercise autonomy by making informed care decisions that reflect their goals, values, and preferences. Clinicians demonstrate respect for autonomy by providing information and guidance that enable patients to make knowledgeable decisions; honoring patient choices and implementing them in care plans; preserving patient confidentiality; and protecting the security of patient information.

It is important to recognize that the notion of autonomy encompasses a range of conceptions, some highly individualistic and somewhat isolating, others more relational and compatible with communitarian values. The heightened emphasis our society customarily places on individualism and independence is a largely Western phenomenon and not universally shared. Despite our prevailing focus on self-governance, not everyone is comfortable with or capable of pure autonomy. Patients with diminished or fluctuating cognition are likely to rely on spouses or adult children for help in care planning. Others may come from cultures that favor decision making by the family rather than the individual. For these patients, authentic decision making is an exercise shared with trusted others and reflects *supported* or *delegated* autonomy.

Ultimately, respecting patient autonomy does not mean elevating it to a position where it trumps all other considerations. While it is usually legally and ethically appropriate to honor the wishes of a capable patient, it is also necessary to consider the ethical principles that give rise to other, often competing, obligations.

Beneficence

The principle of beneficence underlies obligations to provide the best care for the patient and balance the risks or burdens of care against the benefits. Promoted goods typically include prolonging life, restoring function, relieving pain and suffering, and preventing harm. Beneficence is the principle with arguably the greatest resonance for caregivers, whose traditional mission is to heal and comfort, and notions of nurturing and protecting are reflected in caring for those who are most vulnerable. Perceptions of benefit and best interest are not purely scientific, however, but involve expectations, goals, and value judgments. Recognition that patients and their doctors may differ in these assessments has been at least partly responsible for the noticeable shift from physician paternalism to greater emphasis on patient choice.

Nonmaleficence

At the very core of the healing professions is the principle of nonmaleficence, captured in the ancient maxim, "First, do no harm." This principle grounds obligations to avoid the intentional infliction of harm or suffering, recognizing that conceptions of harm, as of good, are inextricably tied to individual values and interests. Most, if not all, therapies carry the potential for some risk as well as benefit, and it would not be feasible to limit the therapeutic arsenal to treatments that are entirely benign. Nevertheless, the benefits of recommended treatments are expected to outweigh the possible harms, and physicians are required to discuss that calculus with their patients, comparing the burdens and risks to the anticipated goods. Likewise, the duty to prevent foreseeable harm requires investigators to disclose the benefits and risks of proposed research to potential subjects and institutional review boards.

Justice

Justice or equity refers to those principles of social cooperation that define what each person in the society or member of a group is due or owed—in short, what is fair. The several types of justice all share the basic notion of treating similar cases similarly and dissimilar cases dissimilarly. Most relevant to medical ethics is distributive justice, which concerns the norms and standards for allocating benefits and burdens across a given population. Distributive justice demands that the benefits, risks, and costs of actions—in this case, access to resources related to physical and mental health—be apportioned fairly and without discrimination on both societal and institutional levels. According to the principle of distributive justice, there should be ethically defensible reasons for why certain individuals or groups receive benefits or endure burdens that other individuals or groups do not.

∎

The four ethical principles discussed above—autonomy, beneficence, nonmaleficence, and justice—have assumed a central place in much of bioethics literature, theory, and clinical analysis. Our very brief tour just touches the surface and you are encouraged to consult Beauchamp and Childress for an in-depth treatment. Because these principles have validity and can be useful in thinking through ethical issues, they are referred to frequently in the following chapters. As a cautionary note, however, it is important to resist the temptation to employ principles in a mechanical fashion. If applicable and used with judgment and sensitivity, they can inform sound ethical reasoning. If used rigidly without reference to context and narrative, principlist ethics can lead to a distorted and unhelpful analysis.

It is equally useful to consider clinical situations in terms of key ethical concepts, such as decisional capacity, power imbalances, decision-making authority, access to health care, pain and suffering, confidentiality, truth telling, informed consent, the family's role in decision making, the patient's best interest, forgoing treatment, and quality of life and death. These and other ethical issues will be referred to in analyzing clinical situations throughout the curriculum in part I and discussing the clinical cases in part II.

THE ROLE OF CULTURE, RACE, AND ETHNICITY IN HEALTH CARE

How people confront decisions about health care is shaped in large part by the beliefs, attitudes, and values inherent in the cultures with the greatest formative influence on them. Choices about advance care planning, approaches to decision making, disclosure of information, life-sustaining interventions, and palliation are often informed by culturally determined notions of self-governance and destiny, truth telling and protection from harm, the power of language to reflect or create reality, filial obligation, the meaning of suffering, religion and spirituality, historical discrimination, and mistrust of health care or the health care system.

The following brief examples are offered to illustrate how culture, race, and ethnicity can influence health care. Studies have found that European Americans, who tend to value independence and self-empowerment, are more likely than others to favor advance directives, full disclosure of health information, and limited treatment at the end of life. In contrast, African Americans have demonstrated reluctance to delegate decision-making authority through advance directives, objection to limiting treatment, and preference for aggressive life-sustaining technology, including cardiopulmonary resuscitation. Hispanics have been shown to defer to physician judgment, value decision making by the family rather than an appointed health care agent, and place great importance on how the family is affected by the patient's illness. Asian and Middle Eastern cultures typically prefer to protect patients from knowledge about serious illness or impending death, and favor family rather than individual decision making. Native American cultures tend to reject advance care discussions because they might bring on the envisioned health problems. Reports of these studies emphasize the need for balance in interpreting them. Overreliance on the findings risks cultural stereotyping, while indifference to cultural distinctions risks assuming that all patients share Western attitudes and values (Morrison and Meier, 2004; Kagawa-Singer and Blackhall, 2001; Hopp and Duffy, 2000; Blackhall et al., 1999; Shepardson et al., 1999; Morrison et al., 1998; Berger, 1998; Pellegrino et al., 1992).

The same commentators also point out that cultural determinants influence the values and attitudes of physicians as well as those of their patients. The result is the potential for misperception and miscommunication when the parties to the clinical interaction come from different cultural backgrounds. A valuable ethics committee function can be educating care providers about the personal and cultural differences that influence the clinical dynamic and affect patient care. Consider, for example, a series of grand rounds or in-service presentations on how cultural background can inform patient and provider comfort with notions of autonomy, privacy, advance directives, informed consent, and disclosure.

CONFLICTING OBLIGATIONS AND ETHICAL DILEMMAS

The several ethical principles discussed above confer on clinicians multiple ethical obligations—duties that are grounded in moral norms and must be fulfilled unless there are competing and more compelling obligations. Not surprisingly, these obligations frequently collide.

The tension between and among ethical principles may create dilemmas for clinicians when their obligations are in conflict. Ethical dilemmas usually occur in two types of situations. In some instances, an act can be seen as both morally justified and unjustified, but the arguments supporting each position are inconclusive. This troubling contradiction makes it difficult for the individual to determine the appropriate course of action. Examples would be abortion and assisted suicide, both of which invoke competing ethical norms. In other instances, an individual may be required to respond to different moral imperatives and cannot do one without violating the other. For example, care professionals are required to respect and promote the autonomy of their patients *and* to protect and enhance their well-being, to provide care to those who need it *and* to be responsible stewards of limited resources. Resolving these dilemmas requires clinicians and ethics committees to scrutinize carefully the competing interests and obligations, identify the likely consequences of the available choices, and weigh the benefits and risks to those involved.

Let us return to Ms. Lawrence, the patient who is refusing blood transfusion. The dilemma here concerns the tension between Dr. Thomas's obligation to honor his patient's autonomous decision about blood transfusion and his obligations to prevent harm and provide what he believes is the most beneficial care. On the surface, it seems that he cannot possibly meet one obligation without violating the others, yet he must take decisive action. Because the principles involved are so central to professional practice and the consequences in this case so profound, the goal must be to protect both Ms. Lawrence's rights and her well-being. The ethics committee member(s) can function usefully in a consultative role as these issues are considered.

The first responsibility is to confirm that Ms. Lawrence is capable of making decisions about her care and to ensure that she and Dr. Thomas have clarified the clinical situation, the care goals, the therapeutic options, and their likely consequences. As discussed in later chapters, the exercise of patient autonomy, through informed consent and refusal, depends on the patient's decisional capacity, the quality of the information provided by the physician, and the trust underlying the therapeutic relationship. An ethics consultation can create the opportunity for the patient and appropriate members of the care team to engage in these important discussions.

The next step is to consider the ethical issues, including Ms. Lawrence's right to make care decisions based on her goals and values, and confirm that her refusal is the product of her deeply held religious convictions, rather than coercion or misinformation about blood transfusions. The discussion should explore alternative options and resources, including nonblood therapies and transfer to other institutions that specialize in treatment without transfusion. Ms. Lawrence, her family, and the clinical team must be reassured that her refusal will in no way compromise the rest of her care.

Resolving the conflict between the obligation to respect the patient's autonomy and the obligations to promote her best interest and protect her from harm will require a careful collaborative assessment of her decision making, including how she weighs the benefits and burdens of the proposed treatment. While it is neither necessary nor appropriate to argue her out of her religious beliefs, the ethics consultant is obliged to be certain that her decision to forgo a life-saving intervention is informed, carefully considered, voluntary, and settled. If Ms. Lawrence genuinely believes that surviving with a blood transfusion would be morally unacceptable, then, for her, the benefits of the intervention would be significantly outweighed by the burdens of the outcome. Under those conditions, her refusal of transfusion should be honored while she receives all other appropriate care and support. In this time-consuming and exacting process, the ethics committee consultant is a valuable resource, providing all parties with information, ethical analysis, practical guidance, and support.

It should be remembered, however, that not only the patient's autonomy is at stake. Dr. Thomas and his colleagues also bring to this situation their professional obligations and personal values. Not unreasonably, surgeons and/or anesthesiologists in this circumstance are likely to be very uneasy about attempting surgery under conditions that restrict their ability to provide optimal care. Even though the patient has agreed to and assumed the risks of surgery without blood transfusions, the doctors will argue that they would be knowingly putting her at what they consider unacceptable risk. Doing so would erode both their competence and professional integrity. Under these restrictive conditions, many surgeons and anesthesiologists would prefer to transfer Ms. Lawrence to colleagues or other institutions more comfortable with her limitations, agreeing to operate only if alternatives were not available.

REFERENCES

Ahronheim J, Moreno JC, Zuckerman C. 2000. *Ethics in Clinical Practice.* 2nd ed. Gaithersburg, MD: Aspen Publishers.

Annas GJ. 1991. Ethics committees: From ethical comfort to ethical cover. *Hastings Center Report* May–June 21(3):18–21.

Arras JD, Steinbock B, London AJ. 1999. Moral reasoning in the medical context. In Arras JD, Steinbock B, eds. *Ethical Issues in Modern Medicine.* 5th ed. Mountain View, CA: Mayfield Publishing Co., pp. 1–40.

Beauchamp TL, Childress JF. 2001. *Principles of Biomedical Ethics.* 5th ed. New York: Oxford University Press.

Beauchamp TL, Walters L, eds. 2003. *Contemporary Issues in Bioethics.* 6th ed. Belmont, CA: Wadsworth-Thomson Learning.

Berger JT. 1998. Culture and ethnicity in clinical care. *Archives of Internal Medicine* 158:2085–90.

Blackhall LJ, Frank G, Murphy ST, Michel V, Palmer JM, Azen SP. 1999. Ethnicity and attitudes towards life sustaining technology. *Social Science & Medicine* 48:1779–89.

Fletcher JC. 1991. The bioethics movement and hospital ethics committees. *Maryland Law Review* 50: 859–94.

Hopp FP, Duffy SA. 2000. Racial variations in end-of-life care. *Journal of the American Geriatrics Society* 48(6):658–63.

Jonsen AR. 1998. *The Birth of Bioethics*. New York: Oxford University Press.

Joint Commission on Accreditation of Healthcare Organizations. 1999. *Comprehensive Accreditation Manual for Hospitals*. Oakbrook Terrace, IL: Joint Commission on Accreditation of Healthcare Organizations.

Kagawa-Singer M, Blackhall LJ. 2001. Negotiating cross-cultural issues at the end of life: "You've got to go where he lives." *Journal of the American Medical Association* 286(23):2992–3001.

Levine RJ. 2003. Informed consent: Some challenges to the universal validity of the Western world. In Beauchamp TL, Walters L, eds. *Contemporary Issues in Bioethics*. 6th ed. Belmont, CA: Wadsworth-Thomson Learning, pp. 150–55.

Lo B. 2000. *Resolving Ethical Dilemmas: A Guide for Clinicians*. 2nd ed. Philadelphia: Lippincott Williams & Wilkins, pp. 140–46.

Mappes TA, Degrazia D. 2001. *Biomedical Ethics*. 5th ed. Boston: McGraw Hill, pp. 1–55.

Miller B. 1995. Autonomy and the refusal of life-sustaining treatment. In Arras JD, Steinbock B, eds. *Ethical Issues in Modern Medicine*. 4th ed. Mountain View, CA: Mayfield Publishing Co., pp. 202–11.

Moreno JD. 1998. Ethics committees and ethics consultants. In Kuhse H, Singer P, eds. *A Companion to Bioethics*. Malden, MA: Blackwell Publishers, pp. 475–84.

Moreno JD. 1995. *Deciding Together: Bioethics and Moral Consensus*. New York: Oxford University Press.

Morrison RS, Meier DE. 2004. High rates of advance care planning in New York City's elderly population. *Archives of Internal Medicine* 164(22):2421–26.

Morrison RS, Zayas LH, Mulvihill M, Baskin SA, Meier DE. 1998. Barriers to completion of health care proxies: An examination of ethnic differences. *Archives of Internal Medicine* 158(22):2493–97.

O'Neill O. 2002. *Autonomy and Trust in Bioethics*. Cambridge: Cambridge University Press.

Powell T, Lowenstein B. 1996. Refusing life-sustaining treatment after catastrophic injury: Ethical implications. *Journal of Law, Medicine & Ethics* 24:54–61.

Pearson SD, Sabin J, Emanuel EJ. 2003. *No Margin, No Mission: Health-Care Organizations and the Quest for Ethical Excellence*. New York: Oxford University Press.

Pellegrino ED. 1992. Intersections of Western biomedical ethics and world culture. In Pellegrino ED, Mazzarella P, Corsi P, eds. *Transcultural Dimensions in Medical Ethics*. Frederick, MD: University Publishing Group.

Protection of Human Subjects, 45 CFR 47.107; see also 45 CFR 46.112 (1990).

In re Quinlan, 70 N.J. 10, 355 A.2d 647 (1976).

Rosner F. 1985. Hospital medical ethics committees: A review of their development. *Journal of the American Medical Association* 253(18):2693–97.

Ross JW, Michel V, Pugh D. 1986. *Handbook for Hospital Ethics Committees*. Chicago: American Hospital Publishing.

Ross JW, Glaser JW, Rasinski-Gregory D, Gibson JM, Bayley C. 1993. *Health Care Ethics Committees: The Next Generation*. Chicago: American Hospital Publishing.

Rothman DJ. 1991. *Strangers at the Bedside: A History of How Law and Bioethics Transformed Medical Decision Making*. New York: Basic Books.

Schneider CE. 1998. *The Practice of Autonomy: Patients, Doctors, and Medical Decisions.* New York: Oxford University Press.

Shepardson LB, Gordon HS, Ibrahim SA, Harper DL, Rosenthal GE. 1999. Racial variation in the use of do-not-resuscitate orders. *Journal of General Internal Medicine* 14(1):15–20.

Solomon MZ. 2005. Realizing bioethics goals in practice: Ten ways "is" can help "ought." *Hastings Center Report* 35:40–47.

Spencer EM, Mills AE, Rorty MV, Werhane PH. 2000. *Organization Ethics in Health Care.* New York: Oxford University Press.

Teel K. 1975. The physician's dilemma: A doctor's view. What the law should be. *Baylor Law Review* 27:6–9.

Thomasma DC. 1993. Assessing bioethics today. *Cambridge Quarterly of Healthcare Ethics* 2:519–27.

Thomasma DC, Monagle JF. 1998. Hospital ethics committees: Roles, membership, structure, and difficulties. In Monagle JF, Thomasma DC, eds. *Health Care Ethics: Critical Issues for the 21st Century.* Gaithersburg, MD: Aspen Publishers, pp. 460–70.

Toulmin S. 1981. The tyranny of principles. *Hastings Center Report* (December):31–39.

Wear S, Katz P, Andrzejewski B, Haryadi T. 1990. The development of an ethics consultation service. *HEC Forum* 2:75–87

Wolf SM. 1991. Ethics committees and due process: Nesting rights in a community of caring. *Maryland Law Review* 50:798–858.

2 Decision Making and Decisional Capacity in Adults

||| Mrs. Klein is an 89-year-old woman admitted from home five days ago with cellulitis of the legs. Despite her discomfort, she has cooperated with her diagnostic work-up and treatment and consented to all interventions related to the cellulitis. She was able to provide accurate information about her medical history, which was corroborated by her niece. According to both women, Mrs. Klein has been very healthy and self-sufficient all her life, a state she attributes largely to "keeping my distance from doctors and hospitals." Her goal, expressed repeatedly since admission, is "to go home and take care of my cats."

Mrs. Klein's admission blood tests revealed anemia that suggests slow internal bleeding. Despite repeated attempts to explain the dangers of unchecked bleeding and the importance of identifying the source, she has consistently refused consent for a GI series. When asked why she is opposed to a diagnostic work-up, she replies, "Darling, you look, you'll find. No more tests or treatments. Just get me back on my feet so I can go home to my cats."

After several days, the attending physician requests a psychiatric consult to do a capacity assessment, suggesting that the patient is not capable of making decisions in her best interest and cannot be discharged under these circumstances.

Why does no one question Mrs. Klein's capacity to consent to treatment, only her capacity to refuse?

We now embark on a discussion of the issues most frequently brought to ethics committee attention—how and by whom health care decisions are made. Ethical principles require that decisions about care and treatment be made by the decisionally capable patient (the subject of this chapter), following adequate discussion of the benefits, burdens, and risks of the therapeutic options (the subject of the following chapter). When the patient is not able to participate in this process, the responsibility for making care decisions must be assumed by others.

The quality of the decision-making process and the validity of the resulting consent or refusal are directly related to the clarity of physician-patient communications; the patient's understanding of the information presented; the physician's attention to patient values and preferences; and the patient's trust in the physician that encourages questions and full discussion. Although decisional capacity and consent are thus inextricably linked, for logistical purposes they are discussed separately in this curriculum. This chapter examines decision making and capacity, while chapter 3 sets out the ethical basis and significance of the consent process.

HEALTH CARE DECISIONS AND DECISION MAKING

Health care in general and bioethics in particular deal with decisions requiring attention to patient needs and preferences in the context of medicine's capabilities and limitations. These decisions involve deeply personal ideas about life and death; the meaning of health, illness, and disability; and the importance of self-image, self-determination, and trust. While the patient has the greatest stake in these decisions, others, including family members and care professionals, bring their perceptions and concerns to the discussion. Indeed, it is the value- and interest-based nature of care decisions that makes them so complex and often difficult to negotiate.

DECISION-MAKING CAPACITY

It is tempting to suggest that, like obscenity, decisional capacity is something that cannot be precisely defined but we know it when we see it. While we may sense that a patient is or is not able to make decisions, intuition is not enough to guide an evaluation with such important implications. In the health care setting, the exercise of autonomy is promoted or hindered by the assessment of decisional capacity, which effectively includes or excludes patients from making decisions about their care. Determining the patient's ability to understand the issues, consider the consequences of different options, and communicate these thoughts to professionals is key to supporting autonomy. Without this set of cognitive capacities, patients will need assistance in making and articulating choices. Indeed, as noted below, even capable patients can benefit from assistance in making autonomous decisions. Excluding a decisionally capable patient from making choices violates autonomy; treating an incapacitated patient "as if" she were capable makes her vulnerable to the consequences of deficient decision making. Thus, the clinical assessment of decisional capacity is critical to determining whether the patient can participate in care decisions and provide informed consent and refusal.

Capacity and Competence

Although the terms *capacity* and *competence* are often used interchangeably, in the health care setting there are important distinctions that go beyond semantics. Competence is a *legal* presumption that a person who has reached the age of majority has the requisite cognition and judgment to negotiate most *legal* tasks, such as entering into a contract, making a will, or standing for trial. Incompetence is a functional assessment and determination by a court that, because the individual lacks this ability, she should be deprived of the opportunity to do certain things. Because the legal system is and should be rarely involved in medical decisions, it is customary to refer to the patient's decisional capacity, a *clinical* determination about the ability to make decisions about *treatment* or *health care*.

Elements of Decisional Capacity

Decisional capacity refers to the patient's ability to perform a set of cognitive tasks, including

- understanding and processing information about diagnosis, prognosis, and treatment options
- weighing the relative benefits, burdens, and risks of the therapeutic options
- applying a set of values to the analysis
- arriving at a decision that is consistent over time
- communicating the decision

Decisional capacity thus encompasses several skills, including understanding, assessing, valuing, reasoning, and articulating the factors relevant to a choice. Capacity can be seen as an index of a person's *ability* to exercise autonomy by making decisions that reflect personal preferences, values, and judgments at a given time. This is not the same, however, as the person's *willingness* to make autonomous decisions. Having capacity *enables* but does not *obligate* patients to act independently. Despite our good intentions, we cannot drag people kicking and screaming into self-determination and, in many instances, insisting that patients make decisions abandons them to their own autonomy.

Frequently, capacitated patients look to family, friends, and trusted others to help them exercise autonomous decision making. Patients demonstrate *supported* autonomy when they rely on others for advice in making choices ("I want my son to help make the decision"). Some patients, especially those who are elderly or from cultures in which self-determination is not a central value, demonstrate *delegated* autonomy. These patients often entrust to others the authority to make decisions on their behalf ("Talk to my daughter and do whatever she thinks is right"). Here, autonomy is expressed in the voluntary choice to delegate rather than independently exercise decision-making authority. Patients with capacity who benefit from the advice, guidance, and support of clinicians and trusted others can be said to demonstrate *assisted* autonomy. The ethics committee can perform a useful service by clarifying for the care team—through clinical consultations, in-service presentations, or informal conversations—the several ways in which patients can make authentic decisions.

Decision-specific and Fluctuating Capacity

Capacity is not global, but decision-specific, referring to the ability to make *particular* decisions. A patient may have the ability to decide what to have for lunch but may be incapable of weighing the pros and cons of surgery. For this reason, nothing is less helpful than a chart note that says, "Patient lacks capacity to make decisions." The misleading implication is that the patient lacks the capacity to make *all* decisions, effectively excluding her from making *any* decisions.

In fact, many patients have the capacity to make some decisions and not others. For example, a lower level of capacity is required to appoint a health care proxy agent (appreciation of the likelihood that someone will have to make decisions on her behalf and consistent designation of the same person) than to make the often complex decisions the proxy agent will eventually make. Thus, the appropriate response to the question, "Does this patient have capacity?" is "For what decision?" Likewise, a request for a capacity assessment is most helpful when it specifies the decision(s) at issue, such as "Please evaluate the patient's capacity to make decisions about discharge." Distinguishing among the specific decisions facing the patient and assessing her capacity to make them offers her the opportunity to make the widest range of choices within her ability.

Just as capacity is not global in its application to all decisions, it is not always constant. Depending on their age, cognitive abilities, clinical condition, and treatment regimen, patients may exhibit fluctuating capacity, demonstrating greater ability to make decisions at some times than others. For example, elderly patients, who are especially prone to "sundowning," often exhibit greater alertness, sharper reasoning, and clearer communication earlier in the day. Recognizing this tendency allows care providers to approach patients for discussion and decisions when they are at their most capacitated, thereby increasing their opportunities for autonomous action.

To return to the case of Mrs. Klein, the 89-year-old patient with cellulitis of the legs, a critical threshold question is whether, in making a decision to refuse the diagnostic work-up and return to her home, the patient is exercising decisional capacity. If her decision is an informed and voluntary one that appreciates the implications and accepts the consequences, it should be honored, despite the caregivers' concerns that it is not in her best interest. Nevertheless, efforts to persuade her to reconsider and consent to suggested treatments are still appropriate, especially if the potential risks of nontreatment and the benefits of treatment are significant.

Disagreement with medical recommendations is not by itself evidence of a lack of decisional capacity. Mrs. Klein's decision may be foolish and ill advised, but it is not necessarily the product of a misperception or delusion. Continued discussion will be necessary to confirm her understanding and the consistency of her decision with characteristic behavior and prior choices. She has led an independent life that she attributes partly to avoiding doctors and hospitals. Her present decision to refuse the work-up, therefore, conforms to a pattern of life choices that, until now, have served her relatively well.

Care providers, including health care institutions, have an ethical and legal obligation to arrange for a safe discharge for their patients. Ethical concerns arise when capable patients make decisions that run counter to their best medical interests. Here, clinicians' obligations to respect patient autonomy may be in tension with their obligation to promote Mrs. Klein's well-being and protect her from harm.

One way to address these conflicting obligations is to ensure that, when capable patients are discharged, especially under less-than-optimal circumstances, they are encouraged to accept appropriate nursing and other home care services. In contrast, allowing patients who lack capacity to elect an unsafe discharge is a form of patient abandonment. Whatever the patient's level of decisional capacity, involved family should be encouraged to participate in discharge planning, follow-up care, and advance care planning for future health care decision making.

Intervention by the bioethics consultation service or committee is often requested in cases of uncertain patient capacity, usually when questions arise about consent for or refusal of recommended treatment. These issues and the role of ethics intervention in resolving them are discussed further in chapter 3.

ASSESSMENT AND DETERMINATION OF CAPACITY

III Mr. Herbert is back again. He is a 38-year-old man who is confined to a wheelchair because of bilateral amputations resulting from untreated leg ulcers. Mr. Herbert has had multiple admissions to treat his repeatedly infected areas of skin breakdown. Once the wounds have been cleaned and repaired and the infection is under control, he signs himself out against medical advice (AMA) to return to his fifth-floor walk-up apartment, where he has a thriving business dealing street drugs. He insists that, with his buddies to carry him up and down and his girlfriend to help him with meals and activities of daily living (ADLs), he can manage just fine. He acknowledges that his recovery might be better if he remained in the hospital longer or if he came to the clinic regularly, but, if he is not home, his business will be picked up by other dealers. He insists that he is willing to risk future infections, although he is confident that "you guys will always get me back on my game." Nevertheless, each time he returns, he is in worse shape and it is harder to resolve his medical problems.

The Importance of Determining Capacity

Decisional capacity requires more than the ability to articulate choices. As discussed in chapter 5, young children can be very vocal and sincere in expressing their wishes, but their choices would not be considered thoughtful judgments. The obligation to respect autonomy and the integrity of the informed consent process depend on the patient's ability to understand the facts and appreciate the consequences of treatment options. The presumption is that adult patients have the requisite capacity and, absent contrary evidence, decisions about treatment and nontreatment defer to patient wishes. Moreover, this deference usually extends to all capacitated decisions, including those that providers may think reflect poor judgment or are not in the patient's best interest. Yet troubling and potentially harmful decisions, such as patient rejection of recommended care, must be carefully explored because they may well reflect misunderstanding and lack of trust, rather than informed and considered choices.

III Mrs. Rodriguez is a 69-year-old woman transferred from a nursing home in a semicomatose state and respiratory failure. She was admitted to the intensive care unit (ICU) and intubated to provide ventilatory support. Her multiple medical problems include congestive heart failure, non-insulin-dependent diabetes, and several prior episodes of pneumonia.

After several weeks, the care team recognized that Mrs. Rodriguez would not be able to breathe without ventilatory assistance and recommended that a tracheotomy be done to promote safety and comfort. Because she was still unresponsive, the procedure was explained to her daughter, who provided consent. The next day, Mrs. Rodriguez unexpectedly became more alert and responsive. The critical care resident expressed concern because he believed the patient was indicating opposition to the tracheotomy.

The ear nose and throat (ENT) attending argued that the endotracheal tube made it impossible to determine what, if anything, the patient was trying to communicate and, in any event, she did not have the capacity to make decisions about her care. He insisted that the trach, which would be in the patient's best interest, be performed in accordance with the daughter's consent. The critical care attending asked Mrs. Rodriguez a series of yes-no questions that she could answer by nodding or shaking her head. Her nonverbal but consistent responses, which indicated that she understood the purpose of the tracheotomy and agreed that it should be performed, were considered a ratification of the consent provided by her daughter.

Would Mrs. Rodriguez's capacity have been considered sufficient for her to consent to the tracheotomy without her daughter's involvement? Why might a higher level of capacity be required for her to refuse the procedure?

One useful strategy for approaching decisional capacity is a sliding scale, which assesses the required level of capacity according to the seriousness of the decision. As the risks associated with a decision increase, the level of capacity needed to consent to or refuse the intervention should also increase. For example, a decision about whether to go to physical therapy before or after lunch carries a low risk of harm. This decision could safely be made by a patient with diminished capacity because the consequences of either choice are relatively benign. In contrast, a decision about whether to undergo a life-saving amputation or enroll in an experimental trial of chemotherapy requires the ability to understand and weigh the significant benefits, burdens, and risks of the proposed intervention. Asking a patient with uncertain capacity to take responsibility for a choice this serious would abandon her to the consequences of her deficient decisional ability. Clinically, the sliding scale provides heightened scrutiny when the potential outcomes of decisions require clinicians to be confident that patients fully appreciate the implications of their choices. Mrs. Rodriguez's low level of capacity was considered sufficient to ratify her daughter's consent because she concurred with the plan her care professionals and family agreed would benefit her. If she had refused the recommended procedure, however, it is likely that further assessment of her decisional capacity would have been indicated.

The danger in the sliding scale approach is that of paternalism, the tendency to treat otherwise capable adults as though they were children in need of others to make decisions for them. While it is not necessary that the family and care team agree with the patient's decision, choices considered irrational or harmful to the patient are likely to be challenged or at least closely scrutinized to protect incapable and, therefore, vulnerable patients from making decisions not in their best interest. The fact is, we only question the capacity of people who do not agree with us. Think about it—when was the last time you saw a capacity consult called to evaluate a patient who had just agreed with the doctor?

Capacity assessments, therefore, require a conscious effort to look beyond the decision we would make for ourselves or even recommend for the patient. If we focus exclusively on the *content* or the *outcome* of the decision rather than the decision-making *process,* we risk disempowering people who make risky or idiosyncratic choices. An important safeguard is assessing the decision in terms of *how* it is made, evaluating the patient's ability to manage the several skills required for capable decision making. Likewise, it is necessary to distinguish *questioning capacity* and *finding incapacity.* While treatment refusals or other questionable decisions may *trigger* a capacity assessment, they do not automatically *confirm* incapacity.

Who Assesses Decisional Capacity?

Given the importance of assessing decision-making capacity, the desire for a precise method of measurement is understandable. Unfortunately, it's not that simple. Decisional capacity is an index of patient ability to make decisions and, therefore, involves cognitive processes. Nevertheless, its assessment requires more than a test of mental acuity or a psychiatric exam. The Mini Mental Status Exam (MMSE), often used to evaluate cognitive ability, is useful in gauging "orientation of the subject to person, place, and time, attention span, immediate recall, short-term and long-term memory, ability to perform simple calculations, and language skills" (Lo, 2000, pp. 84–85). The MMSE is less helpful, however, in assessing an individual's ability to understand, weigh alternatives, and appreciate consequences—the skills required for capacitated decision making. This evaluation is more effectively done through one or more discussions that reveal the patient's grasp of the decision's context and implications.

Likewise, simply calling a psych consult does not get the job done. While psychiatric consultation may be helpful in assessing decisional capacity, it is not always necessary or sufficient. To be sure, psychiatric intervention can be invaluable in engaging patients in discussion, eliciting and interpreting their concerns, and identifying mental illness, cognitive impairments, and interpersonal conflicts that can mask or interfere with decisional capacity. Even a skillful psychiatric consultation, however, captures only a snapshot of the patient's thinking at a specific moment rather than over time. Ultimately, the clinicians who observe and interact with the patient day to day—especially nurses, residents, and medical students—may be better positioned to evaluate the quality and consistency of the patient's decision-making ability. For this reason, assessing decisional capacity should be considered part of the clinical skill set of care professionals and the responsibility of the medical team. Reinforcing this aspect of the caregiver role can be a valuable ethics committee function.

DECIDING FOR PATIENTS WITHOUT CAPACITY

Usually, health care decisions are made by capable patients with the advice and support of their caregivers and families. Frequently, however, treatment decisions must be made for patients who lack the capacity to make decisions for themselves. These may be persons who were formerly but are no longer capacitated or individuals, such as newborns or the severely retarded, who never had an opportunity to form values or preferences.

Making medical decisions for others raises a series of questions involving the patient's clinical needs and treatment options, what is known of the patient's care wishes, and the appropriate delegation of decision-making authority. Answering these difficult questions is often complicated by disagreements between and among the patient's family and care providers. Mediating these conflicts and facilitating decision making for incapacitated patients are among the most frequent and effective interventions by the ethics committee. The theory and skills important to clinical consultation are discussed at greater length in part II.

Standards of Decision Making

The standards of health care decision making rely on the patient's voice as the central and most authentic source. When that voice is temporarily or permanently unavailable, those who act on behalf of the patient have only indirect access to her wishes and values. Three standards are customarily invoked in an attempt to get as close as possible to what would be the patient's decision, each concentric circle drawing on less direct information from the patient.

- Prior explicit articulation is the previous expression of a capacitated person's wishes, the most reliable information about her preferences. *"What do we know* about this person's wishes based on what she has said or written?"
- Substituted judgment is a decision by others based on the formerly capacitated person's inferred wishes. "Knowing what we know about this person's behavior, values, and prior decisions, *what do we think she would want* in these circumstances?"
- Best interest standard is used to arrive at a judgment based on what a reasonable person in the patient's situation would want. This standard is used when the incapacitated person never had or made known treatment wishes and her preferences cannot be inferred. Others weigh the benefits and burdens to the patient of a proposed intervention or care plan. *"What do we believe* would best promote this person's well-being in these circumstances?"

Decision Making for the Formerly Capacitated

The notion that only the explicit statement of a capable patient can inform treatment decisions has proved to be double-edged—both a protection of the patient's right to consent or refuse and a barrier to decision making when the patient's wishes are unknown or inaccessible. Among the clinical setting's greatest challenges is the patient who was formerly but is no longer capable and/or communicative, making it difficult to determine or honor her wishes. In this category are the elderly demented and patients of any age with terminal illness or irreversible injury that has impaired their decision-making ability. In response to the needs of the formerly capacitated, two approaches that invoke the three decision-making standards have developed—advance directives and surrogate decision making.

Advance Directives

||| Mrs. Stern is a 74-year-old woman admitted from home for surgical repair of a hip fracture. Although she is in the early stages of dementia and has mild coronary artery disease, she has

been healthy and fairly independent until her recent fall. She has lived alone since her husband's death three years ago, but her daughter, Mrs. Keller, lives nearby and they either visit or speak daily.

On admission, despite her considerable discomfort, Mrs. Stern was alert, understood her medical condition, and was able to provide consent for the surgery. During the postoperative period, however, she has been increasingly agitated and confused. When recent blood tests indicated anemia, she was unable to discuss the need for a transfusion. She asked that the doctors talk to her daughter, who provided the necessary consent.

Mrs. Stern is scheduled to be discharged to a nursing home for rehabilitation in preparation for her eventual return home. She is expected to make a good recovery from her surgery and should be able to resume her normal activities with some assistance. Her doctors anticipate that, once she is in familiar surroundings, she will be less agitated and confused. Because her dementia is likely to progress, however, she will find it increasingly difficult to make independent decisions, including those related to her health care. For that reason, the care team is encouraging the execution of an advance directive that will enable care decisions to be made on her behalf when she is no longer able to make them herself.

If Mrs. Stern is determined to lack the capacity to make care decisions, is she capable of executing an advance directive? Would different levels of capacity be required to execute a living will and appoint a health care proxy agent?

Advance directives are legal instruments intended to secure an individual's ability to set out prospective instructions regarding health care. Conceived during the 1970s, they responded to the concern that patients who were unable to speak for themselves might be subjected to unwanted medical interventions, especially at the end of life. The 1990 federal Patient Self-Determination Act (PSDA) requires any health care facility receiving federal funds to offer patients the opportunity to execute advance directives and assistance in doing so. Although all fifty states have statutory and/or case law governing advance directives and all states honor them, their standards and restrictions differ. While advance directives are helpful whenever substitute decision making is required, they are most often invoked in making decisions at the end of life. For that reason, they are discussed further in chapter 6.

Advance directives commonly come in two varieties—living wills and health care proxy appointments. In different ways, they provide direct expression of the patient's wishes, enabling caregivers to rely on the most immediate of the decision-making standards. The living will is a written set of value-neutral instructions about the particular medical, surgical, or diagnostic interventions the individual *does* or *does not* want under particular circumstances, usually at the end of life. The structure of the document generally has a trigger phrase, such as, "If I am in an irreversible coma, . . ." or "If I am unable to recognize or relate to my loved ones and my doctors say that I will not recover, . . ." followed by the list of instructions related to the specified circumstances.

Patient wishes may also be communicated orally when the patient is unable to execute a written document. In these instances, the patient's verbally expressed instructions can be documented by a health care provider or other individual. If properly documented and witnessed, these statements are considered formal advance directives in several states.

Because the living will presents the explicit articulation of the patient's prior capacitated wishes, it can provide helpful guidance to family and clinicians about what she would want in the current circumstances. It is significantly limited by the fact that it is a static piece of paper written when the person could not accurately anticipate her future medical condition. In addition, these documents do not always mean what they say. The person whose living will says," I don't ever want to be on a respirator" probably does not mean, "I don't want to be on a respirator for four hours if it gives me ten more years on the tennis court." What she probably means is, "I don't want to live out the rest of my life on a respirator." But living wills typically do not provide for that kind of nuance. Finally, this type of advance directive usually refers only to end-of-life care. The result is a set of instructions that reflect what the patient *believed* and *tried to communicate* at a particular time about what she *thought she would want* under different circumstances at a later time. Because of their limitations, living wills are most useful for someone who does not have trusted friends or family to make decisions in the event of her incapacity.

The preferred advance directive is the health care proxy, sometimes called a durable power of attorney for health care decision making. This document enables a capable individual to legally appoint another person—an agent—to make health care decisions on her behalf after capacity has been lost. The agent is authorized to make any and all health care decisions the individual would make, not just those about end-of-life treatment.

The health care proxy is recommended over the living will because it authorizes decision making in the event of temporary or permanent incapacity and permits greater flexibility in responding to unanticipated or rapidly changing medical conditions. The agent is generally required to honor the patient's previously expressed wishes in making care decisions. If those instructions do not apply to or are inconsistent with the patient's current health needs, however, the agent is empowered to use his knowledge of the patient's wishes, values, and decision history to exercise substituted judgment in making choices that promote the patient's best interest. This scope of authority presupposes a patient-proxy relationship characterized by trust, familiarity with the patient's wishes and values, and the agent's willingness to exercise judgment and make hard decisions in the patient's interest.

Mrs. Stern is a good example of a patient who lacks the capacity to make health care decisions, yet is capable of appointing a trusted person to make decisions for her. Her current illness and hospitalization have exacerbated the agitation and confusion of her early-stage dementia, making it difficult or impossible for her to understand and decide about her medical treatment adequately. Moreover, she does not want to assume this responsibility, preferring to delegate decision-making authority to her daughter.

Thus, while she may not have the capacity to make decisions about her current treatment or articulate instructions about future care in a living will, she does understand the notion that someone will have to make decisions for her and she consistently designates the same trusted person for that task, meeting the criteria for health care proxy appointment.

Deciding for Patients without Capacity or Advance Directives

Advance directives appear to provide all the authorization and safeguards necessary to communicate and implement prior care wishes effectively. You might reasonably think that every capable person would have one. Unfortunately, you would be wrong. Even though people are encouraged to express their health care preferences prospectively through the designation of a health care agent or the execution of a living will, only 15 to 25 percent of adults in the United States have an advance directive. Thus, decisions for most patients who lack capacity are made by unofficial surrogates—people who assume the decision-making role without specific legal appointment or the guidance of documented patient wishes. In some states, a surrogate's authority to make health care decisions for someone else may be based on statutory or case law. More often, an informal surrogate is asked by the medical team to participate in making treatment decisions. The people who fill this void and act on behalf of incapacitated patients include family, close friends, trusted others. In their absence, care providers and courts, who are essentially strangers to the patients, may assume this responsibility.

Without the patient's explicit instructions in an advance directive, health care decisions made by surrogates are necessarily based on the remaining two decision-making standards—either substituted judgment (when the patient's wishes can be inferred) or the best interest standard (when the patient did not have or did not articulate treatment preferences). Clinicians and families of patients unable to participate in care discussions or decisions work to determine a course that meets medical, legal, and ethical imperatives. Goals and plans of care are considered in light of the patient's condition and prognosis, the benefits, burdens, and risks of the therapeutic options, and what is known about her wishes or best interests. Depending on the laws of the state in which the patient is treated, family and trusted others may have greater or lesser latitude in drawing on their knowledge of and concern for the patient in making decisions on her behalf. In helping to guide substitute decision making, ethics committee consultants need to be familiar with the scope of authority that their states accord to informal surrogates.

Decision Making for Patients Who Never Had Capacity

Those who never had the opportunity or ability to form values or preferences include newborns and severely retarded adults. As discussed in chapter 5, decisions for the endangered or profoundly disabled newborn are almost always made by the parents who are presumed, by tradition and law, to act in the best interests of their child.

However, courts tend to override parental refusals of specific life-saving interventions, especially if the child can be returned to reasonable health.

Mentally retarded adults, like infants and young children, are considered to need decision making by others because they are and have always been incapable of reasoned judgment. As in the case of salvageable newborns, courts tend to overrule requests to withhold or terminate beneficial treatment.

Addressing the needs of never-capacitated patients does not raise the question, "What does or did this person want?" Because there is no way of knowing what these individuals would have wanted and there is no history of past decision making to use as a guide, the best interest standard is invoked to inform care decisions on their behalf. In these instances, the analysis is based on the objective assessment of what would be most likely to benefit or promote the well-being of a hypothetical patient in the same circumstances, similar to the legal reasonable person standard discussed in chapter 3. In the clinical setting, the best interest standard might consider mitigating pain and suffering, prolonging life, restoring and enhancing comfort, and maximizing the potential for independent functioning.

Sometimes, in an attempt to represent the patient's interests, care providers and surrogates create what amounts to a fiction of substituted judgment. For example, they might ask, "What would this imperiled newborn or profoundly retarded adult want if he could want anything?" Careful review of the decision-making standards reveals the fallacy in this approach. Precisely because this patient has no history that would permit inference about his wishes, substituted judgments cannot be made. Rather, decisions on his behalf must be based on the best interest standard, drawing on what *others* believe would be best for him.

REFERENCES

American Bar Association. 2004. ABA public education: Health care advance directives. What is a health care advance directive? [On-line]. www.abanet.org/publiced/practical/directive_whatis.html (last accessed May 8, 2006).

American Hospital Association. 1985. *Values in Conflict: Resolving Issues in Hospital Care. Report of the Special Committee on Biomedical Ethics.* Chicago: American Hospital Association.

Beauchamp TL, Childress JF. 2001. *Principles of Biomedical Ethics.* 5th ed. New York: Oxford University Press, pp. 98–103.

Berger JT. 2005. Patients' interests in their family members' well-being: An overlooked fundamental consideration within substituted judgment. *Journal of Clinical Ethics* 16(1):3–10.

Breslin JM. 2005. Autonomy and the role of the family in making decisions at the end of life. *Journal of Clinical Ethics* 16(1):11–19.

Buchanan AE, Brock DW. 1989. *Deciding for Others: The Ethics of Surrogate Decision Making.* Cambridge: Cambridge University Press.

DeRenzo EG, Panzarella P, Selinger S, Schwartz J. 2005. Emancipation, capacity, and the difference between law and ethics. *Journal of Clinical Ethics* 16(2):144–50.

Drane J. 1984. Competency to give an informed consent: A model for making clinical assessments. *Journal of the American Medical Association* 252(7):925-27.

Emanuel EJ, Emanuel LL. 1992. Four models of the physician-patient relationship. *Journal of the American Medical Association* 267(16):2221-26.

Gillick MR. 2004. Advance care planning. *New England Journal of Medicine* 350(1):7-8.

Kennedy GL. 2000. Legal and ethical issues. In *Geriatric Mental Health Care.* New York: Guilford Press, pp. 282-317.

Lo B. 1990. Assessing decision-making capacity. *Journal of Law, Medicine & Ethics* 18(3):193–203.

Lo B. 2000. Decision-making capacity. In *Resolving Ethical Dilemmas: A Guide for Clinicians.* 2nd ed. Philadelphia: Lippincott Williams & Wilkins, pp. 80-87.

Lo B, Steinbrook R. 2004. Resuscitating advance directives. *Archives of Internal Medicine* 164:1501–6.

Mezey M, Teresi J, Ramsey G, Mitty E, Bobrowitz T. 2000. Decision-making capacity to execute a health care proxy: Development and testing of guidelines. *Journal of the American Geriatrics Society* 48(2):179–87

Patient Self-Determination Act, 1990. 42 U.S.C. §1395 cc(a).

Post LF. 2007 (in progress). Substituted decision making. In Capezuti E, Siegler G, Mezey MD, eds. *The Encyclopedia of Elder Care.* 2nd ed. New York: Springer Publishing Co.

Post LF, Blustein J, Dubler NN. 1999. The doctor-proxy relationship: An untapped resource. *Journal of Law, Medicine & Ethics* 27:5–12.

Powell T. 2005. Voice: Cognitive impairment and medical decision making. *Journal of Clinical Ethics* 16(4):303–13.

Powell T, Lowenstein B. 1996. Refusing life-sustaining treatment after catastrophic injury: Ethical implications. *Journal of Law, Medicine & Ethics* 24:54–61.

Sabatino CP. 1994. 10 legal myths about advance medical directives. ABA Commission on Legal Problems of the Elderly. [On-line]. www.abanet.org/aging/myths.html.

Schneider CE. 1998. *The Practice of Autonomy: Patients, Doctors, and Medical Decisions.* New York: Oxford University Press.

3

Informed Consent and Refusal

||| Mrs. Stack is a 67-year-old woman admitted with rectal bleeding, chronic renal insufficiency, diabetes, and blindness. On admission, she was alert and capacitated. Two weeks later, she suffered a cardiopulmonary arrest, was resuscitated and intubated, and was transferred to the medical intensive care unit (MICU) in an unresponsive and unstable state. Consent for emergency dialysis was obtained from her son, who is also her health care proxy agent. Dialysis was repeated two days later.

During the past several years, Mrs. Stack has consistently stated to her family and her primary care doctor that she would never want to be on chronic dialysis and she has refused it numerous times when it was recommended. The physician, who has known and treated Mrs. Stack for many years, also treated her daughter who had been on chronic dialysis for some time and had died after suffering a heart attack. According to the physician and the patient's family, Mrs. Stack's refusal of dialysis has been based on her conviction that her daughter died as a result of the dialysis treatments.

Mrs. Stack's mental status has cleared considerably and, despite the ventilator, she is able to communicate nonverbally. Although she appears to understand the benefits of dialysis and the consequences of refusing it, including deterioration and eventual death, she has consistently and vehemently refused further treatments. Her capacity to make this decision is not now in question. Her son, however, wants her to undergo dialysis and insists, "She's feisty and I just have to be tough with her. It's for her own good." He has told his mother, "If you don't have dialysis, I'll have to put you in a nursing home." Finally, after several extended interactions with her son, the patient reluctantly agrees to undergo dialysis. How should her consent be interpreted? What are the care team's obligations?

Let's face it—most clinicians and administrators are less interested than you are in the principle of autonomy or the concept of decisional capacity. What concerns them is the fact that, unless the patient or a surrogate can authorize treatment, the clinical process comes to a screeching halt. Ethics committee involvement is frequently requested in the hope that clarifying and allocating decisional authority will get the process moving again. This brings us to the practical application of this authority.

In the clinical setting, the exercise of autonomy is most fully realized in the doctrine of informed consent and refusal, the legal and ethical embodiment of the right to self-determination in health care. Indeed, the right to determine what is done to one's body, including the right to consent to and refuse medical treatment, is considered so funda-mental that it is protected by the U.S. Constitution and state constitutions, and sup-ported by decisions of the U.S. Supreme Court. In the informed consent process, a decisionally capable individual who understands the benefits, burdens, and risks of a proposed treatment grants explicit permission for or rejects a particular intervention.

EVOLUTION OF THE DOCTRINE OF INFORMED CONSENT

The legal doctrine of informed consent was initially based on the law of battery, holding that any unconsented-to touching, even to promote the patient's well-being, consti-tuted an unlawful act. In time, courts came to reject the rather crude notion that con-sent either did or did not occur. Considered more useful was the standard of negligence, which permits a more nuanced examination of whether a physician-patient discussion revealed the risks and benefits material to the patient's decision about treatment.

By the latter part of the twentieth century, the new dynamic of more robust pa-tient participation had introduced a somewhat adversarial tone. Some patients came to see informed consent as their offensive security against physician overreaching, while some physicians saw it as their defensive protection against charges that they provided inadequate information—the medical equivalent of a prenuptial agreement. As a result of liability concerns, the critical role of informed consent as the expression and protec-tion of patient self-determination in health care decision making has been modified by its risk management function.

ELEMENTS OF INFORMED CONSENT AND REFUSAL

The basic elements of informed consent and refusal include

- decisional capacity
- disclosure by physicians of sufficient information relevant to the decision in question
- understanding of the information disclosed
- voluntariness in acting without compulsion or coercion, and, on the basis of these,
- communication of consent to or refusal of the proposed medical intervention

Each of these elements is essential to the integrity of the process. For example, disclosing information about the proposed treatment is necessary but not sufficient unless the information is both adequate and understood. Likewise, consent that is informed but coerced is invalid.

These elements come together in the following definition: "One can confidently presume that an act is an informed consent if a patient or subject agrees to an intervention on the basis of an understanding of relevant information, the consent is not controlled by influences that engineer the outcome, and the consent given was intended to be a consent and therefore qualified as a permission for an intervention" (Beauchamp, 1997, p. 185). A more elaborated formulation includes *recommendation,* the physician's obligation to go beyond mere disclosure, and *authorization,* the patient's active ratification of the consent or refusal (Beauchamp and Childress, 2001, p. 80). Indeed, it may be helpful and more accurate to think in terms of *assisted* or *advised consent* as the dynamic that links the physician's disclosure and guidance with the patient's understanding and decision making.

Capacity and Consent

As discussed in chapter 2, the relationship between consent and decisional capacity explains the informed consent and refusal process that is so central to the patient-physician interaction. Consent is more than permission to treat; it can be seen as the compact by which a capable patient voluntarily entrusts his care to a clinical professional. Capacity is the set of cognitive, volitional, and affective patient abilities that lends authenticity and validity to the consent and authorizes the professional to enter into and maintain the care-providing compact.

Disclosure of Information

‖ Mr. Porter is a 52-year-old man whose advanced diabetes has resulted in decreased peripheral circulation and gangrene in his lower extremities, particularly severe in his left foot. He has worked as a mail carrier for thirty-one years and, he says proudly, "never missed a day." According to his family, he has resisted seeking medical attention because of his fear that amputation would be recommended, a course he would unquestionably refuse.

It is clear to the surgeon that only amputation of Mr. Porter's left foot will save his life, but that aggressive deep debridement (removal of dead or diseased tissue) of his right foot might possibly prevent the spread of gangrene on that side. When she approaches the patient for consent to surgery, she says, "Mr. Porter, we need to take you to the operating room to clean away all the dead tissue on your feet. If we don't do this, the infection will continue to spread and you could die. Don't worry, we do this all the time in cases like yours."

What is the nature of the interaction? Has the surgeon met her professional obligation? What would be the quality of Mr. Porter's consent?

True informed consent is impossible unless the patient can adequately evaluate his condition and the benefits, burdens, and risks of the therapeutic options. Accordingly, respecting the patient's rights of self-determination requires that he have access to relevant and sufficient information, which gives rise to the professional obligation of disclosure.

The challenge to the physician is determining *what* and *how much* information to provide. In assessing the quality of disclosure for purposes of informed consent, the courts have defined two standards—professional practice and reasonable person. A third standard—subjective—has also been advocated. These standards reflect both the legal criteria for disclosure and the underlying ethical distinctions about who determines the relevance and sufficiency of the information to be disclosed.

The professional practice standard bases adequate disclosure on what the customary practice of professionals in the physician's community would deem appropriate. This standard presumes that the physician, acting in the patient's best interest, is in the best position to determine what information to provide. Because the determination lies with the physician, this somewhat paternalistic standard, also known as the reasonable doctor standard, risks undercutting the patient's autonomous decision making.

In contrast, the reasonable person standard holds that disclosure should be based on what a reasonable person would consider material in making *this* decision. This standard, which is accepted in a minority of states, shifts the determination of what is pertinent from the physician to the patient. In so doing, it supports patient autonomy and elevates the physician's ethical obligation to respect it even over the obligations of beneficence.

The subjective standard looks at what *this* specific patient would consider material in making *this* decision. It is also possible to combine the reasonable person standard with the subjective standard by disclosing what a reasonable person would consider material to the decision, and then providing opportunity for *this* patient to ask questions of particular importance to his situation.

Because the content and process of informed consent should enhance the patient's capacity to make decisions, limiting the professional obligation to mere disclosure of facts is inadequate. In addition to the provision of appropriate information by the physician, informed consent requires that it be *understood* by the patient or surrogate decider. Thus, the obligation has not been met unless the information is presented in ways that are educationally, linguistically, and culturally accessible to the people who will have to use it to make important decisions. Finally, the patient is also entitled to the physician's judgment in the form of recommendations about the clinical options and their likely outcomes in light of the patient's goals and values.

Thus, the core information that physicians are obligated to disclose is generally held to include

- the facts about the proposed diagnostic or therapeutic intervention that patients typically consider relevant in deciding whether to consent
- information about the intervention and its purpose that the physician considers important to the patient's decision
- information about the consequences of nontreatment and alternatives to the proposed intervention
- the physician's recommendation about how the patient might consider the intervention's benefits and risks

‖ Mr. Silver is a 39-year-old man with prostate cancer. Although the disease is confined to his prostate, Dr. Binder knows that, in a patient this young, the cancer is virulent and should be treated aggressively. For this reason, he strongly recommends that Mr. Silver undergo a radical prostatectomy. Mr. Silver has heard about the potential side effects of the surgery, including impotence and incontinence, and he insists that he prefers radiation.

Dr. Binder has explained that the chances of a long-term cure are 30 to 40 percent better with the prostatectomy and that any resulting problems can be surgically corrected later. Mr. Silver is adamant, however, saying, "Unless you can tell me that the odds are overwhelming that I will not be impotent or incontinent, I'll take my chances with the radiation." His wife has told Dr. Binder privately, "I don't care about the side effects and he'll get used to what-ever happens. I just want him alive. We could have many good years ahead of us if he has the surgery."

What would be the quality of Mr. Silver's consent to the prostatectomy if he did not fully appreciate the risks? Does the physician have an obligation to Mrs. Silver that is in conflict with his obligation to his patient?

The notion of patient best interest is far from clear in this case. The conflicting potential outcomes appear to be surviving cancer with sexual and urinary dysfunction versus maintaining those functions at an increased risk of dying from cancer. Depending on their personalities, values, and notions of an acceptable quality of life, reasonable patients, families, and professionals may disagree about which option is preferable.

This case illustrates the tension between the physician's obligation to respect patient autonomy and the obligation to promote patient best interest. Because Mr. and Mrs. Silver define best interest differently, the information Dr. Binder provides will greatly influence how they think about treatment. Mrs. Silver has very real concerns about her husband's welfare and his decision will have a significant impact on her life, affecting the most intimate aspects of their relationship. She is hoping to influence her husband to make the choice that she believes will be better for both of them.

While Dr. Binder can and should try to convince his patient to choose the most beneficial option, he should not manipulate the decision process by withholding critical information. Ultimately, his obligation is to his patient, who, as a capable person, is in the best position to assess the facts and consequences according to his own values, beliefs, and goals, as long as he has the necessary information and recommendation.

Voluntariness

||| Mr. Jenkins is a 28-year-old man with chronic renal disease who has been on hemodialysis for several years. Despite scrupulous attention to his medication, diet, and dialysis regimen, multiple complications have led to his deteriorating condition. Peritoneal dialysis has been ruled out because prior surgeries have left abdominal adhesions. At this point, his doctors believe his only chance for improvement or even survival is a kidney transplant.

Mr. Jenkins' immediate family consists of his pregnant wife and their 3-year-old son, his parents, his 26-year-old sister, and his 19-year-old brother. His parents and sister have been tissue typed and found to be incompatible as donors. His brother has said that, as much as he cares about the patient, he does not want to give up his football scholarship to college, which would be required if he had only one kidney.

At a family meeting, called to discuss options, Mr. Jenkins' parents, wife, and sister pressure his brother to be tested. After forty-five minutes of "How can you be so heartless?" "What is your career compared to your brother's life?" "You're no better than a murderer!", he agrees to be typed. When he is found to be a suitable donor, he says to the physician, "Now I have no choice. I have to donate or I'll be killing my brother and my family will hate me."

Is Mr. Jenkins' consent the product of altruism, family persuasion, or coercion? Does the physician have obligations to Mr. Jenkins that are in conflict with his obligations to the patient? How might the ethical dilemma be resolved, and what might be the role of the ethics committee?

But wait, there's more to consent and refusal. Genuinely autonomous decision making is both adequately informed and free of undue influence that corrupts the authenticity of the choice. Voluntariness refers to the individual's independence in making decisions that are the product of information, analysis, and personal values, not influenced by threat, force, or manipulation. *Independent* decision making, however, is not the same as *isolated* decision making, which would deprive the patient of physician and family recommendations and support. Problematic influences are those that subvert autonomous action by distorting individual choice through coercion or deception.

Influences with detrimental impact on the informed consent process can come from the patient's physician, family, or others in a position to exert compelling pressure. Voluntariness can be overtly sabotaged by relentless badgering, threats of family disruption, or emotional manipulation. An example would be, "Undergoing this treatment is the only way to save our marriage." Voluntariness can also be undermined when the physician says, "I won't continue to care for you if you don't do what I say."

What distinguishes problematic from beneficial influences are the quality, intent, and manner of the attempt to alter the decision. Interactions that provide additional information, encouragement, and support may modify the patient's choice by enhancing his decision-making powers. If, however, the influence is the product of deception that withholds or distorts information, if it denies or diminishes choice, if it appeals to fear rather than reason, it is likely to be controlling rather than supportive action. Continual attention to the purpose, process, and impact of external influences is necessary to preserve the integrity of the consent process.

THE NATURE OF INFORMED CONSENT

Informed Consent as an Interactive Process

By its nature, true informed consent is a process, not a moment in time, a perfunctory discussion, or a signed document. Meaningful consent is voluntarily and knowledgeably *given* by the patient, not *secured* or *imposed* by the staff as part of an assignment. Consent is not something the physician extracts from or does to the patient—"You need to get consent from Mrs. Simon" or "I consented Mr. Thomas." This attitude violates the autonomy of the patient and makes the signed consent form a trophy rather than the documentation of a process of communication, education, understanding, and trust.

The physician should begin the process by determining what the patient knows and whether he wants to participate in decisions about his care. Ongoing discussion should confirm his decisional capacity, his preferences and values, his appreciation of his condition, and the implications of his choices. Unless and until the patient is found to lack the ability to make his own decisions or he makes a capacitated and *voluntary* delegation of his decision-making authority to someone else, the patient is the person with whom the physician communicates.

The informed consent process, thus, assumes greater significance than simple physician disclosure of information and patient permission for treatment. It is an interaction between patient and physician, often including the family or trusted others, that promotes the exchange of relevant information and the provision of guidance and support that facilitates effective decision making.

While this process is necessary each time consent is required for an intervention, these discussions are not isolated events. As this chapter and the ones that follow demonstrate, the collaborative nature of the therapeutic relationship requires ongoing physician engagement in the decision-making process, including

- working with the patient and/or family to determine the goals of care based on the patient's condition, prognosis, and health care wishes
- developing a plan of care based on the goals that meets the patient's medical needs and is consistent with the patient's known wishes or the family's informed understanding of what is best for the incapacitated patient
- providing care that benefits the patient without imposing unnecessary suffering or prolonging the dying process, and discontinuing interventions that have not demonstrated clinical effectiveness
- regularly providing the patient and family with sufficient information to enable them to understand the progress and purpose of treatment, and appropriately revise care goals
- determining what elements of the care plan present genuine choices for patient and family decision making, and guiding and supporting those decisions

Sharing the Burden of Decision Making

The prevailing emphasis on patient autonomy risks diminishing the importance of the caregiver role in making difficult decisions. Treatment decisions require a grasp of often complex medical information, as well as insight into the patient's personal goals and values. As discussed in chapter 6, decisions about end-of-life care, in particular, are emotionally wrenching and their memory is long-lasting. Both professionalism and compassion dictate that the burden of making them be shared by those responsible for the care.

The suggestion is sometimes made that the full disclosure necessary for informed consent requires that physicians offer all possible treatment options for consideration. We argue that respecting patient or surrogate choice also recognizes that *some* care decisions *do not require and should not impose the burden of patient or family consent.* Presenting patients and families with false choices diminishes the exercise of their autonomy and abdicates the professional's responsibility to exercise clinical judgment. False choices are offered when patients and families are asked to reject interventions that have no clinical indication.

When reversal of or improvement in the patient's condition is no longer possible, it is appropriate to limit the therapeutic options to those with likely benefit. Interventions that are physiologically impossible or outside the standards of medical practice should not be proposed. These distinctions are addressed further in the discussion of medical futility in chapter 6. When specific treatments, such as dialysis, antibiotics, or vasopressors, are no longer effective, it is disingenuous to present them as options and hope that patients and families will be savvy enough to make the decisions that physicians already know they want. When there are *no real options*, physicians can and should determine *which interventions should be offered for consideration.* This does not mean disempowering patients and families. It means assuming the responsibility for making the judgments only physicians can make and then promoting the authentic choices reserved for patients and families.

Reflecting the tension between respecting patient autonomy and promoting patient well-being, physicians walk a fine line between supporting and usurping health care decision making. Patients and families depend on professional guidance in making care decisions and depriving them of clinical judgment, advice, and support can be seen as a form of abandonment. Even real choices should not be presented as value-neutral when one approach is clearly better, and physicians should be encouraged to clearly recommend what they believe to be the most appropriate course.

Guiding patient decisions should not be confused with paternalism, which demeans the capable adult and constricts the exercise of self-determination. Yet, patients and their surrogates have different levels of comfort assuming responsibility for treatment choices and caring physicians provide more or less structure as needed. Recognizing this delicate balance, commentators have suggested various approaches to providing information and decision-making support. For example, Emanuel and Emanuel (1992) offer four models of physician-patient interaction, representing different degrees of control and collaboration. Ultimately, providing genuine choices and thoughtful recommendations enhances patients' capacity to act in ways that promote both their autonomy and their well-being.

EXCEPTIONS TO THE CONSENT REQUIREMENT

The requirement for informed consent before treatment may be suspended in three narrow circumstances.

1. Emergency Care—Informed consent is not required when patients are unable to participate in care decisions, information about their wishes is not available, and delaying treatment would place their lives or health in peril. No one would seriously suggest that surgery to stop bleeding wait until an unresponsive accident victim regains consciousness and is able to provide consent. In such circumstances, consent is presumed based on the assumption that patients would want emergency treatment.

2. Therapeutic Exception—In very rare instances, physicians may believe that the disclosure of information about diagnoses or prognoses will cause clinically unstable patients to suffer immediate, direct, and significant harm. *Only in these limited and extreme circumstances* are physicians justified in withholding potentially harmful information from patients until such time as their clinical condition permits disclosure. The reasons for withholding the information must be detailed in the medical record and, whenever possible, the information must be disclosed to the patient's family or other trusted surrogate. Justifications for nondisclosure on this basis must be carefully scrutinized to ensure that it is the

patient's well-being, not the physician's comfort, that is being protected. As noted in the discussion of truth telling in chapter 4, inappropriately invoking this exception to the disclosure obligation must be avoided because it threatens the trust so essential to the therapeutic relationship.

3. Waiver of Consent—Corresponding to the right of informed consent is the patient's right not to be burdened with unwanted information or the pressure to make decisions *if he understands the consequences of giving up the opportunity to make decisions about care.* Electing not to know and delegating decisional authority to another person can be an authentic exercise of autonomy. But there must be an affirmative declaration by a capacitated patient that he wishes not to be involved in treatment decisions. The fact that he asks few questions or says, "Don't bother me with this now" is not the same as explicitly saying that he does not want to know or decide. Delegation of decision-making authority is not something that should be inferred, but something that must be confirmed. The right not to receive information is further addressed in the discussion of truth telling and disclosure in chapter 4.

Thus, effective consent provides ethical as well as legal authorization for the physician to treat. In contrast, assent, a notion with particular relevance in pediatrics, reflects the patient's *agreement* with a treatment plan rather than *authorization* of it. Only when the conditions of informational disclosure, understanding, and voluntariness have been met in the context of decisional capacity can the patient's consent or refusal be considered truly informed and authentic.

Returning to the case of Mrs. Stack, the 67-year-old woman with chronic renal insufficiency, a critical element in the ethical analysis is the assessment of decisional capacity. In her immediate postarrest and intubated state, she clearly lacked the ability to make decisions. Nevertheless, she was known to have had this capacity prior to admission and, during her hospitalization, she was found to have regained it sufficiently to understand the benefits of dialysis and the consequences of not receiving it. Because physicians are usually obligated to respect the wishes of capable patients, determining Mrs. Stack's decisional capacity and her wishes is of paramount importance.

In this case, Mrs. Stack's primary physician and family believe that her repeated refusal of dialysis has been based on her belief that her daughter died *because* of the treatments. Thus, it may legitimately be asked whether Mrs. Stack's reasons for refusing are based on an adequate comprehension of the risks and benefits of dialysis or on misunderstanding. Some have argued that a patient's decision to refuse treatment should be discounted if it is based on emotional, irrational, or false views. In general, however, coercing or disregarding otherwise decisionally capable patients should be avoided and efforts should focus on assisting them to make decisions based on accurate information and comprehension of the medical risks and benefits.

When the patient's ability to understand her medical condition and make choices is uncertain, consistency and durability of decisions can often substitute for capacity. Mrs. Stack's refusal of dialysis has been consistent over time, an important factor in assessing the quality of her decision making. While her refusal may be based on a misunderstanding, this durability indicates that she is comfortable with her position and speaks in favor of respecting her choice.

The patient's son threatens her with nursing home placement if she refuses dialysis—an odd ploy, because she is not likely to survive for long without the treatments. Despite the possibility that he has pressured her into accepting treatment, some types of influence are ethically acceptable because they do not rise to the level of coercion. Therefore, even if the son persuades his mother to change her mind, it does not necessarily invalidate her decision to accept dialysis. Caregivers should confirm the patient's change of mind and satisfy themselves that it is truly informed and voluntary. One approach is to observe discussions between the patient and her son, if they do not object. Another safeguard is to review Mrs. Stack's decision with her when her son is not present.

REFERENCES

Ackerman TF. 2001. Why doctors should intervene. In Mappes TA, DeGrazia D, eds. *Biomedical Ethics*. 5th ed. Boston: McGraw Hill, pp. 80–85.

Arnold R, Lidz C. 2001. Informed consent: Clinical aspects of consent in health care. In Levine C, ed. *Taking Sides: Clashing Views on Controversial Bioethical Issues*. 9th ed. Guilford, CT: Dushkin/McGraw-Hill, pp. 4–11.

Beauchamp TL. 1997. Informed consent. In Veatch R, ed. *Medical Ethics*. 2nd ed. Sudbury, MA: Jones and Bartlett Publishers, pp. 185–208.

Beauchamp TL, Childress JF. 2001. *Principles of Biomedical Ethics*. 5th ed. New York: Oxford University Press, pp. 77–98.

Brock D. 1993. Informed consent. In *Life and Death: Philosophical Essays in Biomedical Ethics*. New York: Cambridge University Press, pp. 21–54.

Brody H. 1989. Transparency: Informed consent in primary care. *Hastings Center Report* 19(5):5–9.

Emanuel EJ, Emanuel LL. 1992. Four models of the physician-patient relationship. *Journal of the American Medical Association* 267(16):2221–26.

Garrett TM, Baillie HW, Garrett RM. 2001. Principles of autonomy and informed consent. In *Health Care Ethics: Principles and Problems*. 4th ed. Upper Saddle River, NJ: Prentice Hall, pp. 29–56.

Katz J. 2003. Informed consent—Must it remain a fairy tale? In Steinbock B, Arras JD, London AJ, eds. *Ethical Issues in Modern Medicine*. 6th ed. Boston: McGraw-Hill, pp. 92–100.

Lo B. 2000. *Resolving Ethical Dilemmas: A Guide for Clinicians*. 2nd ed. Philadelphia: Lippincott Williams & Wilkins, pp. 19–29.

Meisel A, Kuczewski M. 1996. Legal and ethical myths about informed consent. *Archives of Internal Medicine* 156:2521–26.

President's Commission for the Study of Ethical Problems in Medicine and Biomedical and Behavioral Research. 1982. *Making Health Care Decisions: The Ethical and Legal Implications of Informed Consent in the Patient-Practitioner Relationship* (Vol. 1: Report). Washington, DC.

Schneider CE. 1998. *The Practice of Autonomy: Patients, Doctors, and Medical Decisions*. New York: Oxford University Press.

Shalowitz KI, Wolf MS. 2004. Shared decision-making and the lower literate patient. *Journal of Law, Medicine & Ethics* 32(4):759–64.

State of Tennessee Department of Human Service v. Mary C. Northern, Court of Appeals of Tennessee, Middle Section, Feb. 7, 1978. In Steinbock B, Arras JD, London AJ. 2003. *Ethical Issues in Modern Medicine.* 6th ed. Boston: McGraw-Hill, pp. 283–87.

Transcript of proceedings: Testimony of Mary C. Northern. In Steinbock B, Arras JD, London AJ. 2003. *Ethical Issues in Modern Medicine.* 6th ed. Boston: McGraw-Hill, pp. 287–90.

Veatch RM. 2001. Abandoning informed consent. In Levine C, ed. *Taking Sides: Clashing Views on Controversial Bioethical Issues.* 9th ed. Guildford, CT: Dushkin/McGraw-Hill, pp. 12–18.

4 Truth Telling: Disclosure and Confidentiality

Arguably, the most valuable health care resource is information. Clinicians depend on its accuracy in making their diagnoses and prognoses. Patients rely on its adequacy in evaluating their options and arriving at their decisions about care. Families wait for news of their loved ones' changing conditions.

But beyond lab data and examination findings, clinical information defines the very nature of the therapeutic relationship, involving notions of self-image, privacy, autonomy, power, and trust. How clinical information is elicited, protected, and shared is a matter of ethical concern for professionals, especially when their obligations conflict.

The idea that care professionals should tell their patients the truth seems self-evident and uncontroversial. Previous chapters have devoted considerable space to the discussion of the importance of *informed* decision making and the trust that is so central to the therapeutic relationship. Like most other aspects of the clinical interaction, however, truth telling can become complicated when patient autonomy, beneficence, and non-maleficence collide.

III   Mr. Nunez is a 46-year-old Hispanic man suffering from terminal esophageal cancer. He speaks no English, but his wife, who is bilingual and constantly at his bedside, translates for the care providers. This way of relating to Mr. Nunez—through his wife—is not recent. For the nine months that Mr. Nunez has been coming to the hospital for treatment, Mrs. Nunez has essentially directed his care and determined what he is to be told. Believing that she is acting in his best interest, his care providers have honored her wishes, but they are increasingly uncomfortable.

It has become clear that Mrs. Nunez is not translating everything that she is being told. In particular, she seems to be censoring information about the seriousness of Mr. Nunez's condition. When asked about this, Mrs. Nunez has made it very clear that she does not want her husband told that he is dying of cancer. He knows that he has a growth on his esophagus but not that he has cancer. Indeed, according to her, he does not even understand what cancer is. Mr. Nunez has also recently been enrolled in a phase I/II cancer research protocol, consent for which has been given by his wife.

Mrs. Nunez is adamant that her husband not be told about his diagnosis or prognosis. She seems to believe sincerely that, if he were to find out the truth, he would do violence to himself and possibly to her. When asked why she thinks this, she cites an incident in which the patient threatened to harm himself if his condition were found to be more serious than he thought. Although she has been assured that patients usually benefit from understanding their conditions, she insists that nothing can be gained for Mr. Nunez by telling him the truth. She concedes that he occasionally asks questions, but claims that she has been able to satisfy him with evasive or deceitful answers. When asked whether she would agree to have Mr. Nunez told the truth when he is finally too weak to harm himself, she emphatically replied, "No! Never! I can't imagine what it would be like for him to know that he is dying. I won't have this!" Although she describes her husband as "like a baby," there is no reason to believe that the patient could not comprehend the nature and seriousness of his condition. His cognitive status cannot be confirmed, however, because Mrs. Nunez has forbidden a psychiatric evaluation.

Members of the care team are conflicted about the limits on their ability to interact with Mr. Nunez. Several strongly believe that he is being deprived of his rights to information, while others suggest that his wife knows him better than they do. The oncology fellow notes that "in certain countries, such as Japan, patients are not routinely told the truth about their diagnoses as a way of protecting them from stress, but at least they are not tortured by being enrolled in research that is not likely to benefit them."

How and by whom should this patient's best interests be defined? Do Mr. Nunez's rights conflict with his best interest? What arguments support disclosure or nondisclosure in this case?

JUSTIFICATIONS

Honesty and trustworthiness as core interpersonal values derive from the moral imperative of veracity. Three justifications that have been advanced to support the obligation of veracity have particular relevance to the clinical setting. They are "respect owed to others . . . fidelity and promise-keeping . . . [and] relationships of trust between persons . . . necessary for fruitful interaction and cooperation" (Beauchamp and Childress, 1994, p. 396).

1. Respect for others is reflected in the ethical principle of autonomy. The capable individual's right to be self-determining imposes on clinicians the obligation to provide adequate information for informed health care decision making.
2. Fidelity and the keeping of promises are central elements in the trust-based relationship between patient and clinician. This fiduciary bond creates an implicit contract that both parties will be honest and will honor their commitments.
3. Productive therapeutic interactions rely on the truthful management of information. The effective clinician-patient relationship depends on the exchange of accurate and complete information about symptoms, diagnosis, prognosis, and treatment options, as well as confidence that care plans will be followed and patient wishes will be honored.

In this context, the uneasiness of the professionals caring for Mr. Nunez is understandable if they believe that withholding information undercuts his autonomy, erodes their trusting relationship, and inhibits effective clinical management. Only the strong likelihood that disclosure would be harmful to the patient can justify withholding information about his condition. This very rare therapeutic exception to the disclosure obligation is discussed below.

DISCLOSURE

Ethical Obligation

As discussed in chapter 3, collaborative decision making and informed consent depend on the reasonable disclosure of necessary or material information. Patients and their authorized surrogates are ethically and legally entitled to information that enables them to understand the likely course of the medical condition, evaluate the therapeutic options, and make choices consistent with patient goals and values.

Disclosure invokes respect for the patient's right to information that promotes effective decision making and the ethical imperatives to maximize benefits and minimize harms. Yet, as the case of Mr. Nunez illustrates, these same principles create tension between and among professionals' obligations. The analysis weighs the benefits of disclosing information that enhances patient understanding and self-determination against the potential harms of anxiety and stress that disclosure may cause.

Because laboratory and examination findings are controlled by the care team, particularly the medical staff, disclosure of clinical information is at the discretion of the physician. Access to medical information is thus an inherently unequal process that places the patient at a potential disadvantage in decision making. This imbalance confers on doctors the disclosure obligation.

Arguments for Disclosing Information

ǀǀǀ Ms. Kim, a 23-year-old woman, presents with an isolated case of first-bout optic neuritis. The ophthalmologist, Dr. Frank, is concerned about whether to inform her that multiple sclerosis (MS) may develop in the future. His dilemma arises because, at the time the optic neuritis presents, the likelihood of subsequent development of MS is uncertain. Until recently, it was thought that the degree of association between optic neuritis and MS was around 11 percent. Increasing evidence, however, suggests that the association may be as high as 80 percent.

The arguments in favor of disclosure are both ethical and practical. To know the truth about one's current and future medical condition is essential to a sense of self-mastery, especially as that condition changes and possibly deteriorates. Lack of information impairs decision making about health care and other life plans. Even when treatment options are limited, knowing what to expect allows patients to understand and prepare for what lies ahead.

Dr. Frank's concern is that disclosing the possibility of MS could cause Ms. Kim needless anxiety about an illness that she may never develop. Moreover, because MS cannot be prevented or cured, the information will not afford her any protection. On the other hand, it can be argued that she has the right to prepare herself for the heightened likelihood that she may develop a debilitating condition that would inevitably affect her ability to function independently. This knowledge may be an important influence in making decisions about lifestyle, career, family, and finances, as well planning treatment that could potentially delay the onset of or mitigate symptoms of MS. Finally, if Ms. Kim discovers this information independently, her trust in Dr. Frank may be eroded by the belief that he was not honest about her risks.

ǀǀǀ Evan Barry was 17 years old when he was diagnosed last year with renal cell carcinoma. His right kidney was removed and he began several rounds of chemotherapy. Early this year, he came to the emergency room complaining of shortness of breath and chest pain. He seemed to be unaware of his diagnosis and could not explain the scar from the kidney surgery. A chest X ray showed metastases to his lungs.

Evan was transferred from the ER to the adolescent unit and given gamma interferon. The physicians on the adolescent floor were puzzled by his apparent ignorance of his condition. When they approached his mother, Mrs. Barry was equivocal about what her son had been told. She said that she had been candid with Evan when he was first diagnosed but, when the physicians encouraged further discussions during the current admission, she adamantly refused to allow anyone to talk with him about his diagnosis and treatment. She expressed fear that he would be devastated and become suicidal, although she acknowledged that he had never attempted or threatened suicide.

Staff on the adolescent unit believed that Evan was frightened and isolated by the lack of information and communication. One of the residents carefully asked questions to probe the extent of his knowledge about his cancer. Evan said tearfully that he did not know what was wrong with him and that the doctors always spoke with his mother, not with him. He also said, "My mom is very worried about me but it makes her sad to talk about my problems and I don't want to upset her even more."

The team agreed that, although the lack of information was probably very frightening for Evan, he seemed to be protecting his mother by not asking questions. Concern was expressed that, as a capable adult who appeared to want and need information and support, he should be told the truth.

What are the care providers' conflicting obligations and how can they be resolved? What benefits and risks should be considered? Who should determine what Evan is told?

Truth telling goes to the core of trust-based relationships, especially those among family members and between the patient and care professionals. Shielding patients from the truth is generally an imperfect undertaking, requiring the collusion of others, including staff, family, and friends, in a conspiracy of silence. Uncertainty about what the patient knows and discomfort with the deception often result in caregivers and even family avoiding contact with the patient. It is not unusual to hear, "I was so sure that I would give it away that I just didn't want to be around him."

Yet, patients—even children and adults with a history of not wanting to know—sense when things are being kept from them and may avoid discussion as a way of accommodating those protecting them. Evan, for example, is reluctant to ask questions about his condition because he knows that talking about it upsets his mother. The result is a cycle of increasingly difficult efforts for mother and son to protect each other from acknowledging their sadness and fear. The burden of the deception itself, thus, can be a barrier to communication. Perhaps the most damaging aspect of withholding information is that the patient is isolated at precisely the time when close and supportive relationships are critical. In short, although the obligation of truth telling is not an absolute, it is something that requires a compelling reason to disregard.

Conflicting Obligations

The tension arises when clinicians feel that their obligations require them to either disclose information that the patient may not want or withhold potentially problematic information, all in the name of promoting the patient's well-being. The challenge is determining what the patient should know to receive needed care without undue stress and have his autonomy respected.

As you might suspect at this point, disclosure is not simply a matter of rattling off the results of lab tests or physical examinations. Effective disclosure is a clinical skill that depends on physician judgment and communication as well as knowledge. Too much information can be as harmful as too little. The difference between truth telling and truth dumping is the difference between providing specific material information that facilitates decision making and indiscriminately overloading the patient with facts in the interests of completeness. An unbroken monologue of clinical data can be counterproductive, leaving the patient with glazed eyes and little recollection of what was said. Far more useful is breaking up the explanation every few sentences with, "Does that make sense?" or "What else can I tell you that would be helpful?" Patients often indicate what they want to know, and perceptive clinicians can be guided by their spoken or unspoken signals.

Truth dumping also occurs when information is disclosed without the accompanying explanations or guidance that frame the decisions patients or surrogates must make. "Let me tell you what all this means and then we can figure out the reasonable choices you might consider." Finally, patients need to be reassured that they are not expected to absorb everything all at once. "I know that this is a lot to take in right now and we will talk again. When you think of questions, it might be a good idea to write them down so that we can address them next time."

Patients have both the right to receive information and the right *not* to receive it. Some people, especially those who are elderly, anxious, easily confused, or from cultures that do not place a high premium on individual autonomy, find it burdensome and even frightening to learn about their conditions and be asked to make treatment decisions. For example, while persons from European American backgrounds typically value full disclosure of medical information, those from Asian and Middle Eastern cultures tend to protect patients from knowing about illness or impending death. For them, authentic decision making in the clinical setting is expressed in the capacitated request *not* to be informed and the voluntary delegation of decision-making authority to trusted others. Implicit is a long-standing or culture-based comfort with the practice of decision making by surrogates. Likewise, Mr. and Mrs. Nunez may be an example of families that have their own decision-making patterns that may be effective and comfortable, rather than paternalistic or coercive. Decision making, like other interpersonal dynamics, comes in assorted shapes and sizes entitled to respectful attention. But, as noted in chapter 3, a waiver of informed consent is something that must be explicitly confirmed, not inferred, to demonstrate respect for the patient and protect his autonomy.

Arguments for Not Disclosing Information

The more common disclosure dilemmas concern withholding information from patients who have not waived that right, usually justified by notions of shielding them from harm. Disclosure, especially of bad news, is one of the most difficult clinical tasks, and evasion or awkwardness is often the result of efforts to avoid inflicting pain. Physicians often protect themselves and—they think—their patients by resorting to euphemism. "The patient has a grim prognosis" becomes "the patient is not doing well." "The patient is dying" becomes "the patient is failing." Sometimes it sounds as though, if the patient and care team only tried harder, she would not be dying.

Rather than comfort, however, deliberate vagueness creates confusion, anxiety, and unrealistic expectations. It is not uncommon for a family to react with frustration and seemingly unreasonable demands when told that, although the patient is *not doing well,* aggressive treatments should be limited. The family argues that she could be doing *better* if only the care team were doing *more* rather than *less.* The importance of compassionate candor is emphasized in the discussion of medical futility and forgoing treatment at the end of life in chapter 6.

Sometimes, discomfort in discussing bad news with the patient persuades care professionals that disclosure would be *harmful,* when in fact it might only be *distressing.* The risk is that the therapeutic exception, noted in chapter 3, may be expanded beyond its strict definition (exception to the disclosure obligation when the information itself would cause *immediate, direct, and significant harm* to the patient) and applied to situations in which the information would be upsetting, but not dangerous. Whenever clinicians consider withholding information, especially from capable patients, they need to question who is being protected, whether the protection is truly warranted, and what the cost will be to the trust between doctor and patient. This dilemma, which requires balancing the ethical obligations of respect for autonomy, beneficence, and nonmaleficence, often triggers a bioethics consultation to explore the benefits and risks of disclosure to the patient.

Pressure also comes from families—parents of young children, grown children of aging parents, or concerned spouses like Mrs. Nunez—not to share information with the patient. The reasons are usually "The news will kill him" or "You will take away all hope." The first objection indicates the need to reassure anxious relatives that the patient will not be burdened with information that he does not want or cannot safely assimilate. The second objection speaks to expectations and the importance of hope. As further discussed in chapter 7, bad news or even a terminal diagnosis need not signal a future so bleak that deception is justified. It is frequently necessary to redefine what can be hoped for—perhaps not long life or unlimited function, but rather increased comfort or a peaceful death surrounded by loved ones.

Let us consider how these issues relate to Mr. Nunez. His caregivers are faced with conflicting obligations in determining what he should be told about his condition.

Because they have been prevented from interacting with him directly, they have no independent assessment of his capacity, emotional stability, or desire for information. All communications have been filtered through his wife, whose motives may be well meaning but overprotective, or possibly not in his best interest. The care professionals need to clarify with Mrs. Nunez that providing her husband with good care requires that they interact with him directly. She should be reassured that harmful or unwanted information will not be forced on him but that his perceptions and wishes will be skillfully assessed as part of his clinical evaluation.

When withholding information is suggested, it is necessary to determine the patient's capacity, understanding of the clinical situation, and desire for information. The first step is to use the patient's preferred language, in this case, Spanish. One approach might be, "Mr. Nunez, the examinations and tests will be giving us information about your condition and then some decisions will have to be made about your treatment. Some patients want to know all the information and some don't. What would make you comfortable? Whom would you like us to talk to? Do you want us to discuss these things with you or with someone else?" Capable patients can then elect to participate in the process or voluntarily delegate that responsibility to another person. Even if Mr. Nunez explicitly says, "I don't want to know and I want my wife to make decisions for me," he should be kept in the communication loop by being asked periodically, "Do you have any questions? Is there anything we can tell you?" A wish not to be burdened with information or decision making should not deprive patients of attention in other ways.

DISCLOSURE OF ADVERSE OUTCOMES AND MEDICAL ERROR

‖ Mrs. Allen, a pregnant woman with diabetes, had been encouraged to undergo amniocentesis to determine the fetus's lung development in order to plan induction of her delivery. Because there is a window of safety in delivering diabetics, this procedure is considered standard of care. During the amnio, the umbilical cord was nicked, resulting in bleeding and requiring an immediate caesarean section.

The neonatology house staff has requested an ethics consult to discuss whether the parents should be told the reason for the emergency delivery and, if so, whether the information should come from the obstetric team or the neonatologists.

Adverse Outcomes and Medical Error

Disclosure of bad news is difficult under any circumstances. Disclosure of bad news when things go wrong is a clinician's worst nightmare, but it is one that must be confronted for the sake of patients and professionals. We begin with some important definitions. *Adverse outcomes* are unintended negative results of medical care that create actual or potential harm to the patient. These untoward occurrences may be the result of carelessness or ineptitude, or they may reflect foreseen but unavoidable risk even when standard of care was practiced. The former—*medical errors*—are considered avoidable, while the latter are generally seen as unavoidable. Distinguishing between these types of adverse outcomes may be problematic, although standard of care is sometimes used as an important criterion.

Other analyses distinguish between *system* and *individual or human* errors, attributing some adverse outcomes to problems in the health care delivery system and others to the actions of individual providers. This approach reflects the notion that "no one person [is] responsible, because it is virtually impossible for one mistake to kill a patient in the highly mechanized and backstopped world of a modern hospital" (Belkin, 1997, p. 28). The 2000 Institute of Medicine report, *To Err is Human: Building a Safer Health System,* generated considerable interest in disclosure of information as a key to managing and preventing adverse outcomes. As a result, oversight and accrediting bodies, clinicians, and institutions are adopting the concept of health care delivery as a system-wide interlocking dynamic that can either allow or prevent error. In analyzing adverse events, this perspective focuses on organization *processes* rather than individual performance.

Scope of Disclosure

Disclosure includes but is not limited to the requirements of informed consent, which permit *prospective* analysis of proposed interventions. Armed with adequate information, the patient can proceed to make decisions about future care. Full disclosure that promotes patient self-determination and protection also includes *retrospective* analysis of unintended consequences. This aspect of disclosure suggests that, in addition to patients' need for information to enhance care planning and decision making, there is also a desire just to understand what did or will happen to them. Taken together, the *preview* and *review* aspects of the disclosure obligation can be seen in the patient's need to *act* and to *know*.

Obligation of Disclosure

The obligation to disclose adverse outcomes rests on both ethical and legal foundations. Recognizing the need to ensure the provision of adequate information, courts have imposed fiduciary obligations of disclosure on physicians. Judicial reasoning is that these obligations exist when "one party is dependent on another for information or knowledge that only the first party possesses" (Vogel and Delgado, 1980, pp. 66–67). In the clinical setting, the physician is the person most likely to have and control information about an untoward event or medical error, heightening the professional obligation of disclosure. The patient who has suffered an undisclosed adverse event is doubly vulnerable—not only is she unaware of the actual or potential harms she faces and how to prevent or mitigate them, she may not know the nature of the event or even that it has occurred. Her reliance on the physician for information that will minimize harm and/or help her cope with the consequences creates an ethical imperative for timely and full disclosure of the adverse event. This obligation has received explicit attention in the various codes and opinions that provide ethical guidance and analysis for physicians.

A related basis for the disclosure obligation can be found in the values underlying informed consent. This analysis views informed consent as a compact entered into by physician and patient. The doctor says, in effect, "Here is the information you need, including the possible risks." The patient says, in effect, "I understand what you have said and I consent to the test or treatment *because I trust that you have told me everything I need to know* in order to make a decision." Implicit in the patient's response is, "I trust that you will exercise all due care in treating me. *I further trust that, if any foreseen or unforeseen harms should occur, you will disclose that information so that I can understand and manage the negative consequences.*"

Seen in this light, the values underlying informed consent support the disclosure obligation. The patient is able to balance the benefits, burdens, and risks in advance of treatment, and also mitigate potential harms and protect herself from further harms after an untoward event has occurred. Rather than a passive recipient of treatment, the patient becomes a fully equal partner in planning for and managing the outcomes of care.

Barriers to Disclosure

Given the ethical and legal justifications, it seems hard to argue with the notion that information about untoward occurrences should be made available to patients or their surrogates. It will not be surprising, however, that physicians are very reluctant to discuss negative outcomes with patients and families. Reasons for avoiding disclosure include the difficulty of determining whether the event was medical error, the belief that the information will only be upsetting, and the omnipresent fear of legal action.

Liability to medical malpractice suits is cited by physicians as the chief barrier to disclosure of unintended occurrences. Doctors' understandable risk aversion makes them uneasy about admitting error or other behavior that might have contributed to patient harm. That said, you should know that legal action does not inevitably follow adverse events, including those caused by negligence. Instead, whether litigation is instituted appears closely related to how physicians handle discussions with patients about untoward outcomes, including disclosure of information about actual or potential harm (Liebman and Hyman, 2004; Gallagher et al., 2003; Goldberg et al., 2002). Concerns about who assumes the duty of disclosure and bears responsibility are especially difficult in an academic medical center, with its multiple levels of interdisciplinary staff and different authority structures.

Perhaps even more threatening to physicians than the specter of malpractice litigation is the personal devaluation that accompanies acknowledging adverse events. This may include "a loss of personal confidence and self-esteem, diminished professional authority and reputation, as well as a loss of referrals and income" (Baylis, 1997, p. 338). The inability to cope with untoward outcomes appears to stem less from blatant physician callousness or dishonesty than from belief in the widespread myth of infallibility and total control that define the perfect healer. This image, born in medical schools, nurtured throughout medical careers, and sold to the public, is shared by physicians and their patients, leading to unrealistic expectations, unreasonable disappointments, and unbridgeable gaps in communication.

Growing recognition of these issues has prompted six states (Florida, Nevada, New Jersey, Oregon [voluntary participation], Pennsylvania, and Washington) to enact disclosure laws requiring that patients or their surrogates be notified of adverse events, typically according to specified procedures and within specified time limits (Liebman and Hyman, 2006). One response to these statutory requirements and the potential that other states may enact similar legislation has been the Project on Medical Liability in Pennsylvania, using trained mediators to strengthen physicians' skills in communicating difficult news and establishing mediation as an alternative to proposed litigation (Liebman and Hyman, 2004).

CONFIDENTIALITY

III Mr. Miller is a 42-year-old man who came to the emergency room with iritis and whose work-up was positive for syphilis. When Dr. David discussed the diagnosis with Mr. Miller, the patient requested that Dr. David not disclose the infection to his wife or report it to the state department of health. He said that he must have contracted the condition during a one-time extramarital encounter on a recent business trip. He also stated that he has not had sexual contact with his wife since that time and that he will undergo treatment before doing so.

Another aspect of information management central to the therapeutic relationship is the ethical obligation of confidentiality, which also derives in part from the moral imperatives of veracity and privacy. "Confidentiality is present when one person discloses information to another, whether through words or an examination, and the person to whom the information is disclosed pledges not to divulge that information to a third party without the confider's permission" (Beauchamp and Childress, 2001, pp. 305–6). In that sense, confidentiality, like truth telling, invokes the patient's trust in and reliance on the health care professional's integrity. Although the common perception is that confidentiality binds only the patient and physician, the professional obligation also covers other clinicians, including chiropractors, clinical social workers, dentists, nurses, podiatrists, and psychologists.

Justifications for Protecting Confidentiality

III Mr. Gordon, a 43-year-old man, is picked up by the police on Saturday evening and rushed to the nearest emergency room after passing out on a mid-town sidewalk. ER physicians detect a high level of alcohol in his blood and a urine toxicology screen reveals opiates. Upon regaining consciousness, Mr. Gordon provides his past medical history, which is unremarkable, and says that his occupation is city sanitation truck driver. He acknowledges that he used alcohol and cocaine earlier in the evening, and reminds the physicians that they have a duty not to disclose to others confidential patient information.

What obligations do physicians have to Mr. Gordon and others, and how can they be reconciled? What ethical principles and additional factors should be considered?

The notion that the therapeutic interaction creates a zone of protected information can be supported by the three justifications for veracity discussed earlier.

Respect for persons underlies patients' right to control who has access to their heath care information and requires that medical records and communications in the clinical setting be protected from unwarranted disclosure. If personal information can be seen as a reflection of the most intimate aspects of an individual's life, then control of that information can be seen as a form of self-determination that requires provider respect. Protecting confidentiality also prevents the harms that result from unauthorized disclosure of sensitive information, such as HIV status or psychiatric history.

Fidelity and promise keeping are reflected in the bond of trust that requires professionals to hold in confidence information learned in the clinical interaction. This justification is based on the moral imperative to honor a duty or promise regardless of the results. It holds that, without explicit patient waiver, the clinician is bound by the confidentiality inherent in the relationship. The argument also encompasses the notion of secrets, those pieces of our private selves we give in trust to others with the implicit or explicit understanding that they will be held in confidence.

The effectiveness of the clinical relationship and the resulting quality of the health care provided depend on an atmosphere of trust that promotes the candid and complete exchange of information. This justification rests on the need to encourage patients to provide all relevant facts about their medical history and symptoms, no matter how private or potentially embarrassing, to facilitate accurate diagnosis and effective treatment. This utilitarian rationale argues that, without an obligation of strict nondisclosure, patients would avoid seeking or fully cooperating in treatment.

Barriers to Confidentiality

It would seem that nothing could be more ethically compelling than the promise to protect what patients reveal about themselves. Like truth telling, confidentiality seems a clear and simple duty that professionals owe their patients. But, like other ethical imperatives, the confidentiality obligation is neither absolute nor always easy to honor.

So what gets in the way of protecting patient confidences? Medical information is generated in the health care setting as a product of the therapeutic interaction between clinician and patient; it is also generated in the pharmacy, the research lab, the autopsy room, the insurance office, the medical classroom, and the hospital elevator. It goes into reports, books, lectures, legal briefs, and computers, from which it is accessed by countless people for countless valid and not-so-valid reasons.

The treating relationship is only one context in which medical confidentiality is raised. The dramatic change in health care delivery has altered what used to be a confidential relationship between patient and family doctor. Medical treatment has moved from the home to the institutional setting; multiple disciplines and subspecialties, legal and government bureaucracies, and third-party payers now converge on each case; and computers connect all parties to the clinical interaction. The result is that the number of people with legitimate and nonlegitimate access to medical information has increased geometrically. A 1982 article reported that medical information about a patient, whose case was not unusual or complex, was necessarily available to at least seventy-five people who provided direct or support health care services (Siegler, 1982). We can safely assume that access to patient information and the parties who want it have expanded significantly since then. The contemporary clinical setting has greatly enhanced the efficiency and efficacy of communication among care providers, while compromising the privacy of patients' medical information. Concerns about the security of patient information prompted the inclusion of stringent regulations in the 1996 federal Health Insurance Portability and Accountability Act (HIPAA).

Consent to care with a loss of some measure of privacy is either explicitly obtained, through signed releases upon entering the hospital, or presumed, but the consent is never to be considered unlimited. For example, although it should be explained upon admission, it is generally understood that treatment in a teaching hospital includes having one's records, examinations, and therapies available for observation and study by students and house staff. Most patients expect that their cases will be discussed formally and even informally to obtain the benefit of other opinions and to provide teaching examples. They neither expect nor deserve to have their personal or medical information shared in public hospital areas or social situations. Likewise, patients should have control over who has access to their medical information through updates in their clinical condition. As a precaution against inadvertent unwanted disclosure, it may be helpful to say early in the patient's hospital stay, "You seem to have a lot of family and friends who are concerned about you. Please know that we will not be discussing your medical condition with anyone unless you specifically request that we do so."

In addition to those who use medical information for treatment purposes, such data are routinely used by medical researchers, law enforcement agencies, attorneys (requesting their own clients' records or those of other patients in connection with medical malpractice or personal injury), insurers (life, health, disability, and liability), employers, and creditors. Although these secondary users are routinely required to access information though formal requests for patient record releases, they may not always follow procedure. Finally, there are potential users of medical information who have nothing to do with the patient's health care, including those with commercial, political, and media interests.

So, are confidentiality and privacy obsolete or decrepit, as some commentators (e.g., Siegler, 1982) suggest? Given the formidable barriers and incentives in the current health care setting, is it possible or even desirable to manage the flow of information? The goal of providing state-of-the-art care increasingly requires quick access to medical data by multiple parties. The protection of third-party interests is receiving heightened attention. The obligation of confidentiality is being reshaped by its exceptions and its boundaries are increasingly porous. Yet, the ethical core remains intact and worth preserving. The contours may be redrawn, but the central values deserve protection through policies and regulations that respond to current clinical and legal imperatives.

Justifications for Breaching Confidentiality

Even people with little experience in the health care setting know and rely on the sanctity of clinician-patient confidentiality. Based on well-established ethical and legal justifications, this obligation normally precludes professionals from disclosing information learned in the course of diagnosis or treatment. Precisely because this ethical mandate is so central to the clinical relationship, exceptions are justified only when disclosure of confidential information is essential to preventing significant harm to other vulnerable individuals, especially those at unsuspected risk. In these select instances, the patient's right to confidentiality is considered to be outweighed by the obligation to protect those who are not in a position to protect themselves.

The following two situations that justify breaching confidentiality illustrate the conflicting ethical obligations when competing claims are made for physician fidelity. In both circumstances, the needs of the nonpatients are elevated because their vulnerability is heightened by their very ignorance of the risks they face.

1. Providing information that prevents harm to *identified* third parties at risk (e.g., partner notification). This exception reflects the opinion in *Tarasoff v. Regents of University of California,* a 1976 case in which the court held that a psychotherapist who had prior knowledge of a patient's intention to kill his unsuspecting girlfriend had a duty to warn her. This reasoning has been incorporated into the laws of many states in addressing the needs of those who have been unwittingly exposed to HIV/AIDS or sexually transmitted disease. When the infected patient refuses to inform sexual or needle-sharing partners, notification is considered essential to enable those known to be at risk to be tested and treated.

2. Providing information that prevents harm to *unidentified* others at risk (e.g., public health or public safety reporting). In some instances, the potential danger is to the general population, rather than to specified individuals. To protect the

public health and safety, state laws commonly require that health care providers report certain findings, including suspected cases of child abuse and neglect; wounds that are the result of gun shots, knives, or other pointed instruments; burn injuries of specified severity; and cases of reportable communicable diseases specified in state health laws.

In the case of Mr. Miller, Dr. David is in a difficult position. He knows that confidentiality is the bedrock of the patient-physician relationship, assuring the patient that he can share accurate and sensitive information with the doctor without fear of disclosure. Not only does the assurance of confidentiality promote trust, it facilitates full and candid communication that is vital to successful diagnosis and treatment. Fear that sensitive or embarrassing information, such as a diagnosis of sexually transmitted disease (STD), will be disclosed may dissuade Mr. Miller from providing critical facts or even seeking necessary treatment.

Sometimes, however, withholding information poses risks to others outside the physician-patient relationship. In this case, Mr. Miller's wife is at risk of contracting syphilis and she is especially vulnerable because she has no reason to suspect that she is at risk. By taking action early through testing and, if necessary, treatment, she may be able to avoid the dire consequences of syphilis and perhaps other STDs. To protect vulnerable persons, public health has traditionally intervened by contact tracing and partner notification. Clinicians are required by law to report most STDs by patient name to public health officials so that they can trace and notify partners at risk. Public officials try to maintain the anonymity of the index case as much as possible. But if Mrs. Miller's only sexual partner has been her husband, it may be difficult or impossible to prevent her from figuring out how she was exposed.

Despite pressure from Mr. Miller, it is ethically and legally unacceptable for Dr. David to cooperate with the request to withhold information that can prevent harm to an identified person at risk. Dr. David should counsel Mr. Miller about the importance of disclosure, including the legal requirements and the risks of nondisclosure, and encourage him to tell his wife. It may be helpful if he offers support in the disclosure process.

Mr. Gordon's case raises somewhat different issues. Here, the concern is whether the physicians have a responsibility to report the fact that a person who drives a sanitation truck for the city is known to have used alcohol and illegal drugs. In this analysis, the justifications underlying the confidentiality obligation would be weighed against the possible harms to unidentified persons—the public—who have no reason to believe that they are at risk. Relevant factors would include the potential for harm, the likelihood that it could be prevented, alternatives to breaching confidentiality, and the legal requirements of the state in which the situation occurs.

While no one would encourage Mr. Gordon to abuse alcohol or drugs, it can be argued that his behavior on this occasion does not place others at immediate or inevitable risk. In this case, the patient's substance-related loss of consciousness occurred on a weekend evening, not during work hours, and not while he was driving a truck or any other vehicle. It would be important to know whether his use of alcohol and drugs is substantial or minimal, and whether it occurs daily or only occasionally. This information, which is relevant to his health care as well as the safety of others, is much more likely to be revealed to his caregivers if Mr. Gordon is assured that it will be kept confidential.

In terms of state law, the patient's only illegal behavior is his use of narcotics. Health care professionals should not be expected to compromise their obligations to their patients by functioning as agents of the law enforcement or judicial systems. Accordingly, all states presume a general rule of patient confidentiality, carving out selected specific instances when that obligation must be breached to protect others from harm.

If Mr. Gordon suffered from epilepsy, he would be required by all states to report his condition to the motor vehicle bureau and, if he worked as a school bus driver, his physicians would have a heightened incentive to discourage his driving. The argument might also be made that, if Mr. Gordon did not report his epilepsy, his doctors would have an ethical obligation to do so. None of those conditions apply here, however, and his care professionals are likely to respect his confidentiality, while counseling him about responsible behaviors.

REFERENCES

American College of Physicians. 1993. *Ethics Manual.* 3rd ed. Philadelphia: American College of Physicians. Cited in Witman AB, Park DM, Hardin SB. 1996. How do patients want physicians to handle mistakes? *Archives of Internal Medicine* 156(22):2565–69.

American Medical Association, Council on Ethical and Judicial Affairs. 1997. Patient information: Opinion E-8.12, Issued March 1981, updated June 1994. *Code of Medical Ethics.* Chicago: American Medical Association.

Ahronheim JC, Moreno JD, Zuckerman C. 2000. *Ethics in Clinical Practice.* 2nd ed. Gaithersburg, MD: Aspen Publishers.

Baylis F. 1997. Errors in medicine: Nurturing truthfulness. *Journal of Clinical Ethics* 8(4):336–40.

Beauchamp TL, Childress JF. 1994. *Principles of Biomedical Ethics.* 4th ed. New York: Oxford University Press, p. 396.

Beauchamp TL, Childress JF. 2001. *Principles of Biomedical Ethics.* 5th ed. New York: Oxford University Press, pp. 283–319.

Belkin L. 1997. How can we save the next victim? *The New York Times Magazine,* June 15, pp. 28–70.

Berger JT. 1998. Culture and ethnicity in clinical care. *Archives of Internal Medicine* 158 (19):2085–90.

Bok S. 1983. The limits of confidentiality. *Hastings Center Report* February:24–31.

Cullen S, Klein M. 2000. Respect for patients, physicians and the truth. In Munson R, ed. *Intervention and Reflection: Basic Issues in Medical Ethics.* 6th ed. Belmont, CA: Wadsworth, pp. 435–42.

Freedman B. 2003. Offering truth: One ethical approach to the uninformed cancer patient. In Steinbock B, Arras JD, London AJ, eds. *Ethical Issues in Modern Medicine.* 6th ed. Boston: McGraw-Hill, pp. 76–82.

Gallagher TH, Waterman AD, Ebers AG, Fraser VJ, Levinson W. 2003. Patients' and physicians' attitudes regarding the disclosure of medical errors. *Journal of the American Medical Association* 289(8):1001–7.

Goldberg RM, Kuhn G, Andrew LB, Thomas HA. 2002. Coping with medical mistakes and errors in judgment. *Annals of Emergency Medicine* 39(3):287–92.

Greenberg MA. 1991. The consequences of truth telling. *Journal of the American Medical Association* 266(1):66.

Institute of Medicine, Committee on Quality of Health Care in America. 2000. *To Err Is Human: Building a Safer Health System.* Washington, DC: National Academy Press.

Jansen LA,, Ross LF. 2000. Patient confidentiality and the surrogate's right to know. *Journal of Law, Medicine & Ethics* 28:137–43.

Joint Commission on Accreditation of Healthcare Organizations. Patient Rights and Organization Ethics Chapter (RI), Standard RI.1.2.2; Intent of Standard RI.1.2.2. *Comprehensive Accreditation Manual for Hospitals.* Oakbrook, IL: Joint Commission on Accreditation of Healthcare Organizations.

Kagawa-Singer M, Blackhall LJ. 2001. Negotiating cross-cultural issues at the end of life: "You've got to go where he lives." *Journal of the American Medical Association* 286(23):2993–3001.

Kohn LT, Corrigan JM, Donaldson M, eds.1999. *To Err is Human: Building a Safer Health System.* A report from the Committee on Quality of Healthcare in America, Institute of Medicine, National Academy of Sciences. Washington, DC: National Academy Press.

Krumholz A., Fisher RS, Lesser RP, Hauser WA. 1991. Driving and epilepsy: A review and reappraisal. *Journal of the American Medical Association* 265(5):622–26.

Levinson W., Roter DL, Mullooly JP, et al. 1997. Physician-patient communication: The relationship with malpractice claims among primary care physicians and surgeons. *Journal of the American Medical Association* 277(7):553–59.

Liebman CB, Hyman CS. 2004. A mediation skills model to manage disclosure of errors and adverse events to patients. *Health Affairs* 23(4):22–32.

Liebman CB, Hyman CS. 2006. Prescription for improving the way health care and legal systems deal with unanticipated outcomes in medical care. Presentation , the Association of the Bar of the City of New York, May 24, 2006.

Novack DH, Detering BJ, Arnold R., et al. 1989. Physicians' attitudes toward using deception to resolve difficult ethical problems. *Journal of the American Medical Association* 261(20):2980–85.

Pellegrino ED. 1992. Is truth telling to the patient a cultural artifact? *Journal of the American Medical Association* 268(13):1734–35.

Ptacek JT, Eberhardt T. 1996. Breaking bad news: A review of the literature. *Journal of the American Medical Association* 276(6):496–502.

Quill TE, Townsend P. 1991. Bad news: Delivery, dialogue, and dilemmas. *Archives of Internal Medicine* 151(3):463–68.

Ruddick W. 1999. Hope and deception. *Bioethics* 13(3/4):343–57.

Siegler M. 1982. Confidentiality in medicine—A decrepit concept. *New England Journal of Medicine* 307:1518–21.

Sigman GS, Kraut J, La Puma J. 2003. Disclosure of a diagnosis to children and adolescents when parents object. In Beauchamp TL, Walters L, eds. *Contemporary Issues in Bioethics.* 6th ed. Belmont, CA: Wadsworth-Thomson Learning, pp. 133–38.

Stein J. 2000. A fragile commodity. *Journal of the American Medical Association* 283(3):305–6.

Surbonne A. 1992. Truth telling to the patient. *Journal of the American Medical Association* 268(13): 1661–62.

Tarasoff v. Regents of the University of California, 551 P.2d 334 (Cal. 1976).

Thomasma DC. 2003. Telling the truth to patients: A clinical ethics exploration. In Beauchamp TL, Walters L, eds. *Contemporary Issues in Bioethics.* 6th ed. Belmont, CA: Wadsworth-Thomson Learning, pp. 128–32.

Vincent C. 2003. Understanding and responding to adverse events. *New England Journal of Medicine* 348(11):1051–56.

Vogel J., Delgado R. 1980. To tell the truth: Physicians' duty to disclose medical mistakes. *UCLA Law Review* 28:52–94.

Wu AW, Cavanaugh TA, McPhee SJ, et al. 1997. To tell the truth: Ethical and practical issues in disclosing medical mistakes to patients. *Journal of General Internal Medicine* 12(12):770–75.

5

Special Decision-making Concerns of Minors

DECISIONAL CAPACITY AND MINORS

If you think that assessing adults' ability to make and take responsibility for decisions is challenging, keep reading. Children and adolescents present a whole other set of issues related to their emerging cognitive abilities, self-awareness, and moral authority. Because minors are usually considered incapable of assuming responsibility for their health care, conflicts about treating this vulnerable population will likely come before your ethics committee.

As discussed in chapter 2, the concept of decision-making capacity involves notions of autonomy and moral responsibility. Autonomy refers to self-governance, which requires that, at the very least, the individual has a *self* to govern. In this sense, autonomy implies a more or less integrated set of personal values and preferences that are recognizable and generally well-established. Moral responsibility refers to a person's capacity to be accountable for his actions and suggests qualities of stability, consistency, and foresight. These qualities develop as part of the maturation process that begins in young childhood and continues through adolescence into adulthood.

Children

‖ Timmy, a healthy 3-year-old child, is scheduled for a tonsillectomy this morning. His parents have done everything they can to prepare Timmy for the surgery, including reading him books about going to the hospital, "operating" on his stuffed rabbit, and packing all his favorite toys. Despite their presence and reassurance, however, Timmy becomes increasingly agitated. He resists all contact with any medical personnel, including the nurses, the surgeons, and Dr. Lewis, the anesthesiologist.

Although Dr. Lewis tries to explain what she is doing and what will happen, Timmy keeps screaming, "No! No!" He struggles to climb off the stretcher and spits out the Versed that the nurse tried to mask with apple juice. In order to proceed, Dr. Lewis must hold him down and sedate him with an injection. When Timmy is sufficiently sedated and offers no resistance, Dr. Lewis brings him to the operating room, where the surgery proceeds without incident.

Following surgery, Timmy is returned to the main recovery room and then to the pediatric ambulatory area, where his parents are waiting for him. He still screams when he sees clinical personnel but, except for continuous crying, there are no postoperative problems.

Anyone who has spent time with young children knows that they do and do not want things, sometimes loudly, often inconsistently, and almost always vehemently. The sincerity with which they voice their wishes, however, should not be confused with the judgment necessary for responsible decision making. Timmy genuinely does not want to be in the hospital and efforts by his caregivers or even his parents to reason with him will not change his mind. He is unable to appreciate the need for surgery or the prospect of feeling better once his tonsils are removed. He cannot be placated by promises of ice cream when the operation is over. He is incapable of thinking about anything except his current fear and his desperate desire to be elsewhere.

Because of their immaturity, young children lack the attributes associated with autonomy and self-governance—that is, they do not have decision-making ability. The same is largely true of older children, although they may have preferences that can and should be accommodated in treatment plans. The younger the child, the less problem we have in saying, "This is a person for whom most decisions must be made by others because he has not developed the cognitive ability, experience, or judgment necessary to reason or the opportunity to form values and preferences that will inform his decisions."

As noted in chapter 2, however, decisions run along a continuum from low to high risk. Certainly, even young children are able to make some choices—"Do you want to wear the red or the blue shirt today?"—and giving them opportunities to do so helps them develop decision-making skills. As the consequences of the decisions become more significant—selecting suitable television programs, eating nutritious food, using seat belts—the intervention of adults becomes increasingly important. The need for adults to act on behalf of young children becomes especially clear when the decisions have critical outcomes and long-lasting consequences, as in the health care setting.

Adolescents

||| James Bell is a 16-year-old adolescent admitted to the hospital with pain in his right leg. He is a tall, good-looking young man who is an honor roll student and involved in numerous school and community activities. His main claim to fame is his prowess in several sports and he is hoping to get an athletic scholarship to college. He lives with his mother, with whom he appears to have a good relationship.

After examination and tests, a diagnosis of osteosarcoma of the right femur was made. The hematology-oncology and orthopedic doctors met with James and his mother two days ago to discuss the diagnosis, prognosis, and treatment options. All the professionals recommended amputation of the leg rather than local excision, because amputation has been shown to increase the survival rates. James and his mother were both shocked and distressed by the news. When the options were explained, Mrs. Bell asked many questions, but James was silent. Finally she said to James, "There doesn't seem to be any question that amputation will give you the best chance to beat the cancer. I know it will be hard, but I think this is what we have to do." James replied, "No way! No way they're cutting off my leg! I'll agree to the local treatment, but that's it." When the doctors and his mother tried to persuade him, he said, "I'd rather die with my leg than live without it! You can't make me do this!" He has remained adamant, despite several attempts to explain the important benefits of amputation.

Can adolescents be considered to have the capacity to make health care decisions, especially those with serious consequences? Who does or should make health care decisions for adolescents? What else would be important to know about James' decision and reasoning? What is the relationship between consent and assent? Should surgery proceed over James' continued objections?

As anyone who has ever been or known an adolescent is aware, these issues become dramatically more complex during the teenage years. Along the decision-making continuum, adolescents occupy a position that is legally and ethically ambiguous. By the age of 14, the normal child demonstrates a capacity to reason, including the ability to understand the causes and effects of illness, that is both as good and as flawed as it will be in adulthood. It will come as no surprise, however, that adolescent capacity to make autonomous decisions is enormously variable, partly because it is tied to the growing ability to make authentic statements about values and commitment. As the individual develops in experience and judgment, he edges closer to assuming control of and responsibility for his own decisions and correspondingly greater weight is given to his values and wishes.

The challenge in evaluating this ability is to consider the relevant factors and skills in their appropriate context. The law, as a crude instrument, makes blunt distinctions necessarily based on somewhat rigid and arbitrary standards. Thus, we have those eagerly awaited milestone ages at which people are finally allowed to drive, vote, drink, and serve in the armed forces. Likewise, determining the ability to make decisions that provide *legally* binding consent is based on easily defined characteristics, such as the age of majority, marital or parental status, or economic self-sufficiency.

In contrast, the ethical analysis of adolescent decision-making capacity is more complex, multifactorial, and nuanced. In assessing the capacity of an adolescent to make decisions that will be given *moral* weight, it is necessary to look beyond cognitive skills to consider

- personal values
- patterns of decision making and behavior, including risk taking
- biological and emotional maturity
- life experience, including health care and treatment experience
- appreciation of cause, effect, and consequence
- notions of the future, including life plans

While both adult and adolescent decision making combine these factors, adolescent decisions are typically the product of greater uncertainty and insecurity, less experience, more volatile emotions, immature self-image, unrealistic appraisal of risks and consequences, susceptibility to peer pressure and the desire to conform, and greater focus on the present than the future. These characteristics have direct implications for the capacity to make decisions, especially those with high stakes consequences. For example, an adolescent patient with chronic or serious illness may exhibit greater knowledge and more mature judgment about treatment decisions than would be displayed by a peer who has not had the same debilitating experience.

James has been presented with a prospect that would devastate a person twice his age. He is forced to confront his own mortality decades too soon. If that were not enough, he is asked to accept a drastic alteration in body image and the loss of what makes him special—his athletic prowess. No wonder he's reeling. As a newly diagnosed cancer patient, he is doing what many adults initially do in his situation—rejecting more unwanted information.

At 16, James is approaching adulthood. He may very well have the cognitive ability to understand his situation and consider his treatment choices. What he may not have is the experience and judgment necessary to make decisions with long-term consequences. To the extent possible, he should be given the opportunity to be an active participant in planning his care. His involvement will be critical to the success of his treatment and recuperation, as well as rebuilding his body image and sense of self-determination.

To assess his ability to participate, James' caregivers will need to know much more about his maturity, his ability to solve problems and consider alternatives, and his experience with illness and loss. It is not uncommon to hear people, especially adolescents, reject something by saying, "I'd rather die" as a way of expressing the strength of their feelings. Most often, however, they have little or no real sense of death or the implications of such a choice. It is also important to clarify James' reasons for refusing.

If he does not understand or believe the seriousness of his condition, he needs further explanation. If he is looking at short-range issues, such as his appearance, his popularity with his friends, his altered athletic ability, he may benefit from spending time with other adolescents in his situation.

A history of other illness and treatment will also affect his ability to deal with his current situation. For example, a 16-year-old who has lived for years with chronic and debilitating illness, endured rounds of unsuccessful radiation and chemotherapy, or rejected one or more transplanted organs may be well positioned to say, "Enough. I know what this is about and it's not the way I want to live for whatever time I have left." In contrast, James is newly diagnosed with an illness that has the potential for remission or cure. Despite the significant burdens of the proposed amputation, they may be vastly outweighed by the long-term benefits.

Perhaps James has been exposed to others—his father, other relatives, or even friends —in similar situations. If so, their clinical outcomes and successful or unsuccessful coping strategies will likely influence his response to his illness. If not, his lack of preparation for this unexpected assault will complicate his ability to absorb the implications of his diagnosis, prognosis, and treatment options.

Ideally, James, his mother, and his caregivers will be able to collaborate in a process of education and support while making these difficult decisions about his future. As discussed below, although he is unable to provide legally binding consent, his assent to treatment will be critically important. If he remains unpersuaded by the benefit-burden analysis and adamantly opposed to amputation, however, it may be necessary to proceed with surgery over his objections. Ultimately, the gravity of his condition and the potential for life-saving treatment, the clinical judgment of his caregivers, and the experience and devotion of his mother will assume greater weight than his choice in making decisions with profound and lasting consequences of this magnitude.

CONSENT FOR MINORS

How and by whom decisions are made has special significance in the health care setting. Because the law almost always considers minors to lack the judgment and experience necessary for responsible decision making, it generally denies them legal power and requires the consent of one or both parents or a legal guardian to authorize medical care. Sometimes, however, the law departs from this requirement when it appears that the young patient's best interests will be served by having others assume decision-making authority.

Newborns

The neonatal intensive care unit (NICU) is the scene of both high drama and devastating choices. The care of newborns has changed enormously over the last few decades. Because of technological advances, substantial medical progress has been made in the care of very premature, seriously ill, and handicapped neonates. In addition, decision making about the treatment of such infants has become more collaborative, including clinicians, parents, and other family members, and occasionally lay persons who work outside the NICU. Careful scrutiny is increasingly important because, while new techniques enable health professionals to maintain the lives of infants who would otherwise not survive, this rescue is often at the cost of significantly diminished prospects for a meaningful life.

These issues began to attract public attention and governmental regulation in 1982, when a baby born with Down's syndrome and an opening between the esophagus and trachea was permitted to die without life-saving intervention. The parents' concern about the potential for some degree of mental retardation made them refuse the recommended surgical repair, a decision upheld by the state court. The case of Baby Doe generated considerable publicity, the outrage of right-to-life groups and advocates for the developmentally disabled, and a controversial response by the U.S. Department of Health and Human Services. This case and its regulatory results are discussed further in part VI.

The ethical principles that guide neonatal intensive care decisions include beneficence, nonmaleficence, and justice. Beneficence and nonmaleficence create the professional obligation to provide care for the newborn that maximizes benefit and minimizes harm. Moreover, because the infant is the patient, his interests must be assessed independently of the interests of the family. Beneficence is also invoked as a guiding principle for parents, obligating them to make decisions that will promote the welfare of their baby. Conceptions of benefit and harm may be defined differently by health professionals and parents, however, creating conflicts in the NICU over how or even whether to treat. Justice requires that treatment decisions be based on the infant's best interests, without considerations of race, ethnicity, or ability to pay.

Taken together, these ethical principles create the obligation that newborns, who are especially vulnerable, receive heightened protection. Decision making for critically ill and handicapped infants is complicated by two factors. First, prognostication can be very uncertain in the early neonatal period and may not be clarified until numerous aggressive measures have been instituted. Second, decisions to provide, withhold, or withdraw aggressive life-sustaining measures frequently involve quality-of-life judgments. Because parents and clinicians may have very different notions of what constitutes an acceptable or unacceptable quality of life for the child, consensus on these deeply personal issues is often difficult to achieve. The resulting collision of principled obligations can create painful conflict for those who care for and about the infant.

Our society's deference to parental decisions rests on respect for family integrity, the presumption that parents act in their child's best interests, and the need to have a designated authority to make such decisions. Accordingly, parental decisions about the care of newborns are routinely honored unless they contradict the clinical judgments of the care team. Typically, when physicians recommend a course of treatment that is clearly in the newborn's best interests, parents agree. In rare cases, parents make decisions that are likely to harm their child and not provide compensating benefit. Decisions that put children at unjustified risk are considered abuse of parental authority and usually trigger outside intervention.

Between these two extremes, many decisions made by parents fall into a gray area, where it is not at all clear whether the choice will benefit their newborn. In these cases of uncertainty, parental decisions tend to be respected. The difficult issues that arise in the NICU place significant ethical responsibilities on caregivers, including

- putting the child's interests at the center of decision making
- involving parents in the decision-making process
- providing parents with full and accurate information about their child's condition, prognosis, and treatment options
- providing parents with guidance, support, and time to decide on care goals and plans
- being willing to make care recommendations
- letting parents know that it is appropriate to forgo treatment when the burdens clearly outweigh the benefits

When conflicting values and interests complicate decisions about neonatal care, hospitals are increasingly referring these cases to infant bioethics review committees for special attention.

Children

||| Melissa is a one-month-old infant admitted with a severe infection that has resulted in significant and irreversible brain damage. She is currently on a ventilator and cannot suck, so a tracheostomy and a gastrostomy will be necessary to support her respiration and nutrition. She responds only to painful stimuli, such as the frequent blood draws necessary to monitor her infection. According to the treating team, her condition will not improve because, as the attending explained to her mother, "the infection has destroyed Melissa's brain."

Melissa's mother, Ms. Green, is a 45-year-old deaf woman who has eleven children, most of whom are in foster care and several of whom are in the process of being adopted. It is not clear why the children have been taken from her, but she maintains contact with some of them. Melissa's father is reportedly a violent man with a drug problem and Ms. Green apparently left him because he abused her.

Ms. Green has told the sign language interpreter that this is her last chance to be a mother because she rarely has a chance to see her other children. She enjoys coming to visit Melissa anytime she pleases, "touching her, holding her, and feeling like a real mom." She does not want to let her baby go and she will not consent to anything, such as a recommended do-not-resuscitate (DNR) order, that would prevent the doctors from keeping Melissa alive. Even when the pain and lack of benefit to Melissa are explained, Ms. Green remains adamant that aggressive treatment be continued.

How should Ms. Green's capacity to make decisions about Melissa's care be assessed? What factors might impair her ability to make decisions in Melissa's best interest?

As in other instances of surrogate choice, care issues related to young children concern who makes decisions, according to what standards, and with what review. Legally, the first question is almost always resolved in favor of the parents, who are responsible for upbringing and welfare because they are presumed by tradition and law to act in their child's best interests.

Note that this presumption of parental authority distinguishes health care decision making for a minor from decision making on behalf of an incapacitated adult. In the latter case, the power to make treatment choices may be accorded to the patient's family or assumed by the court only when the adult patient has been *shown* to be incapable of choosing. In contrast, recognition that children lack the capacity to make their own health care decisions *presumptively* confers this authority on parents or guardians unless they are specifically disqualified by a determination of unfitness.

Ms. Green's capacity to make decisions for her daughter requires careful scrutiny because of her apparent inability to understand Melissa's medical condition, prognosis, and limited treatment options. While her impaired hearing may hinder her understanding of the clinical situation, her deafness should not be the deciding factor. Her diminished capacity may be the result of several factors, including her deafness, possibly limited intelligence, and/or the stress of caring for a critically ill child.

These problems may be complicated by Ms. Green's apparent inability to appreciate her child's best interests or that they may be in conflict with her own interests. If her focus is on extending her opportunity to function as a mother rather than on what benefits her child, she may not be the best person to be making care decisions for Melissa.

▍▍▍ Larry is a 12-year-old who was struck by a car and has been brought to the trauma ER. There, it was discovered that he has a severe renal injury with significant internal bleeding. When his parents arrive, they tell the physicians that, because they and Larry are Jehovah's Witnesses, transfusion of blood or blood products is out of the question.

How should the religious convictions of Larry's parents influence the decision about his receiving potentially life-saving blood transfusion? What weight should be given to Larry's religious beliefs?

Just when you thought parental authority was secure from interference, the issues become more complicated. The rights granted parents or guardians, as well as the restrictions placed on those rights, are rooted in an ethical perspective that assigns top priority to the interests of the child. In this view, widely shared in our culture, parents are entrusted with the well-being of their children and charged with specific duties, including the provision of food, clothing, shelter, basic education, and health care.

Within the parameters set by these duties, parents may make choices based on their own values and beliefs about what is best for their children. So far, so good. Note, however, that parental authority is not unlimited because it is constrained by parental responsibility. When parents abuse their authority—for example, by refusing consent for clearly beneficial medical treatment—the child's interests trump even the well-established presumption of parental rights.

Accordingly, the law deviates from the almost automatic deference to parents in the context of decisions about health care when the child's welfare or life is at stake. In such cases, the law requires physicians to act on behalf of the child and permits the state to intervene. For example, a standard exception to the requirement of parental consent for medical treatment is emergencies, when delaying treatment would threaten the child's life or health. Likewise, all states provide for removing children from abusive or harmful environments or situations in which they are deprived of necessary medical treatment. In addition, parents are prevented from interfering with needed medical care and can be criminally prosecuted for failing to provide that care.

Courts have agreed that parents may not withhold life-saving treatment from a child who is neither terminally ill nor permanently comatose. Treatment refusal has not been permitted even when the therapy is painful and only marginally effective if it is determined that the child will die without it. When the contested treatment is elective or carries substantial risks, however, courts are more likely to accede to parental refusal. Although decisions continue to vary, the trend appears to be limiting parents' authority when their decisions conflict with generally accepted medical judgment. Judicial intervention is less likely when parents are providing some kind of professionally accepted treatment. Several illustrative legal cases are summarized in part VI.

Court intervention usually involves authorization, at the request of health care providers, to perform a particular surgical procedure or course of medical treatment over parental objection. Because these cases focus on a specific, usually life-saving, therapeutic objective, courts are likely to override parents' refusal, which is usually based on religious or philosophical belief. In these singular instances, traditional deference to parental decision-making authority gives way to the determination by others of what is best for the child. For example, courts have ordered children inoculated over their parents' religious objections.

Similarly, parents who are Jehovah's Witnesses are not permitted to refuse life-saving blood transfusions for their children. Members of this faith believe that receiving blood or blood products places their souls in eternal jeopardy, making it worse to survive after transfusion than to die without having received the blood. This deeply held belief should be honored when it is expressed by capable adult patients who understand and accept the risks posed by their religious commitments. In contrast, a child who is too immature to have developed settled religious convictions or make autonomous decisions that place his life at risk cannot be permitted to assume this responsibility.

Given the extent of Larry's injuries and internal bleeding, he appears to be at risk of serious harm and possibly death if he is not transfused. The likelihood and magnitude of the harm if he does not receive blood mean that his parents' decision to withhold transfusion is not in his medical interest. Under most circumstances, this would justify overriding their refusal to consent to transfusion. In this case, however, Larry is approaching the age when he might be considered to have settled religious beliefs and values. If he is able to express an informed conviction about being a Jehovah's Witness, it becomes more complicated to support paternalistic intervention to transfuse over his objections. One recommendation would be to interview him without his parents present to evaluate his maturity, understanding, and the strength of his religious convictions.

Finally, courts tend not to order treatment for children who are comatose, for whom death is imminent, or for whom the marginal benefits of treatment are outweighed by its burdens. In these situations, courts have held that the decision to forgo treatment was in the children's best interest.

Just as there are limits to parental rights to refuse treatment, there are also limits to parental rights to insist on treatment. When specific interventions are determined by the care team to be inappropriate or ineffective, when the burdens and risks clearly outweigh the benefits, physicians have an obligation to protect their young and vulnerable patients from measures that are not clinically indicated.

It is important, however, to recognize and address the motivation behind much of what may appear to be unreasonable parental demands. The job of parents is to stand between their children and danger, to protect them from injury and illness. When, despite their best efforts, their children are sick or hurt, parents may direct their efforts toward ensuring that everything possible is done to promote recovery. Whether the therapies they propose are standard of care or unconventional, they are likely to feel the obligation to advocate strongly for anything that holds out even the slimmest prospect of success. It is understandable, therefore, that they perceive refusal to provide the requested treatments as yet another barrier to fulfilling their nurturing responsibilities.

As discussed further in chapter 6, demands for treatment should trigger a discussion with parents that begins by exploring what "do everything" means, clarifying their expectations of the proposed therapies, and explaining the likely course with and without the treatment. The focus should be on the care that *will* be provided rather than what will not, emphasizing that the shared goal is to provide only care that will benefit the child and maximize comfort and quality of life. Whenever possible, parents should be involved as collaborators in care planning as a way of helping them retain their role as guardians of their children's well-being.

Adolescents

III Nora is a 17-year-old young woman initially seen in adolescent health clinic, referred by a pediatric nephrologist for primary care and contraceptive counseling. She has a history of urinary tract problems diagnosed two years ago after proteinuria was discovered on routine urinalysis. She has been taking Cozaar for the proteinuria.

Nora told the clinic physician, Dr. Gonzalez, that she became sexually active six months ago and has been intimate with the same male partner, Joe, who is 21 years old. She says they have always used condoms except once, which is when she became pregnant last year. At her mother's insistence, she terminated the pregnancy immediately.

During her clinic visit, Nora requested Depo Provera for contraception. Her last menstrual period had been six weeks earlier and she was awaiting her next menses. Routine blood work was ordered, including a test to rule out pregnancy before giving her the first Depo injection at her next period. Test results indicated an early pregnancy.

The clinic social worker made several unsuccessful attempts to schedule an appointment to discuss options, but Nora missed each appointment. Finally she came to the clinic twelve weeks after her last period. Dr. Gonzalez had a lengthy discussion with Nora about the potential risk to the fetus because, throughout the pregnancy, she has been taking Cozaar, a medication contraindicated in pregnancy. Nora insisted that she understood the possibility of prematurity and/or birth defects, but said that she wanted to keep this pregnancy. She promised to discuss the situation with Joe over the weekend. She was explicit about not wanting her mother to know, because "she made me have an abortion the last time." She was told to discontinue the Cozaar and return to the clinic on Monday.

When Nora and Joe met with the social worker, they communicated their decision to keep the pregnancy. Their plan is not to tell her mother until after Nora has moved in with Joe. It is also apparent that Nora has not told Joe about the risk of birth complications.

How should Nora's capacity to make decisions about this pregnancy be assessed? What factors should be considered? Is her mother required to be involved in these decisions?

Adolescents, who are neither children nor adults, stand with a foot in each world. Their intellectual and emotional development is greater than that of young children, yet most are not fully mature. While their cognitive skills are growing and they are likely to have a well-developed set of preferences and moral values, they still lack the experience and judgment of adults.

Because the legal age of majority in almost all states is 18, adolescents are technically minors for most purposes. The few exceptions, provided for in state law, are the ability of the emancipated minor and the mature minor to make legally binding decisions. For example, a minor who has given birth may relinquish the child for adoption.

The age of and criteria for consent to health care vary by state, and the law has relaxed the customary requirement for parental consent by carving out specific situations in which adolescents may make decisions about their treatment. The trend began in 1976 with a line of cases in which the U.S. Supreme Court held that minors who are sufficiently mature should be able to authorize abortions without parental consent or notification. Subsequent cases permitted teens access to contraception and statutes provided access without parental consent to treatment for substance abuse and sexually transmitted diseases.

These pragmatic exceptions to the parental consent requirement apply in situations in which it is imperative that teens are treated for their own good and as a matter of public health. The underlying concept recognizes that some highly sensitive health care circumstances have serious implications for young patients and others. In these situations, adolescents are more likely to seek and, therefore, receive health care if they can consent to it without involving or notifying their parents. This utilitarian reasoning is similar to the justification for confidentiality, discussed in chapter 4.

The mature minor doctrine is based on the notion that some minors have the cognitive ability and maturity to make informed decisions about their care. This doctrine, given force in many states' case or statutory law, provides for minors to consent to care in the following circumstances:

- The minor is an older adolescent (e.g., older than fourteen or fifteen years)
- The minor is capable of giving an informed consent
- The care is for the benefit of the minor
- The care does not present a high level of risk
- The care is within the range of established medical opinion (English, 1999, p. 86)

Minor treatment statutes address the societal obligation to protect adolescents and provide access to care, rather than a societal recognition of adolescent maturity and decisional capability. The reasoning behind them is similar to a sliding scale, making it more likely that adolescents will be permitted to make care decisions that do not carry great risks. In this way, these laws reflect the dual goals of protecting society and promoting minors' best interest.

Statutes in every state, known as minor consent statutes or medical emancipation statutes, authorize minors to consent to care based either on their *status* or on the specific *service* they are seeking. The categories of minors authorized by one or more states to consent to medical care based on their *status* are:

- Emancipated minors [often defined using one or more of the following criteria]
- Married minors
- Minors in the armed forces
- Mature minors
- Minors living apart from their parents
- Minors over a certain age
- High school graduates
- Pregnant minors
- Minor parents (English, 1999, p. 85)

Central to this legal framework is the notion that, because these minors are no longer under effective parental supervision, parental consent is not a sensible precondition to accessing care.

The categories of *services* for which one or more states authorize minors to give consent are:

- Emergency care
- Pregnancy related care
- Contraceptive services
- Abortion
- Diagnosis or treatment of venereal or sexually transmitted diseases
- Diagnosis or treatment of reportable, infectious, contagious, or communicable diseases
- HIV/AIDS testing or treatment
- Treatment or counseling for drug or alcohol problems
- Collection of medical evidence or treatment for sexual assault
- Inpatient mental health services
- Outpatient mental health services (English, 1999, p. 85)

Because these statues are state-specific and their provisions differ, clinicians treating adolescents should be very familiar with the laws of the jurisdiction in which they provide care. Likewise, if your ethics committee addresses issues of adolescent health care, knowledge of the relevant laws and regulations in your state would be important. The take-away message is that the range of adolescent decisional capacity and the range of health care issues requiring decisions demand a heightened level of scrutiny and a constant balancing of rights and interests.

CONFIDENTIALITY AND DISCLOSURE

‖ Donna is a 15-year-old who has come to the clinic for her annual physical prior to the beginning of school. Her mother, who accompanied her, remains in the waiting room during the exam. Donna appears healthy and active. In addition to a demanding scholastic schedule, she is on the track team and participates in several extracurricular and community activities. Although she appears bright and pleasant, she is clearly uneasy about something. Finally, at the end of the examination, she tells Dr. Jin that she and her boyfriend have recently begun having sex and she feels it would be responsible for her to be on birth control pills. She asks for a prescription, but insists that the doctor not tell her mother about her sexual activity or her request for contraception. Dr. Jin's discussion with her about sexual relations and contraception indicates that her decision is not coerced and that she understands its implications.

When Dr. Jin leaves the exam room, Donna's mother approaches her in the hall and says, "Doctor, I suspect that Donna's boyfriend is pressuring her to have sex. She's just not ready for that and I need to know what is going on. Please tell me if she has discussed this with you."

What are Dr. Jin's obligations to Donna? What are Dr. Jin's obligations to her mother?

Remember when you were 15 and did not want your parents to know about something in your life? Remember when you were afraid that your teenager was growing up too fast? Sorting out the boundaries of adolescent privacy and confidentiality is difficult under any circumstance; it can be especially challenging in the health care setting when so much more is at stake.

Maintaining the confidentiality of adolescents' health information serves many of the same important functions that it does for adults and some that are especially important to the adult-in-training. Patients are more likely to seek treatment, especially for conditions that are sensitive or socially stigmatizing, and, once in treatment, are likely to provide more complete and accurate histories if they know their confidences are secured. Protecting the privacy of adolescents also shields them from embarrassment, discrimination, and potential family disruption or even violence. Finally, honoring their privacy helps adolescents in their critical development of autonomy.

Adolescents' health care confidentiality is guarded by the protections built into federal and state constitutions, statutes and regulations, court decisions, and professional ethical standards. However, these safeguards are never absolute and the ambiguous status of adolescents adds to the difficulty of determining what information should be protected or disclosed, to whom, and under what circumstances. Some state statutes pair adolescents' right to consent to treatment with their right to decide about information disclosure. Others require disclosure of health care information over the adolescent's objection in certain situations, including specific disclosure to parents, mandatory reporting of physical or sexual abuse, or disclosure when the adolescent poses a severe and imminent danger to herself or others.

Dr. Jin's obligations to Donna's mother are the same as they would be to the concerned family of any patient—to provide her daughter with the most appropriate health care in light of her medical needs, her appreciation of her condition, her options and their implications, and her wishes. Here, the ethical analysis would balance the likely benefits of protecting Donna's confidences (strengthening the trust in the therapeutic relationship and promoting further beneficial patient-physician interaction, preventing unwanted pregnancy, and facilitating autonomous decision making) against the likely risks (erroneously presuming that Donna is making a voluntary and mature decision about sexual activity, and inhibiting mother-daughter discussion about a sensitive topic that might benefit from parental guidance).

If Dr. Jin's clinical assessment indicates that maintaining Donna's confidentiality would promote her best interest, her ethical obligations would not include disclosure of information about contraception that Donna wishes to remain between herself and her doctor. It would be appropriate, however, for her to explore with Donna the potential advantages of confiding in her mother and the possible ways to do it.

SPECIAL PROBLEMS OF THE ADOLESCENT ALONE

lll Andy was 15 when he learned he had rhabdomyosarcoma of the spine. With his specific form of cancer, cure is highly unlikely. Andy's mother is an alcoholic who has been in and out of substance abuse treatment for years. Throughout his illness, she has not been available for support or help in decision making. Andy's father also has not been present in his life. Andy did rely heavily on a close friend of his mother's who, unfortunately, is no longer available to him.

Before his illness, Andy was a bright, athletic young man who enjoyed many activities. He has tried to make the best of his situation. He underwent surgery to remove the tumor and also had radiation therapy and chemotherapy, but none of the treatments was totally effective. He has never achieved remission and his pain has increased. Because of his mother's absence, the health care providers have discussed Andy's treatment options with him, although they actually have made most of the day-to-day decisions.

A significant turning point in Andy's illness occurred when his mother refused to move from her walk-up apartment into an available ground floor apartment. His deterioration has made it impossible for him to negotiate the stairs, and his mother's resistance to relocating means that he can never return home. Since he is in the last stage of his illness, his doctors have asked Andy to consider whether he wants to continue chemotherapy. Against their recommendation, Andy has declined further treatment.

Should Andy's refusal to continue treatment be honored? Is he capable of making this decision? What responsibilities do Andy's care providers have to him as his disease worsens?

The journey from childhood to adulthood is filled with the potential for growth, achievement, and self-fulfillment. It is also fraught with confusion, uncertainty, and risk. Fortunately, most young people have the security of at least one caring and responsible adult to help them navigate the distance. Some are not so lucky.

A special category of minors is the adolescent alone. These young people are actually or functionally alone because they do not have a supportive relationship with an adult in a birth, foster, adoptive, or chosen family. No trusted adult is consistently available to guide and monitor their passage to adulthood or help them evaluate and make appropriate decisions about medical options.

The number of adolescents alone has increased in the past several years, causing clinicians, researchers, other service providers, and policy analysts to focus on the special problems they present. Some of these young people have been orphaned because their caregiving parent died of AIDS or other diseases, substance abuse, or violence. Some are functionally alone because their parent, grandparent, or other nominal caregiver is mentally ill, addicted to drugs or alcohol, or simply overwhelmed by poverty or other pressures. Some gay and lesbian youth have been ostracized by their families. Some adolescents have run away from homes where adults physically or sexually abused them. Some in foster care may feel that, although they have both biological and foster parents, they have no one to trust with private information and concerns. Some have parents or other adults who drift in and out of their lives, leaving them without the security of a stable relationship.

The adolescent alone occupies an ambiguous legal status, which can present particularly difficult problems regarding consent and confidentiality in health care. A variety of legal mechanisms may justify the provision of care to the adolescent alone based on his own consent in specific circumstances. These include the emancipated minor and mature minor doctrines, as well as state-specific medical consent laws, discussed above. These doctrines are not accepted in all jurisdictions, however, and consent provisions vary from state to state. For this reason, health care professionals are advised to familiarize themselves with the relevant laws in the states where they practice, particularly those that might provide the basis for the adolescent's legally valid consent. In addition, because clinicians and administrators may interpret the doctrines inconsistently, care may be provided differently to these adolescents within the same state or even within the same institution. Finally, even when the laws are consistently understood and interpreted, they do not adequately address the range of ethical issues presented by the care of the adolescent alone.

Many of the ethical principles that apply to adolescents with adult supports also apply to adolescents alone, including principles that govern capacity and informed consent and those related to the right to refuse and demand care. Thus, health care providers should assess any adolescent's capacity to consent in light of the specific decision at issue and its implications, as well as the young person's developmental characteristics, life situation, and medical history. Heightened concern about the adolescent's capacity is appropriate whenever the decision involves long-term negative health or life consequences. When recommended treatment is refused, health care providers should initiate an extensive discussion with the teen and explore mutually acceptable alternatives. As is true in the adult setting, refusal of treatment is not the end, but only the beginning of the discussion with the adolescent patient. Likewise, the same assessment and serious discussion should be initiated by health care providers when the adolescent requests treatment that providers judge to be inappropriate or dangerous.

The obligation to protect patient privacy and confidentiality is as important for the adolescent alone as it is for other adolescents. Breaches of confidentiality may carry particular risks and be especially counterproductive for these vulnerable minors. The result can be their return to the abusive homes from which they fled and the exacerbation of problems that led them to their current difficult situations. At the outset of the clinical relationship, therefore, health care professionals should assure adolescents that confidentiality will be protected except in specific limited circumstances, which should be clearly defined.

Finally, when treating an adolescent alone, the natural inclination of many caregivers is to expand their role to meet many of the youth's unmet needs. Although clinicians may feel as if they are acting like family, it should be clear to them and to the adolescent that they are professionals with the skills and the limits of professionals. Far from rejecting the adolescent alone, establishing and reinforcing the boundaries of the therapeutic relationship creates a stable atmosphere of dependability and trust that is so badly needed in their lives.

The special needs and vulnerability of this population make it likely that, if an adolescent alone is receiving care in your institution, the case will come to the attention of your ethics committee. Your familiarity with the ethical and legal issues will enhance the quality of your deliberations and the usefulness of your recommendations to the team caring for the patient.

REFERENCES

Alderman EM, Fleischman AR. 1993. Should adolescents make their own health-care choices? *Contemporary Pediatrics* 10:65–82.

American Academy of Pediatrics, Committee on Adolescence. 1996. The adolescent's right to confidential care when considering abortion. *Pediatrics* 97(5):746–51.

American Academy of Pediatrics, Committee on Bioethics. 1995. Informed consent, parental permission, and assent in pediatric practice. *Pediatrics* 95(2):314–17.

American Academy of Pediatrics. 1994. Guidelines on forgoing life-sustaining medical treatment. *Pediatrics* 93(3):532–36.

Beauchamp TL. 1997. Informed consent. In Veatch RM, ed. *Medical Ethics.* 2nd ed. Sudbury, MA: Jones and Bartlett Publishers, pp. 185–208.

Becker S. 2003. Consent to medical treatment for minors §19.06. In *Health Care Law: A Practical Guide.* San Francisco: Matthew Bender & Co.

Blustein J. 1982. *Parents and Children.* New York: Oxford University Press.

Blustein J. 1996. Confidentiality and the adolescent: An ethical analysis. In Cassidy R, Fleischman A, eds. *Pediatric Ethics: From Principles to Practice.* Amsterdam, The Netherlands: Harwood Academic Publishers, pp. 83–96.

Blustein J, Levine C, Dubler NN, eds. 1999. *The Adolescent Alone.* New York: Cambridge University Press.

Blustein J, Moreno J. 1999. Valid consent to treatment and the unsupervised adolescent. In Blustein J, Levine C, Dubler NN, eds. *The Adolescent Alone.* New York: Cambridge University Press, pp. 100–110.

Brock D. 1993. Informed consent. In *Life and Death: Philosophical Essays in Biomedical Ethics.* New York: Cambridge University Press, pp. 21–54.

Brock DW. 1996. Children's competence for health care decisionmaking. In Ladd RE. *Children's Rights Re-Visioned: Philosophical Readings.* Belmont, CA: Wadsworth Publishing Co., pp. 184–200.

DeRenzo EG, Panzarella P, Selinger S, Schwartz J. 2005. Emancipation, capacity, and the difference between law and ethics. *Journal of Clinical Ethics* 16(2):144–50.

Dubler NN, Stern G. 1991. *Illusions of Immortality: The Confrontation of Adolescence and AIDS.* A Report to the New York State AIDS Advisory Council from the Ad Hoc Committee on Adolescents and HIV.

English A. 1999. Health care for the adolescent alone: A legal landscape. In Blustein J, Levine C, Dubler NN, eds., *The Adolescent Alone.* New York: Cambridge University Press, pp. 78–99.

English A., et al. 1995. *State Minor Consent Statutes: A Summary.* Cincinnati: Center for Continuing Education in Adolescent Health.

Fleischman AR. 1994. Ethical issues in neonatology. In Oski FA, DeAngelis CD, Feigin RD, Washburn J, eds. *Principles and Practice of Pediatrics.* Philadelphia: Lippincott Williams & Wilkins, pp. 339–42.

Furrow BR, Johnson SH, Jost TS, Schwartz RL. 1991. *Health Law: Cases, Materials and Problems.* 2nd ed. St. Paul, MN: West Publishing Co., pp. 1183-92.

Hastings Center Research Project on the Care of Imperiled Newborns. 1987. Imperiled newborns. *Hastings Center Report* 17:5–32.

Menikoff J. 2001. *Law and Bioethics: An Introduction.* Washington, DC: Georgetown University Press, pp. 298–99.

Mlyniec WJ. 1996. A judge's ethical dilemma: Assessing a child's capacity to choose. *Fordham Law Review* 64:1873–1915.

Paradise E, Horowitz RM. 1994. *Runaway and Homeless Youth: A Survey of State Law.* Washington, DC: American Bar Association Center on Children and the Law.

Quinn MM, Dubler NN. 1997. The health care provider's role in adolescent medical decision-making. *Adolescent Medicine* 8(3):415–25.

Rosato JL. 1996. The ultimate test of autonomy: Should minors have a right to make decisions regarding life-sustaining treatment? *Rutgers Law Review* 49(1):1–103.

Ross LF. 1997. Health care decisionmaking: Is it in their best interest? *Hastings Center Report* 27(6): 41–45.

Schneider CE. 1998. *The Practice of Autonomy: Patients, Doctors, and Medical Decisions.* New York: Oxford University Press.

Weir RF, Peters C. 1997. Affirming the decisions adolescents make about life and death. *Hastings Center Report* 27(6):29–40.

Wolfe J, Klar N, Grier HE, Duncan J, Salem-Schatz S, Emanuel EJ, Weeks JC. 2000. Understanding of prognosis among parents of children who died of cancer: Impact on treatment goals and integration of palliative care. *Journal of the American Medical Association* 284(19):2469–75.

6 End-of-life Issues

⦀ Mr. Tofer is a 77-year-old man admitted for resection of a squamous cell carcinoma of the tongue. The surgery was successful but, on the following day, he experienced respiratory distress that required intubation. Because he was not able to be weaned from the ventilator after three weeks, a tracheostomy was performed to place the ventilator tube directly into his trachea, which would be safer and more comfortable than continuing to pass the endotracheal tube down his throat. He has had two subsequent episodes of low blood pressure and is experiencing progressive renal failure. His mental status has deteriorated during the four weeks he has been in the ICU and he is responsive only to painful stimuli, such as suctioning of his tracheostomy.

Mr. Tofer's only family is his nephew, Lawrence. Although they have not had a close relationship, they have maintained contact over the years and Lawrence appears concerned about his uncle. Lawrence is not Mr. Tofer's appointed health care proxy agent and they have never had discussions about care at the end of life.

The renal team met with Lawrence to discuss the plan of care. Dr. Cooper, the renal attending, said that, although dialysis might improve Mr. Tofer's mental status, it would not change his overall grave prognosis. The consensus of the renal team is that the patient is a poor candidate for dialysis and has less than a one percent chance of surviving this hospitalization. Given the considerable risk and the slight benefit, the team would consider dialysis only if the family insisted. Dr. Cooper also recommended a do-not-resuscitate (DNR) order so that, if Mr. Tofer experienced a cardiopulmonary arrest, resuscitation would not be attempted.

What should Lawrence consider in making decisions about his uncle's care? What are the team's responsibilities?

DECISION MAKING AT THE END OF LIFE

If you were wondering when we would get to the really tough issues, the ones that make up the bulk of your ethics committee agenda and clinical consults, this is it. Not surprisingly, some of the most difficult health care choices take place at the end of life. Like much in bioethics, the issues related to dying and death are relatively new and would not have been raised a few generations ago when the health care focus was on attempting to cure or control disease. The response to illness and injury was to try all available measures and hope that something would be effective. Questions about whether the patient was receiving too much treatment or whether life was being unnecessarily prolonged would not have been asked.

Since then, we have managed to greatly expand both our treatment options and our ethical dilemmas. We have witnessed the development of medical and surgical interventions that can often return critically ill patients to health; they can also prevent death, even when improvement is not feasible. Decisions about end-of-life care now require greater scrutiny of the likely outcomes of therapy, including the important distinction between physiologic effectiveness (will the treatment work?) and therapeutic benefit (will the patient be better off because of the treatment?). Recognizing that cure-oriented and life-sustaining measures are not always medically appropriate for or even wanted by patients, bioethics works to facilitate decisions about when to deliver the patient from death and when to let death deliver the patient from us.

Sometimes, dying patients are capable of making or at least contributing to decisions about their care. More often, end-of-life decisions are made when the patient is no longer able to participate in deliberations. As a result, they typically involve efforts by others to determine the care plan that would most effectively meet his clinical needs and promote his well-being. As discussed in chapter 2, any decision making on behalf of an incapacitated patient requires that professionals, families, and other surrogates try to identify what his care wishes would be or determine what would be in his best interest. You already know from your experience in the clinical setting and on the ethics committee that these decisions become infinitely more difficult when the stakes are life and death.

Faced with the need for substitute decision making at the end of life, clinicians routinely turn to family members, who are presumed by tradition, and often by law, to know and act in the patient's best interest. As a rule, both medicine and law are more comfortable providing than withholding treatment, and considerable authority is customarily granted to family in *consenting* to treatment. Decisions about *limiting* treatment are far more problematic, however, and some states restrict the ability of non-appointed surrogates, even next of kin, to authorize the withholding or withdrawing of life-sustaining treatment.

The profound consequences of the choices, uncertainty about decision-making authority, lack of clarity about patient wishes, and lack of consensus on goals of care make end-of-life decisions among the most challenging in the clinical setting. For this reason, ethics committee consultations are frequently requested as death approaches.

DEFINING DEATH

∥ Gary, a 9-year-old, was admitted to the hospital after infection from an abscessed tooth spread to his sinuses and eventually to his brain. Despite aggressive treatment, his brain swelled in response to the infection, causing increased intracranial pressure. Ultimately, clinical examinations and tests revealed that he met the criteria for brain death. The attending pediatrician and the pediatric neurologist met with Gary's parents to tell them that the massive infection had destroyed his brain and that the condition was irreversible. In an extended discussion, the doctors explained that, because their son's brain had completely stopped functioning, he was no longer alive. His devastated parents refused to accept the determination of death. His mother cried, "Look at him. His eyes are closed and he doesn't answer us, but he's still breathing and his heart is still beating. He just needs more time to get better. You can't take away the machines that are keeping him alive."

What are the obligations of care professionals in planning for care at the end of life? How can the care team help families accept irreversible deterioration, dying, and death?

Although some things should be relatively straightforward, like knowing when a person is dead, this is not always the case. When science was less precise, death was generally agreed to have occurred when the heart and lungs ceased functioning. By the late 1960s, advances in resuscitative techniques and artificial respirators enabled cardiopulmonary function to be maintained even after the brain had stopped working. Ultimately, the traditional definition of death—irreversible cessation of cardiopulmonary function—was supplemented by a definition that accounted for cessation of entire brain function.

The first well-accepted definition of brain death was the product of the Ad Hoc Committee of the Harvard Medical School to Examine the Definition of Brain Death. The committee defined brain death as irreversible loss of total brain function, including "unreceptivity and unresponsivity . . . no movements or breathing . . no reflexes . . . [and] . . . flat electroencephalogram" (Ad Hoc Committee, 1968, pp. 85–86). By the time the committee published its report in 1968, the sophisticated medical technology that permitted measurement of brain waves also enabled organ harvesting and transplantation. The generally recognized motivation for developing brain death criteria was the ability to perfuse organs, the only way to keep them viable for transplantation. Thus, the advances in medical and surgical techniques, the need for transplantable organs, and the unacceptability of taking them from a still-living person prompted a new definition of death.

The Uniform Determination of Death Act (UDDA), adopted in 1980 by the National Conference of Commissioners on Uniform State Laws, expanded the definition of death to include both cessation of circulatory and respiratory function *and* brain death. That dual standard was endorsed in 1981 by the President's Commission for the Study of Ethical Problems in Medicine and Biomedical and Behavioral Research in its report, *Defining Death,* which encouraged all states to adopt the UDDA.

While the brain death definition may have clarified and simplified some clinical determinations, it has also created a category of potential confusion. Terminology is critical and, especially in dealing with families, clinicians should clearly distinguish brain death and other conditions in which the patient is unresponsive.

Brain death is the irreversible cessation of the *entire* brain's ability to function, including the upper brain, which controls the higher functions of cognition and memory, and the brainstem, which controls the body's automatic functions, such as breathing and heartbeat. Because the brain's regulation of vital functions has shut down, the person is considered both clinically and legally dead. While the family comes to terms with the death and considers possible organ donation, mechanical supports may temporarily continue to perfuse the organs and maintain cardiac and respiratory function. It is, however, counterintuitive for grieving families to accept that death has occurred when looking at a body that is warm, is healthy-colored, has a heart beat, and appears to be breathing because the cardiopulmonary system is being mechanically supported.

In contrast to brain death, the patient in a vegetative state has suffered profound *upper* brain damage and has lost cognitive function; yet she retains the *lower* (brainstem) function that controls the systems essential to life. The vegetative state has been further defined as persistent or permanent (PVS), depending on its duration and irreversibility. "When a vegetative state continues beyond thirty days, it is described as 'persistent.' A vegetative state is generally considered permanent three months after anoxic injury and twelve months after trauma" (Fins, 2005, p. 22). The patient has no awareness of herself or her surroundings and no ability to think or interact, but she is alive and not dependent on machines to maintain life. Indeed, as the case of Terri Schiavo demonstrated, if nutrition and hydration are maintained and no additional illness or injury intervenes, patients can live for years in PVS.

The minimally conscious state (MCS) has been described as a condition in which people who have been in a vegetative state for less than a year occasionally progress to demonstrate "unequivocal, but fluctuating evidence of awareness of self and the environment" (Fins, 2005, p. 22). Finally, coma is a label used for temporary or permanent unresponsiveness that may result from a variety of conditions, including illness, injury, or chemically induced unconsciousness.

Because these conditions have such different courses and outcomes, clearly distinguishing among them with careful language is essential to helping families adjust their expectations to the clinical realities. For example, describing a patient in PVS as being "comatose" may unfairly encourage the belief that the responsiveness will return. Likewise, it is extremely unhelpful to tell a family, "Your loved one is brain dead, but we are keeping him alive on machines." Saying this is confusing and hinders acceptance of the patient's death. The term *life support* is also counterproductive in this context because it implies that machines are supporting life. It is more honest and compassionate to explain, "Although your husband is no longer alive, these machines are perfusing his organs and supporting his heartbeat and respirations. Now that death has been confirmed, these mechanical supports are no longer necessary because they are no longer sustaining his life. Unless you are considering organ donation, the mechanical supports should be discontinued so that his body can rest."

Although families often have difficulty accepting the death of their loved ones, some families have specific moral or religious objections to cessation of brain function as a determination of death and may insist that mechanical supports not be discontinued. While brain death regulations are state-specific and institutions adopt their own protocols, in these cases reasonable accommodations should be made for an explicitly specified period of time. These accommodations (e.g., continuing ventilation, nutrition and hydration, and/or medications) should take place in a quiet private room, if possible, but not in the Emergency Department or the critical care unit. Such placement would be counterproductive to the family's acceptance of the death and an unwise use of resources. The clinical staff should emphasize that the accommodations are for the benefit of the *family,* not the now-deceased patient.

If a family without specific moral or religious objections to the brain death determination is still unable to accept the death, reasonable accommodations may be appropriate for a specified time. In this case also, it should be made clear that nothing more can be done for the patient and concern is now focused on the family's adjustment. Efforts to help the family come to terms with the loss may include bioethics consultation, social service intervention, psychiatric counseling, and pastoral care.

ADVANCE HEALTH CARE PLANNING

Advance Directives

The 1976 case of Karen Ann Quinlan raised what came to be known as the "right to die"—actually, the right to refuse treatment—and brought to national attention the risks to a patient whose treatment wishes are unknown in a high-tech, aggressive, cure-oriented health care environment. Although physicians determined that the 21-year-old was in a persistent vegetative state (PVS) and would not recover, they were reluctant to agree to her family's wishes and discontinue life-support measures. In a unanimous landmark decision, the New Jersey Supreme Court held that if there were "no reasonable possibility" that she would ever return to a "cognitive, sapient state," her ventilator could be removed without fear of criminal or civil liability. The *Quinlan* case highlighted the potential for incapacitated patients to be burdened with unwanted treatment, providing the impetus for the development of advance directives that could guide care according to patient wishes.

Subsequent cases, most notably the 1990 case of Nancy Cruzan, sharpened the focus on determining the prior wishes of the incapacitated patient as the guide to making authentic health care decisions. After the 25-year-old woman had been in PVS for seven years, her parents petitioned for an order to discontinue artificial nutrition and hydration. The U.S. Supreme Court, in its only such decision, recognized the protected interest of a capable individual in refusing unwanted treatment, including measures necessary to maintain life. The Court also held that, when life-sustaining treatment is refused on behalf of an incapacitated patient, states may insist that these decisions be based on clear and convincing evidence of what the *patient* wanted, not what others want *for* her.

The cases of Karen Ann Quinlan and Nancy Cruzan, discussed at greater length in part VI, captured national attention for two reasons. First, these were young women in devastating conditions from which they would not recover. Second, and perhaps more significant, decisions about their care were not automatically considered to be the responsibility of those closest to them. In addition to sympathy, these stories prompted many people to say, "Hey, wait a minute. This could happen to me or someone I love. What if no one knows what I would want? What if these decisions are made by doctors or courts or other strangers?"

The answer seemed to be some method of prospectively documenting care instructions to provide clarity and legal authorization for later decision making. Advance directives were developed to provide for treatment preferences, values, and directions to be articulated by a capable person so that they could be communicated and implemented after capacity has lapsed. As discussed in chapter 2, the most common types of directives are living wills and health care proxy appointments.

III Mr. Jennings is a 24-year-old man who has just been brought to the ER after a traffic accident. He has been receiving regular care in the HIV clinic since his initial diagnosis three years ago and, with a CD4 count of 460, his HIV is under good control. He is physically active and was on his way home from playing basketball when his bike was struck by a car. He is unconscious and suffering from a dislocated shoulder and a collapsed right lung.

As the ER team is preparing to intubate Mr. Jennings, his mother and sister arrive with his living will, which says, "If I am ever unresponsive and in respiratory failure, I do not want to be maintained on life support, including ventilatory support." His sister insists, "That may be what he wrote, but it's not what he meant. He's not ready to die. You must do everything to save his life, even putting him on a respirator."

The care team knows that short-term ventilatory support will permit the resolution of the pneumothorax and that Mr. Jennings' chances are excellent for full recovery from his injuries and return to baseline function. The team is concerned that a living will is a legal expression of the patient's wishes and that respecting his autonomy requires that it be honored, even though his clinical condition would benefit from intubation.

And you thought that a living will was the answer to uncertainty about patient wishes.

A living will is a list of instructions reflecting the individual's wishes about the treatments he does or does not want, usually at the end of life. A health care proxy appointment enables a capable person to appoint an agent to make health care decisions whenever capacity has been lost, either temporarily or permanently. The features of both types of advance directive are often combined in one document that provides for the appointment of a primary agent and an alternate agent, as well as the optional articulation of specific treatment wishes.

While advance directives, especially health care proxies, may be used to guide care at any time the patient has lost capacity, they figure prominently in planning care at the end of life. As discussed in this chapter and chapter 7, the approach of death prompts consideration of life-sustaining treatment, palliation, futility, and quality-of-life judgments. Because these issues are most often addressed when the patient is least able to participate, decisions with lasting consequences must be made on his behalf by others based largely on what they believe he would want. Advance directives can provide surrogate deciders with the insight and confidence to act in ways that are consistent with his preferences and/or best interest.

What could be simpler or clearer? As you well know, clinical ethics consultations are often requested to help the care team, families, and health care agents interpret and implement advance directives. Confusion usually concerns the authority of the directives and the meaning of their provisions. Several points should be emphasized. First, both living wills and health care proxies take effect only when the patient has been determined to have lost decisional capacity. The existence of an advance directive, therefore, does not alter the capable patient's decision-making rights; its authority lies dormant unless or until the patient is deemed unable to make health care decisions.

Second, even when decisional capacity has been lost, treatment instructions are implemented only if the patient meets the criteria specified in the directive. Take, for example, a living will that states, "If I am ever terminally ill, permanently unconscious, or unable to recognize or interact with my family, I do not want to be maintained on ventilatory support, dialysis, or artificial nutrition or hydration." Before even considering withholding or withdrawing these life-sustaining measures, a clinical determination would have to be made that the patient is in one of the specified medical conditions.

III Mrs. Becker, an 82-year-old woman, has been sent by the nursing home to the hospital for replacement of her pacemaker. Her significant dementia prevents her from understanding her clinical condition and health care decisions are made for her by her daughters, who are her proxy agent and alternate agent. When the daughters arrive at the hospital, they tell the care team that they will not consent to replacing the pacemaker because they are honoring what they believe to be their mother's wishes. "Our mother was an elegant, fastidious, and very private person. She always said that, if she were ever incontinent and had to wear diapers, she would not want to live. We know that, if she could appreciate her situation now, she would be humiliated and would not want to continue this way."

Mrs. Becker, however, does not realize that she is incontinent or that her condition would have been a source of embarrassment. At the nursing home, she greets everyone with a smile, enjoys eating lunch in the garden and listening to opera, and loves visits from her grandchildren, even if she does not remember their names. Should her previous wishes limit care that would allow her to continue what appears to be an enjoyable quality of life? On the other hand, does her dementia deprive her of the right to determine how she will be remembered?

Third, inconsistencies between the provisions of a living will and the decisions of a health care agent should be assessed in terms of the patient's current and projected clinical status, and the relationship between the patient and the agent. Because advance directives are executed before the medical condition that will trigger their use, they try to anticipate what the patient would want under circumstances that have not yet occurred. Commentators such as Dresser and Robertson (1989) and Blustein (1999) have suggested that patients with dementia may have interests that differ markedly from those they had when they were capable. The argument offered is that they are in effect different people for whom decisions should be based on their current needs rather than their prior wishes.

Mrs. Becker's daughters and caregivers are struggling with this very dilemma. Her incontinence, while previously a distressing notion to her, does not threaten her health or interfere with a current quality of life she appears to find pleasant. Given her otherwise good level of comfort and function, it would be hard to justify forgoing a life-sustaining measure at this time. Yet, her daughters feel that they will have betrayed the trust she placed in them if they disregard her wishes.

One important thing for Mrs. Becker's daughters to clarify is whether they believe that her comments were to be taken literally as instructions or figuratively as an expression of her distaste for the condition of incontinence. In other words, what do they think she would have wanted if she could have envisioned her current, otherwise pleasant, situation? Here, it is useful to consider Dworkin's (1993) distinction between experiential and critical interests. The former are interests in having experiences of certain kinds; the latter are more central and important interests that concern one's long-range goals and the shape of one's life over time. How Mrs. Becker's daughters decide may depend on whether they regard her interest in not being incontinent as so critical to her sense of self that she would not have been able to tolerate her current condition.

The health care proxy is the recommended advance directive because it employs the agent's knowledge of the patient and her authority to interact with the care team and respond to changing clinical conditions. She is able to consider unanticipated or evolving situations, as well as the clinical judgment of the professionals. Precisely because the agent has the advantage of assessing current medical information in light of the patient's values and wishes, her decisions may exceed or even differ from the living will. Even though the living will may be silent about a specific choice, even though the patient may never have discussed her present medical situation, substituted judgment allows the agent to say, "If the patient knew what we know about her condition and prognosis, this is what she likely would decide."

This means that the spirit, as well as the letter, of the directive should be considered in interpreting the instructions and determining whether they apply to the current circumstances. Mr. Jennings' living will, for example, specifies that he would not want ventilatory support if he were "unresponsive and in respiratory failure." Given his HIV status and his reference to being "maintained on life support," it is probable that he was anticipating an end-of-life scenario, permanent unconsciousness rather than an acute event that would respond to a short course of ventilatory support. This assessment is supported by his mother and sister, whose knowledge of his values and preferences is a valuable resource. Thus, the patient's prior wishes as expressed in a living will must be considered in light of the current clinical realities, the expected outcomes, and additional insights about what matters to him.

Two important caveats are in order. Despite early enthusiasm for advance directives, the percentage of people implementing them remains low and, when they are used, their effectiveness in the clinical setting is less than optimal. One problem appears to be the unfortunate link between advance directives and dying. While advance directives are often very helpful in end-of-life decision making, the emphasis should be that they can guide care *whenever* the patient is unable to make his own decisions. Indeed, it is recommended that, when advance directives are discussed with patients, they *not* be presented as end-of-life planning, which may discourage their use. In a perfect world, care professionals would raise the issue as a routine part of the clinical interaction, saying, "I have this discussion with all my patients because I believe that advance directives are an important part of total health care planning. This is not a matter of how old you are or how sick you are; this is a matter of being responsible for how your health care decisions are made." Uncoupling advance directives from end-of-life considerations is likely to make them less threatening, more accessible, and ultimately more useful.

The second barrier to the effective use of advance directives is the lack of understanding about them displayed by patients, families, and care professionals. People often mistakenly assume that, by itself, a detailed list of treatments they do or do not want or the appointment of a proxy agent will get the job done. In fact, what they believe to be informed prospective decisions are likely to be counterproductive if they do not discuss their care preferences with their doctors, families, or proxy agents. People frequently refuse treatments in advance without understanding what they are or how they work. They leave instructions that do not apply to the medical situations in which they ultimately find themselves. They authorize proxy agents who have no idea of their authority, the types of decisions they may have to make, or how to interpret patient preferences. In some instances, agents do not even know that they have been appointed until it is too late to ask the patient, "What would you want?"

Lack of communication and coordination has also been shown to interfere with advance directives accurately influencing care. Even when directives have been executed, they often do not make their way to the acute care hospitals when patients are admitted. Professionals are uncertain how to interpret advance directives and when their provisions are applicable. Physicians are sometimes unable to predict accurately patient treatment preferences and are often unaware that their patients even have advance directives. Research reveals the need for earlier, more frequent, and better doctor-patient communication, focusing on the goals of care rather than specific interventions (Teno et al., 1998; Fischer et al., 1998; Prendergast, 2001; SUPPORT investigators, 1995; Morrison et al., 1995).

Even a carefully executed advance directive is not sufficient if the patient's values and wishes are unknown or unexplained to those who will base decisions on them. People need to talk with their families, caregivers, and trusted others about what is important to them, allowing their values, rather than their scant knowledge of medical interventions, to be the guide. For example, knowing that Mama would agree to temporary treatment but would not want to be permanently dependent on mechanical supports is more useful than a statement about "no dialysis." Understanding that Dad's notion of an acceptable quality of life is being able to interact with others is more helpful than a statement about "no heroic measures."

More often, the explicit authorization and guidance of an advance directive is lacking and treatment decisions require inferences based on recalled comments or behaviors. Unfortunately, these conversations typically take place in the least opportune circumstances—in the acute care setting at the time of a critical event when the unresponsive patient is in multiorgan system failure, the family is under enormous stress, and professionals seek direction in care planning.

Do-not-resuscitate (DNR) Orders

⫿ Mrs. Marcus is a 72-year-old woman with multiple medical problems, who was admitted from a nursing home after being found unresponsive and hypotensive. This is the second time in recent weeks that Mrs. Marcus has been admitted. She was hospitalized for eighteen days with pneumonia and a massive stroke. During that hospitalization, a feeding tube was placed. She was discharged to the nursing home and now readmitted seventeen days later with aspiration pneumonia. She was intubated in the ER and successfully extubated several days later.

Mrs. Marcus's daughter, Deborah, is her health care proxy agent. A living will, executed on the same date as the proxy appointment, stipulates that, if Mrs. Marcus's "brain has ceased to function," she would not want a variety of potentially life-sustaining interventions, including respiratory support, artificial nutrition and hydration, and antibiotics. Although Mrs. Marcus responds only to deep pain and her physicians do not expect her condition to change, Deborah is in favor of continued aggressive treatment, which she hopes will result in her mother's improvement. The attending believes that, if Mrs. Marcus suffers a cardiopulmonary arrest, she could survive a resuscitation attempt but would almost certainly be left in a much worse condition. For that reason, the care team has recommended a do-not-resuscitate (DNR) order to spare Mrs. Marcus an intervention that would increase her suffering without providing benefit.

Deborah refuses to consent to a DNR order because the wording of the living will does not clarify what is meant by the "brain has ceased to function," and she does not think that forgoing resuscitation reflects her mother's wishes. She says that the living will is clear that her mother would not want to linger in a coma. Because she is not yet in that condition, however, Deborah is unwilling to consent to a DNR order or consider less-than-aggressive treatment at this time.

Another type of advance decision making is the do-not-resuscitate (DNR) order. A DNR order means that cardiopulmonary resuscitation (CPR), including mouth-to-mouth resuscitation, external cardiac massage, and/or stimulants, will not be attempted if the patient suffers a cardiopulmonary arrest. Consent to a DNR order can be given either by a capacitated patient or by someone authorized to consent on the incapacitated patient's behalf.

The ethical dilemma is that CPR's ability to prevent death can greatly benefit some patients and greatly burden others. In a young and/or otherwise healthy person, if cardiopulmonary function can be restarted within approximately four minutes, avoiding irreversible damage to brain and other organs, CPR can give back a life. In an elderly, demented, terminally ill person, one who has multiple serious health problems or has suffered severe and permanent damage, CPR can deprive the individual of a peaceful death.

Unfortunately, reports of successful resuscitations and dramatic television and film depictions of heroic rescue have played into popular belief in CPR's life-saving certainty. In fact, the brutal procedure is rarely effective on frail, debilitated, or terminally ill patients and may simply impose suffering and prolong dying. The critical distinction between attempting and successfully achieving resuscitation accounts for efforts to change the term from DNR to the more accurate DNAR (do not *attempt* resuscitation). Because of its profound implications, consent to forgo CPR is explicit and limited, not inferred or automatically transferred from one setting to another. Thus, DNRs must be renewed periodically, a separate nonhospital DNR is agreed to upon discharge to home or another care facility, and a specific discussion is necessary to suspend a DNR order during the perioperative period.

Even experienced physicians know that advising patients or, more often, families that CPR is not recommended is among the most difficult discussions in the clinical setting. No matter how sensitively it is presented, suggesting that life-saving efforts not be undertaken is distressing and frightening, an index of just how hopeless the patient's condition has become. All the physician's judgment, skill, and compassion are required and ethics consultations are often requested to assist in the process.

Rather than an isolated conversation, the DNR discussion should be part of the overall review of the patient's changing clinical condition. Just as other interventions are evaluated in terms of whether they promote the patient's well-being, resuscitation should be subjected to a benefit-burden analysis. Patients, families, and staff should clearly understand that it is the futile or clinically inappropriate *attempt* rather than successful resuscitation that will be withheld. Discussions with Deborah should balance the benefits and burdens of resuscitation to help her view a DNR order as a way to *protect* her mother from a painful but ineffective intervention, rather than *deprive* her of potentially beneficial treatment. Unfortunately, family members like Deborah are not entirely wrong when they fear that consenting to a DNR order signals to the care team that they have given up hope that the patient will improve and are willing to accept less attentive care. Efforts should be directed toward convincing families and educating caregivers that a DNR order permits the forgoing of a single ineffective intervention but will not affect any other treatment, define the goals or plan of care, or limit the team's attention to the patient.

It is unfair to ask families to take full responsibility for the difficult and painful decision to forgo resuscitation. If CPR is not clinically indicated, the physician's clear recommendation, rationale, and support should be central to the discussion. Once the decision has been made, it is often the consent document that may be most distressing, as if putting pen to paper is the act that seals the patient's fate. The most common expression is, "I feel like I'm signing the death warrant." In many cases it is more compassionate to avoid that trauma by obtaining verbal and witnessed consent.

Finally, there are times when, even though the disadvantages of attempting resuscitation have been explained, families cannot or will not authorize a DNR. However well intended, repeated efforts to obtain consent begin to feel like harassment. The issue risks becoming the focus of the clinical interaction and the signed consent perceived as a trophy. In these circumstances, it may be necessary to redirect attention to other care goals that are more important and achievable.

GOALS OF CARE AT THE END OF LIFE

III Mrs. Diller is an 86-year-old woman admitted from home after suffering her second stroke. Following her last stroke, she recovered some mobility and could enjoy some of her favorite activities, such as Bingo. The attending physician, Dr. Tanner, has discussed the case with the neurologist, Dr. Moon, who thinks that it is still too early to predict the potential for recovery because, when strokes are this deep, patients may take longer to improve. She recommends tissue plasminogen activator (TPA), a complex and potentially dangerous therapy that should be instituted immediately. Based on his prior experience with Mrs. Diller and familiarity with her priorities, however, Dr. Tanner favors a care plan that focuses on comfort.

On this admission, Mrs. Diller was responsive and, although she had great difficulty speaking, she insisted that she did not want to "be like this again." Since then, her level of consciousness has deteriorated and she is largely unresponsive, although her family insists that she squeezes their hands when asked. Dr. Tanner has observed the patient squeezing a hand placed in hers, but believes that this is reflexive rather than a response to command.

Before her initial stroke, Mrs. Diller had appointed one of her daughters, Lila, as her proxy agent. Additional instructions in the proxy document include her wish not to be resuscitated if she has a cardiac arrest and not to receive artificial nutrition and hydration if she has a terminal condition or is in an irreversible coma.

Her family describes her as a very independent woman who would be distressed by her current disability but disagrees about the appropriate care plan. Although Lila feels obligated to honor her mother's expressed wishes, she does not want the responsibility of forgoing life-sustaining treatment. Another daughter notes that Mrs. Diller improved considerably after her last stroke and insists that the same thing could happen this time. The patient's brother argues for the TPA advocated by Dr. Moon, while one granddaughter insists that she would not want to be "tortured" with tubes and machines and should be allowed to die in peace. Another granddaughter pleads that, as long as her grandmother can squeeze her hand, she should be kept alive as long as possible.

Perhaps the single most important question in clinical decision making and the one that is central to any ethics analysis is, "What are the goals of care for this patient?" or "What do we intend to accomplish with our diagnostic and therapeutic efforts?" Identifying the care goals, especially at the end of life, requires professionals, families, and, when possible, patients to clearly articulate what they understand and expect. If recovery or substantial improvement is unrealistic in light of a terminal diagnosis and steady deterioration, the goals and plan of care should be revised. If the aim is to relieve suffering and not prolong the dying process, then interventions aimed at cure are inconsistent and serve only to distract from the primary objective.

Regularly reassessing the goals in response to clinical changes permits the care plan to reflect accurately what is both feasible and desirable, especially as death approaches. Critical considerations during this time include the determination that the patient is dying, the initiation or forgoing of particular interventions, and the involvement of additional resources, such as palliative care. As discussed in chapter 7, the relief of pain and suffering is a moral imperative central to the entire clinical interaction, which becomes more prominent at the end of life.

Focusing on the goals of care guards against the risk of resorting to interventions because they are available rather than clinically indicated. The temptation to use every-thing in the therapeutic arsenal makes it easy to justify this treatment, which triggers that one and then, of course, the one that follows. Rather than asking, "What is the goal of this particular intervention?" the patient is better served by asking, "Where does this intervention fit into the overall plan of care? If it advances the agreed-upon goals, we may appropriately begin or continue it. If not, it is probably not indicated."

Keeping the goals at the center of care planning also permits a wider range of treat-ment options, which is especially important at the end of life. Interventions should be evaluated in terms of what they can accomplish for the patient rather than categorized according to conventional labels. For example, surgery, radiation, or antibiotics can be appropriately considered for a dying patient when it is clear that the goal is comfort rather than cure.

Clarifying *whose* goals are being considered is a key element in care planning. A frequent source of ethical tension is the presumption of consensus on care goals when, in fact, the patient, family, and care team may not share the same understanding of the clinical picture or possible outcomes. The patient may want to spare his family the pain of seeing him deteriorate and the emotional and financial burden of his care. His chil-dren may want him to continue aggressive therapy in hopes of a cure. His wife may want him to come home with the focus on symptom management so that his remain-ing time can be spent comfortably finishing his work and interacting with his family. His sister may want to protect him from the knowledge that he is dying. His caregivers may feel that he could benefit from a clinical trial of an experimental protocol.

Mrs. Diller's family and care providers find it hard to agree on a plan of care because of their differing perceptions of her condition, prognosis, and wishes, as well as their own notions of what is in her best interest. Dr. Moon and the patient's brother believe that not pursuing aggressive treatment would be giving up prematurely. Dr. Tanner and one granddaughter urge a focus on comfort measures to protect the patient from treat-ment that would increase and prolong her suffering. As the health care agent, Lila feels bound to honor her mother's expressed preferences, which appear to be forgoing spe-cific life-sustaining treatments. Finally, while differences between physicians' clinical impressions are not uncommon and can be useful in arriving at accurate prognoses, families often find their lack of agreement frustrating.

How the goals of care are articulated and justified will influence the therapeutic and interpersonal dynamics. Inconsistent expectations inevitably lead to descriptions of the family as "unreasonable" or "demanding," and charges that care professionals have not been clear and candid in their explanations or responsive in their treatment. Insuf-ficient attention to what is really being communicated or avoided permits people to mistakenly believe that what they have said has been heard and understood. Your involvement through bioethics consultation can be especially helpful when the parties need to clarify the clinical realities, identify the patient's interests and values, and focus on the goals in developing an appropriate end-of-life care plan.

||| Mr. Giles is a 58-year-old man who has had AIDS for fourteen years, apparently the result of a long history of intravenous drug abuse. He has multiple medical problems, including hypertension, asthma, chronic obstructive pulmonary disease, panic disorder, colitis, stroke, meningitis, and multiple pneumonias, two episodes of which required ventilation. He has been receiving hemodialysis for one year to treat end-stage renal disease. He was admitted from a long-term nursing facility with seizures and changes in mental status. He is nonverbal and only intermittently responsive.

An MRI revealed a brain tumor. Given Mr. Giles' AIDS status, he faces specific risks. Surgery carries a high risk of hemorrhage, which could leave an immediate, severe, and permanent neurologic deficit, such as hemiplegia (one-sided paralysis). Without surgery, his seizures and cognitive changes can be controlled with anticonvulsant medication, but he faces progressive decline in mental status, as well as a slow evolution of hemiparesis (one-sided weakness). Mr. Giles has no family or others involved in his care. Despite encouragement from the nursing facility, he has not completed an advance directive.

An important consideration in setting end-of-life care goals is the quality of the patient's remaining time. For example, it is not uncommon for an intervention to be recommended because it will "improve the quality of life" or for a prognosis to be described in terms of a "poor quality of life." It is worth noting that these subjective, value-laden conceptions are important *personal* evaluations for the patient, family, or other agent, not *medical* assessments for clinicians. Defining beneficence and best interest remains the responsibility of the patient and his surrogates, for whom the requested interventions have the most significance. While the physician can describe the likely range of comfort and function that the patient will experience, it can be argued that only the patient or those who know him well can assess how those projections will be perceived in terms of life quality. When, as in Mr. Giles' case, the patient is without capacity, surrogates, or advance directives, the care team has no insight into his values, wishes, or the quality of life he would consider acceptable. Only in these circumstances are clinicians justified in using the best interest standard to try to assess what plan might benefit the patient.

Setting therapeutic goals should be a fully collaborative effort by the patient or trusted surrogates and the care team, reflecting not only what is possible but what is desirable. This balance calls for articulation and periodic review of the meaning of success, recognizing the subjective nature of quality-of-life assessments. Despite the superiority of professional medical knowledge and skill, the perspective that matters is that of the patient who will experience the life and death that are achieved.

FORGOING LIFE-SUSTAINING TREATMENT

||| Mrs. Lewis is a 72-year-old woman with progressive dementia of unknown etiology, progressive renal failure, and hypertension, admitted with an acute gastrointestinal (GI)

bleed. She has been living at home with her daughter and has received care through the family practice group. She has neither a living will nor a health care proxy.

Prior to admission, Mrs. Lewis could use a walker and a bedside commode. She has not been hospitalized recently and generally manages well at home. While her renal failure has been progressive, her current deterioration may be the result of her acute GI bleed and might be reversible, although the renal attending thinks this is unlikely. Her primary care physician favors a trial of dialysis to see if her renal function improves and her mental status clears, but he doubts the utility of chronic dialysis. Mrs. Lewis's acute bleeding has stopped, but she is not eating and the gastroenterologist has placed a temporary nasogastric tube to provide nutrition. He says that, shortly, a more permanent feeding tube will be necessary for continued nourishment. The chief resident describes Mrs. Lewis as "a little old lady curled up in bed who responds only to noxious stimuli and occasionally utters a single word." He is concerned that dialysis and tube feeding will prolong her dying and increase her suffering.

Her daughter is anxious about making decisions without knowing what her mother would want. In particular, she is concerned about eliminating dialysis from consideration without knowing whether it would be effective.

It's a safe guess that much of your ethics committee agenda and consultation requests concern withholding or withdrawing life-sustaining treatment, especially from patients without capacity. Decisions about deferring or permitting death are difficult for clinicians and administrators; they are painful and often paralyzing for those who act on behalf of their loved ones. If abandoned to make these choices alone, the family or other surrogate is likely to feel solely responsible for the outcome. The lingering regret is likely to be, "If only we had insisted on continued treatment, Mama would be with us today." Clinicians can help make the process more bearable by sharing the burden of making these hard decisions.

Whether end-of-life care choices are made by capable individuals or surrogates, using a benefit-burden analysis as the decision-making model can provide structure, consistency, and support for patients, families, and staff. Central to this analysis is the overarching goal of providing only care that benefits the patient without increasing suffering or prolonging the dying process. When the burdens of an intervention or a course of care are shown to outweigh its benefits, the decision to look for alternatives is more easily and comfortably justified.

One useful strategy is a therapeutic trial. A treatment plan with potential benefits is implemented for a specified period of time, after which its effectiveness is evaluated and it is either continued or discontinued. The key is clearly setting out in advance the proposed length of the trial, as well as the goals, limits, and criteria for success. For example, "Let's try three dialysis treatments during the next seven days. If Mrs. Lewis's renal function and mental status improve, we can consider the benefit of further treatments. If she shows no improvement, we'll know that dialysis is ineffective for her and should not be continued." Consensus on the goals and indices of success encourages the trial of appropriate interventions without the fear that, once begun, they cannot be stopped. Therapeutic trials also provide important reassurance that no potentially beneficial treatments have been left untried.

Productive end-of-life decision making depends on clarity and candor. As discussed in chapter 3, offering false choices when there are no real alternatives frustrates patients and families, and diminishes their exercise of genuine autonomy. Asking, "Should we continue your husband's antibiotics?" or "Do you want us to resuscitate Mama if her heart stops?" is not helpful if it is clear that these interventions are not clinically indicated. It is more responsible and compassionate to say, "The antibiotics we tried are no longer fighting your husband's infection. Because they're not helping him and may be creating other problems, they should be discontinued," or "Let me tell you why we believe that, if Mama's heart stops, attempting resuscitation will not benefit her."

These discussions are never easy, but they can be made less threatening with reassurance that the patient will not be abandoned. When specific interventions will be withheld or withdrawn, the focus should be on those that will be continued or added. It is critical to emphasize that, while the goals of care may change to reflect a greater priority on comfort than cure, the team's commitment to the patient's well-being remains unaltered.

PROTECTING PATIENTS FROM TREATMENT

Decisions about forgoing life-sustaining measures usually arise when death is imminent and continued intervention will not improve the clinical condition but may contribute to suffering. How these issues are resolved depends greatly on how they are framed. Withholding or withdrawing treatment can be seen either as *depriving* the patient of needed care or *protecting* the patient from the burden of ineffective or harmful interventions. When continued treatment will only prolong dying or increase suffering, it is appropriate to help the patient's loved ones give themselves permission to make hard choices, within applicable state law, that will be in his best interest.

An example is considering artificial nutrition and hydration (ANH) at the end of life when the burdens of the intervention will outweigh the benefits. Research has shown that patients with advanced dementia typically stop eating as the end of life nears because their bodies are shutting down and no longer need the nutrition. For these patients, continued tube feeding often creates considerable discomfort, including bloating, gas, nausea, cramping, and diarrhea (Huang and Ahronheim, 2000; Ahronheim, 1996). When the dying process cannot be reversed and an intervention imposes only pain or other distress, it can be argued that discontinuing the treatment—even nutrition and hydration—protects the patient from harm and promotes comfort as death nears.

The frustration and despair of those closest to the dying patient are directly related to their feelings of helplessness as his condition deteriorates. No matter what they do, they cannot prevent the inevitable. But, while they cannot determine *whether* he dies, they can influence *how* he dies. Assessing the care plan according to its relative benefits and burdens, they are able to make decisions that shield their loved one from interventions that create more harm than good. At the end of life, the notion of family as protector can be a powerful and comforting one that can and should be reinforced.

REJECTION OF RECOMMENDED TREATMENT AND REQUESTS TO "DO EVERYTHING"

||| Mrs. Abrams is a 70-year-old woman who came into the hospital for surgical closure of her colostomy. She had been living independently at home and, on admission, she was interactive and fully capacitated. Her medical history includes emphysema from years of cigarette smoking. The surgery was successful but, shortly thereafter, Mrs. Abrams developed abdominal fistulas that required another operation. She was so weakened by her multiple surgeries that she required ventilatory support. Despite strong initial resistance to intubation, she reluctantly agreed to it after discussion with her pulmonologist.

The following day in the ICU, Mrs. Abrams let it be known in no uncertain terms that she wants to be extubated. Her surgeon is playing a marginal role in her care and all important medical decisions are being made by her pulmonologist. Mrs. Abrams' three daughters are deeply troubled by their mother's decision to refuse further intubation. The house staff caring for Mrs. Abrams do not know how to proceed or what is legally and ethically appropriate. They believe that removing the vent would mean almost certain death, which they find personally and professionally very disturbing.

When patient or family decisions conflict with physician recommendations, clinical judgment and skill are tested. Patients often reject proposed interventions likely to be beneficial or even life-saving. While respect for patient autonomy requires that capacitated care decisions be honored, the refusal of treatment should be the beginning, not the end, of the discussion. As discussed in chapter 3, the professional obligation is to ensure that all consents and refusals are informed and thoroughly considered. Because of their profound implications, however, refusals of life-sustaining treatment should receive heightened scrutiny. Special attention should be given to the adequacy of the information presented and the quality of the explanation, possible language or cultural barriers to understanding, and the patient's capacity and appreciation of the consequences of forgoing treatment.

In addressing Mrs. Abrams' request for extubation, the care team should clarify the length of time ventilatory support is recommended, the anticipated benefits, and the likely outcomes of premature vent removal. Carefully probing her concerns should reveal fears and misconceptions that can be addressed. For example, she may be afraid that she will be permanently dependent on ventilatory support, when, in fact, her doctors anticipate that she should be weaned from the ventilator within a few weeks.

Although Mrs. Abrams' ability to communicate will be hampered by the endotracheal tube, adequate time and effort should be invested in assessing her capacity, her goals for care, her expectations, and the consistency of her wishes. Throughout the process, which may take several days, she should be reassured that her request is being carefully considered, especially in light of its significant consequences. A bioethics consultation, including Mrs. Abrams, her daughters, and the care team, can facilitate a clinically, legally, and ethically acceptable resolution. If the patient remains committed to discontinuing ventilatory support, the care plan should focus on promoting her comfort, including measures to minimize air hunger, anxiety, and other symptoms of respiratory distress.

Physicians may also be faced with patient or family instructions to "do everything," including requests for specific interventions judged to be therapeutically inappropriate or otherwise not indicated. At the end of life, family members often feel the need to be good advocates, to ensure that their loved ones are not neglected and that no potentially beneficial treatment is left untried. Especially when they do not know what to anticipate or how much confidence to place in the care professionals, they may insist on all available therapies in the hope that one of them will be effective.

Is the customer or, in this case, the patient or family always right? The short answer is, of course not. Because there is no obligation to provide treatment just because it is requested and because physicians must be guided by their clinical judgment and professional integrity, they should not comply with requests that fall outside the standard of care. That position, however, is only the beginning of the ethics analysis. Like treatment refusals, insistence on inappropriate treatment should trigger further discussion and clarification.

These requests should be seen as an important signal that the parties to the interaction may not share the same understanding of the patient's condition and prognosis, goals of care, available treatment options, and expected outcomes of the proposed interventions. The first question should be, "What does 'everything' mean to you, and what do you expect to happen if we do it?" The focus should be on identifying unrealistic expectations, clarifying the goals of care, the potential for the proposed treatments to achieve those goals, the obligation to prevent suffering without benefit, and further explanation of the recommended plan of care.

MEDICAL FUTILITY

III "He never had time to even catch his breath and already it's come to this." Ari was talking about his father, Dr. Dole, a 54-year-old physician who had diagnosed his own pancreatic cancer just nine weeks ago. He was found to have significant metastases and his condition has deteriorated very rapidly. Now he is in the ICU, intubated and comatose, and his colleagues are finding it increasingly difficult to keep his organ systems from failing. Even with aggressive management, there is reluctant consensus within the medical team that the therapeutic options are running out and nothing further can be done to stem multiorgan failure.

When the critical care team met this morning to discuss Dr. Dole's care, several suggestions were offered for continued and even accelerated interventions. Finally, Dr. Birch said quietly, "Let's face it. This is medically futile."

Judgments about providing or limiting treatment frequently invoke the notion of medical futility. Despite vast literature and vigorous debate, efforts to agree on a determination of futility have been largely unsuccessful. Its narrowest and most useful definition describes the *physiologic impossibility* of an intervention achieving its therapeutic objective. In that strict sense, physicians are excused—even precluded—from burdening patients with treatment that will be clinically ineffective or even harmful.

This narrow and value-neutral definition does not apply, however, to the vast majority of cases in which the notion of futility is raised. Far more often, interventions or care plans are labeled "futile" when they are expected to produce a clinical effect that falls below a specified standard. For example, dialysis may successfully assume the function of failing kidneys, but not contribute to returning the patient to an acceptable overall health status. Depending on the long-range clinical goals, the intervention may be considered futile in achieving the desired objective. Moreover, the differing values and expectations of the patient, family, and care team may prevent consensus on the definition of success, contributing to confusion and conflict in determining the meaning of futility. Finally, notions of futility may have more to do with perceived acceptable quality of life than actual clinical effectiveness.

Care providers faced with new and often competing pressures may misuse the notion of futility in the service of what they see as their ethical responsibilities to patients, families, and society. Mindful of their conflicting obligations to promote the best interests of patients by providing only beneficial treatments, not raise unrealistic expectations, and provide cost-effective care, physicians may label questionably effective interventions "futile" as a way of withholding them. Futility can also function as the trump card to discourage families from insisting on treatment that care providers consider inappropriate. While some physicians see futility determination as the ethical way to manage end-of-life care, others see it as a way to take control of decisions from demanding families.

Labeling inappropriate interventions "futile" distorts the meaning of the term and obscures the message that should be communicated. The more accurate and accessible approach might be to explain that, regardless of what is done, the patient is dying and what matters is the quality of that dying. Invoking futility as a frame for end-of-life issues should be replaced with reality checking—clarifying that the patient is dying, reassessing the goals and expectations of care, defining benefit and burden, and identifying ways to promote physical and emotional comfort.

Seen in this light, further efforts to reverse Dr. Dole's clinical course can be considered medically futile because the interventions are not meeting their physiological

objectives and he is dying regardless of treatment. Continued cure-oriented measures would not only be ineffective, they would be counterproductive and, as discussed in chapter 7, the goals of care are now more appropriately palliative than curative. In other cases, discussion might well reveal that, rather than strict futility, decisions for the dying patient concern quality of life and death.

REFERENCES

Ad Hoc Committee of the Harvard Medical School to Examine the Definition of Brain Death. 1968. A definition of irreversible coma. *Journal of the American Medical Association* 205(6):85–88.

Ahronheim JC. 1996. Nutrition and hydration in the terminal patient. *Clinics in Geriatric Medicine* 12(2):379–91.

Arnold RM. 2002. A rose by any other name. *Journal of Palliative Medicine* 5(6):807–11.

Blustein J. 1999. Choosing for others as continuing a life story: The problem of personal identity revisited. *Journal of Law, Medicine & Ethics* 27(1):20–31.

Brock DW. 1991. Surrogate decision making for incompetent adults: An ethical framework. *The Mount Sinai Journal of Medicine* 58(5):388–92.

Brock DW. 1997. Death and dying. In Veatch RM, ed. *Medical Ethics.* 2nd ed. Sudbury, MA: Jones and Barlett Publishers, pp. 363–94.

Brody H, Campbell ML, Faber-Langendoen K, Ogle KS. 1997. Withdrawing intensive life-sustaining treatment—Recommendations for compassionate clinical management. *New England Journal of Medicine* 336(9):652–57.

Byock I. 1997. *Dying Well: Peace and Possibilities at the End of Life.* New York: Riverhead Books.

Christakis NA, Iwashyna TJ. 1998. Attitude and self-reported practice regarding prognostication in a national sample of internists. *Archives of Internal Medicine* 158(21):2389–95.

Cranford RE. 1995. The persistent vegetative state: The medical reality (Getting the facts straight). In Arras JD, Steinbock B, eds. *Ethical Issues in Modern Medicine.* 4th ed. Mountain View, CA: Mayfield Publishing Co., pp. 172–77.

Cruzan v. Director, Missouri Department of Health, 497 U.S. 261 (1990).

Dresser RS, Robertson JA. 1989. Quality of life and non-treatment decisions for incompetent patients: A critique of the orthodox approach. *Law, Medicine & Health Care* 17(3):234–44.

Dubler NN, Post LF, Barnes B. 1999. Making health care decisions for others: A guide to being a health care proxy or surrogate. New York: Montefiore Medical Center.

Dworkin R. 1993. *Life's Dominion: An Argument About Abortion, Euthanasia, and Individual Freedom.* New York: Alfred A. Knopf.

Fins JJ. 2005. Rethinking disorders of consciousness: New research and its implications. *Hastings Center Report* 35(2):22–24.

Fins JJ, Miller FG, Acres CA, Bacchetta MF, Huzzard LL, Rapkin, BD. 1999. End-of-life decision-making in the hospital: Current practice and future prospects. *Journal of Pain and Symptom Management* 17(1):6–15.

Fisher GS, Tulsky JA, Rose MR, Siminoff LA, Arnold RM. 1998. Patient knowledge and physician predictions of treatment preferences after discussion of advance directives. *Journal of General Internal Medicine* 13(7):447–54.

Gillick MR. 2000. Rethinking the role of tube feeding in patients with advanced dementia. *New England Journal of Medicine* 342(3):206–10.

Helft PR, Siegler M, Lantos J. 2000.The rise and fall of the futility movement. *New England Journal of Medicine* 343(4):293–96.

Huang ZB, Ahronheim JC. 2000. Nutrition and hydration in terminally ill patients: An update. *Clinics in Geriatric Medicine* 16(2):313–25.

Kagawa-Singer M, Blackhall LJ. 2001. Negotiating cross-cultural issues at the end of life: "You've got to go where he lives." *Journal of the American Medical Association* 286(23):2992–3001.

Kalkut G, Dubler NN. 2005. The line between life and death. *New York Times,* May 10, p. A17.

Loewy EH. 1998. Ethical considerations in executing and implementing advance directives. *Archives of Internal Medicine* 158(4):321–24.

Luce JM. 1995. Physicians do not have a responsibility to provide futile or unreasonable care if a patient or family insists. *Critical Care Medicine* 23(4):760–66.

Lynn J, Teno J, Dresser R, Brock D, Nelson HL, Nelson JL, Kielstein R, Fukuchi Y, Lu D, Itakura H. 1999. Dementia and advance-care planning: Perspectives from three countries on ethics and epidemiology. *Journal of Clinical Ethics* 10(4):271–85.

Meisel A, Snyder L, Quill T. 2000. Seven legal barriers to end-of-life care: Myths, realities, and grains of truth. *Journal of the American Medical Association* 284(19):2495–501.

Mezey MD, Cassel CK, Bottrell MM, Hyer K, Howe JL, Fulmer TT, eds. 2002. *Ethical Patient Care: A Casebook for Geriatric Health Care Teams.* Baltimore: Johns Hopkins University Press.

Mezey M, Dubler NN, Mitty E, Brody AA. 2002. What impact do setting and transitions have on the quality of life at the end of life and the quality of the dying process? *The Gerontologist* 42(Special issue III):54–67.

Morrison RS, Olson E, Mertz KR, Meier DE. 1995. The inaccessibility of advance directives on transfer from ambulatory to acute care settings. *Journal of the American Medical Association* 274(6):478–82.

Orentlicher D. 2001. *Matters of Life and Death: Making Moral Theory Work in Medical Ethics and the Law.* Princeton: Princeton University Press.

Post LF. 1999. Decisions to permit death: Whose interests should determine the outcome? *Geriatric Care Management Journal* 9(4):16–23.

Post LF. 2006. Living wills and durable powers of attorney. In Schulz R, Noelker LS, Rockwood K, Sprott RL, eds. *The Encyclopedia of Aging.* 4th ed. New York: Springer Publishing Company, vol. II:668–71.

Post LF, Blustein J, Dubler NN. 1999. The doctor-proxy relationship: An untapped resource *Journal of Law, Medicine & Ethics* 27(1):5–12.

Prendergast TJ. 2001. Advance care planning: Pitfalls, progress, promise. *Critical Care Medicine* 29(2) Supplement N34–39.

President's Commission for the Study of Ethical Problems in Medicine and Biomedical and Behavioral Research. 1981. *Defining Death: A Report on the Medical, Legal and Ethical Issues in the Determination of Death.* Washington, DC: U.S. Government Printing Office.

Quill TE. 2000. Initiating end-of-life discussions with seriously ill patients: Addressing the elephant in the room. *Journal of the American Medical Association* 284(19):2502–7.

In re Quinlan, 355 A.2d 647 (N.J. 1976).

Rhoden NK. 2003. The limits of legal objectivity. In Steinbock B, Arras JD, London AJ, eds. *Ethical Issues in Modern Medicine.* 6th ed. Boston: McGraw-Hill, pp. 368–75.

Schneiderman LJ, et al. 1990. Medical futility: Its meaning and ethical implications. *Annals of Internal Medicine* 112:949–54.

Silveira MJ, DiPiero A, Gerrity MS, Feudtner C. 2000. Patients' knowledge of options at the end of life: Ignorance in the face of death. *Journal of the American Medical Association* 284(19):2483–88.

Singer PA, et al. 2001. Hospital policy on appropriate use of life-sustaining treatment. *Critical Care Medicine* 29(1):187–91.

Sprung CL, Eidelman LA, Steinberg A. 1995. Is the physician's duty to the individual patient or to society? *Critical Care Medicine* 23(4):618–20.

Steinhauser KE, Christakis NA, Clipp EC, McNeilly M, McIntyre L, Tulsky JA. 2000. Factors considered important at the end of life by patients, family, physicians, and other care providers. *Journal of the American Medical Association* 284(19):2476–82.

The SUPPORT Principal Investigators. 1995. A controlled trial to improve care for seriously ill hospitalized patients: The Study to Understand Prognoses and Preferences for Outcomes and Risks of Treatments (SUPPORT). *Journal of the American Medical Association* 274(20):1591–98.

Teno JM, Stevens M, Spernak S, Lynn J. 1998. Role of written advance directives in decision making: Insights from qualitative and quantitative data. *Journal of General Internal Medicine* 13(7):439–46.

Terry PB, Vettese M, Song J, Foreman J, Haller KB, Miller DJ, Stallings R, Sulmasy DP. 1999. End-of-life decision making: When patients and surrogates disagree. *Journal of Clinical Ethics* 10(4):286–93.

Truog RD. 1997. Is it time to abandon brain death? *Hastings Center Report* 27(1):29–37.

Truog RD, Frader JE, Brett AS. 1992. The problem with futility. *New England Journal of Medicine* 326(23):1560–64.

Wicclair MR. 2001. Medical futility: A conceptual and ethical analysis. In Mappes TA, DeGrazia D, eds. *Biomedical Ethics*. 5th ed. New York: McGraw-Hill, pp. 340–50.

Wissow LS, Belote A, Kramer W, Compton-Phillips A, Kritzler R, Weiner JP. 2004. Promoting advance directives among elderly primary care patients. *Journal of General Internal Medicine* 19(9):944–51.

Zeleznik J, Post LF, Mulvihill M, Jacobs LG, Burton WB, Dubler NN. 1999. The doctor-proxy relationship: Perception and communication. *Journal of Law, Medicine & Ethics* 27(1):13–19.

7 Palliation

FROM CARING TO CURING AND BACK AGAIN

Providing comfort, especially at the end of life, is neither a new concept nor a departure from the traditional responsibilities of the caring professions. Until the middle of the twentieth century, the cure of disease and the prevention of death were largely beyond the capability of those who ministered to the sick by trying to relieve their pain. With the development of biotechnology, the obligation to provide care became the obligation to provide cure, and a focus on comfort was reserved for those times when "nothing more could be done." Rather than an inevitability, death was perceived as a failure of skill and the very notion of dying made professionals uncomfortable, even guilty. Increasingly sophisticated science and technology inflated both professional and lay expectations about the power of medicine. The resulting belief that cure is always possible led to a perceived requirement to "do everything" and a sense of defeat whenever patients did not recover or improve.

Palliative care as a discipline has successfully reintroduced the notion that relieving pain and suffering is central to the complete and authentic practice of medicine. Its defining philosophy is that cure and comfort are consistent objectives that may assume greater or lesser prominence, depending on the patient's condition, prognosis, and values. As discussed in chapter 6, the therapeutic continuum seeks a balance of curative and palliative care that responds to the patient's changing condition. When the potential exists for significant improvement, the plan of care emphasizes aggressive curative interventions, supplemented by comfort measures. As the likelihood of remission fades and the patient approaches the end of life, the goal of care shifts and aggressive palliation becomes the primary focus.

This transition, which occurs over time rather than at a given moment, depends on attention to the evolving medical status, the clinical effectiveness of specific interventions, and the wishes and values of the patient and family. Helping patients, families, and professionals to adjust their goals and make decisions in ways that have clinical and ethical validity is the contribution of the bioethics committee.

‖ Mrs. Heller has been a resident of a long-term care facility for many years, during which her chronic obstructive pulmonary disease, diabetes, and osteoarthritis have become more severe. She is now confined to a wheelchair because of the intense pain in her back and hips, which she often describes as excruciating. The mild analgesics, including Tylenol, that have been prescribed do not bring relief and she has become increasingly immobilized, withdrawn, and depressed.

When her nephew, Dr. Agin, visited recently, he was alarmed by the deterioration he saw in his aunt. The person he remembered as vibrant and active was now saying, "I have no life. All I have is pain." When he asked what she would like to be able to do that the pain prevented, he expected her to talk about missing her hiking, gardening, and painting. Instead, she replied, "Sleep. I don't remember the last time I was able to sleep without being awakened by pain."

Dr. Agin has requested a meeting to discuss his aunt's pain management.

THE EXPERIENCE OF AND RESPONSE TO PAIN

Pain

Despite its subjective quality, the experience of pain is very real and can be consuming. As one writer describes it,

> Pain is dehumanizing. The severer the pain, the more it overshadows the patient's intelligence. All she or he can think about is pain: there is no past pain-free memory, no pain-free future, only the pain-filled present. Pain destroys autonomy: the patient is afraid to make the slightest movement. All choices are focused on either relieving the present pain or preventing greater future pain, and for this, one will sell one's soul. Pain is humiliating: it destroys all sense of self-esteem accompanied by feelings of helplessness in the grip of pain, dependency on drugs, and being a burden to others. In its extreme, pain destroys the soul itself and all will to live. (Lisson, 1987, p. 654)

Whatever the clinical setting, medical condition, or technological sophistication, one caregiver mandate remains constant and compelling—the relief of pain. Even when cure is impossible, the duty of care includes palliation. Moreover, this obligation is central to the therapeutic interaction, unquestioned and universal, transcending time and cultural boundaries. Whether the source of the pain is physiological or psychological, its relief is considered a primary moral goal of medicine because of the unique and intimate connection between those who hurt and those who comfort.

Pain and Suffering

A related distinction has been made between pain and suffering. Dr. Eric Cassell (1982) has written about pain as a physiological response of the body and suffering as an existential assault on the person. He describes how one can experience pain without suffering when the goal is a noble or joyous one, using as an example the pain of childbirth. Conversely, a person can suffer without physical pain when he feels the disintegration of his personhood and his sense of control. When pain and suffering *are* closely related, Cassell claims, it is because the patient perceives the pain as overwhelming, uncontrollable, or unending. Emotional isolation may be added by the suggestion that the pain is only imagined. Pain of this kind represents suffering that is a threat, not only to life but to the integrity of the patient's sense of self.

It is impossible to spend any time in a clinical setting without recognizing this distinction. Patients are often asked to endure pain in the pursuit of a cure or remission. In weighing the benefits and burdens of a proposed treatment, the balance of current discomfort for future relief seems ethically appropriate. The calculus is different when the intervention will impose pain or suffering with no benefit. Likewise, suffering without pain is evident in the patient with aphasia that prevents him from communicating with his family, the trained athlete who can no longer care for her most basic physical needs, the father who must accept that his infant will never develop, and the artist trying to create faster than her eyesight is failing.

Responses to Pain

||| Mr. Peters is a 27-year-old African American man with sickle cell anemia, admitted to the ER in sickle cell crisis. He is experiencing severe pain in his thighs, arms, hands, and feet. He is also dehydrated and anemic. An ER resident orders an injection of Demerol for pain and admits him to the hospital.

Following admission, Mr. Peters continues to complain of pain and asks the nurses repeatedly about the medication that has been ordered for him. During morning rounds the next day, the medical team is impressed by how much he knows about his disease and its management. He reports that, most of the time, he is able to manage his pain with an anti-inflammatory drug, such as Motrin. During a sickle cell crisis, however, the only effective pain relief is achieved with intravenous morphine, and he specifies the dosages and schedules that have been successful. He says that, during past hospitalizations, self-administering the morphine with a patient-controlled analgesia (PCA) pump has allowed him to achieve a constant blood level of medication, with supplementary morphine as needed for breakthrough pain.

The attending tells Mr. Peters that Demerol will be available when he requests it to control his pain. She also asks where and from whom he usually receives care, and Mr. Peters names several hospitals where he has been treated during crises. During postrounds discussion, several residents express concern about the patient's detailed request for a particular narcotic in specific dosages. They suggest that this may be drug-seeking behavior by an addict. One resident recounts a similar case during his internship, concluding, "That patient conned us for two days before we caught on. When we cut off her drugs, she left the hospital."

Nothing should be more self-evident than the clinical and ethical imperative to relieve pain. Yet, pain is a complex phenomenon for both patients and care providers in several important ways. First, pain is solitary, experienced only by the patient. Unlike other indications of illness or injury, information about pain is available to the clinician only through the patient's descriptions of and responses to it. This reliance on patient assessment of symptoms makes the evaluation and treatment of pain significantly different from other patient-physician interactions.

Second, although universally acknowledged, the experience and understanding of pain is influenced as much by personal values and cultural traditions as by physiological injury and disease. If the perception of and response to pain are to be understood in a useful way, they should be examined in the context of culture, gender, power, morality, and myth. These factors are especially important in the health care setting, where pain becomes an interpersonal encounter between the sufferer and the reliever. How pain is experienced and expressed by the patient and how it is understood and responded to by the provider largely determine how it is valued and, ultimately, how it is treated.

Both patient and clinician attitudes are affected by their respective personal and cultural values. For example, physicians' clinical judgments about and responses to pain are influenced by group-based factors, including age, gender, race, ethnicity, and physical appearance. The balance of power between provider and patient is yet another theme in the pain management interaction. So long as therapeutic control is vested in the caregiver, the patient remains the passive victim of pain, a supplicant in the standard p.r.n. (as circumstances require) regimen that requires the patient to ask for medication each time it is needed (Post et al., 1996).

Third, both patients and their doctors are influenced by their understanding—often misunderstanding—of pain and the agents for its relief. Studies have shown that physicians are inhibited by their inadequate professional education about analgesia, misconceptions about opioids and addiction, and fears about regulatory and legal liability. Similar misconceptions are shared by the lay public, and Americans have been shown to reject what they believe to be effective medicinal pain relief because they fear overreliance and/or addiction. Reluctance to provide sufficient pain medication has also been related to clinician fears that use of opioids will "kill patients" by depressing respirations and hastening death. These fears, plus concerns about legal liability, are reflected in the stringent laws regulating drug prescription and the suspicions of health care providers who see patient requests for pain relief as drug-seeking behaviors related to addiction. The unsurprising and unacceptable result is the routine undermedication of even terminally ill patients (e.g., Furrow, 2001; Post et al., 1996).

Mr. Peters' case illustrates several of these issues. He comes to the ER requesting morphine, a potent narcotic, and specifying the dosages and intervals that he would prefer. The care team has no prior experience with him and no way of confirming his history of sickle cell or its prior management. Mindful that morphine's effects are euphoric as well as analgesic, and also potentially addictive, the team believes that it must consider the possibility that he is a drug seeker rather than simply a patient in pain. While no explicit mention has been made of his race, it may influence some team members' perception about the likelihood that he abuses drugs. Even if he had not requested a narcotic, by specifying dosages and intervals, Mr. Peters may have seemed "demanding" or "bossy" to some caregivers, who prefer to be in control of the clinical interaction. Individually or in combination, these factors may result in his claims of pain and requests for relief to be discounted.

When dealing with patients in pain, especially pain that is chronic and/or intermittently intense, it is important for caregivers to understand the nature of the discomfort, its effects, and useful ways to respond to it. Assuming that Mr. Peters suffers from periodic sickle cell crises, it is reasonable that he is very familiar with the medications, dosages, and schedules that most effectively treat his pain. Unless and until he demonstrates that his description of symptoms is inaccurate or that he has another motive for his requests, the primary clinical goal should be to relieve his pain as quickly and completely as possible. Collaborating with him in this endeavor has the added benefit of helping him to regain some control over a situation that may well make him feel repeatedly helpless.

III   Mr. Charles is a 32-year-old man with end-stage AIDS. He is wasted, noncommunicative, but responsive to painful stimuli. His rapid breathing, sweating, and restlessness indicate that he is experiencing considerable discomfort. His attending, Dr. Fellows, has written a standing order for Tylenol to be given every four hours, with Demerol to be given "if the patient appears especially uncomfortable."

When Mr. Charles' sister, a nurse, arrives from another state, she is appalled by her brother's condition. She discusses his pain management with Dr. Fellows and asks why he is not receiving constant intravenous morphine. Dr. Fellows replies, "Morphine will depress his respirations and may speed up his dying. I will not be responsible for contributing to his death. We can keep him comfortable by increasing his other medication." She responds, "He's dying now and nothing will change that! Why should he have to die this horribly?"

A critical distinction supporting adequate palliation, especially at the end of life, is the doctrine of double effect, which responds to the ethical tension between the obligations to promote patient well-being and to avoid inflicting harm. The doctrine holds that a single act having two foreseen effects, one good and one bad, is not morally or legally prohibited *if the harmful effect is not intended.* The doctrine requires that three conditions be met: the act itself is not wrong; the good effect is the result of the intentional act, not the result of the bad or harmful effect; and the benefits of the good effect outweigh the foreseen but unintended bad effect. All three conditions are essential to prevent the doctrine from being abused or perverted in an effort to justify actions intended to cause harm.

The doctrine of double effect recognizes that, while the administration of sufficient opioids to manage pain at the end of life risks depressing respirations enough to hasten death, the clinical and ethical mandate to relieve suffering is paramount. Mr. Charles may not be verbally asking for analgesia, but he gives every clinical indication that he is in terrible pain. As his sister points out, he is actively and irreversibly dying, so the question is not *whether* he will die, but *how.* His death is not preventable, but dying in pain is. Under these circumstances, the only thing that can be done to benefit him is to relieve his suffering and make his remaining time more bearable. Using the rationale of the doctrine of double effect, the palliative intervention is both justified and protected. Helping physicians appreciate this distinction so that they can comfortably provide adequate palliation at the end of life is often an important part of ethics committee involvement.

THE MORAL IMPERATIVE TO RELIEVE PAIN

III Carla is a 9-year-old girl who was diagnosed several months ago with Ewing's sarcoma. She has received radiation and chemotherapy, and was recently hospitalized for amputation of her entire left leg. Following surgery, Carla's pain was being successfully managed with a continuous IV morphine drip supplemented by patient-controlled IV morphine to be used when she felt she needed additional pain control. On the third postoperative day, one of her physical therapists told her that she should not activate the patient-controlled morphine until the pain became unbearable because, if she overused narcotics, she would become addicted. An intern who overheard this statement corrected the physical therapist, explaining that addiction is not associated with use of narcotics in the immediate postoperative period and is rarely the result of even chronic use to control severe pain. The intern also reassured Carla, telling her that she should activate the morphine as often as she needed it and that she would not be risking addiction.

Carla's parents, however, became very concerned about the potential danger of addiction and tried to discourage her from using the patient-controlled morphine. When she continued to use the medication, they insisted that her oncologist, Dr. Brader, stop both the continuous IV drip and the patient-controlled morphine. Dr. Brader replaced the morphine with nonnarcotic analgesia, which was much less effective, and Carla began to experience severe pain. Dr. Brader has recommended restarting the morphine to relieve Carla's pain, but her parents are adamant that she not receive any narcotics.

Do the obligations of care professionals include the relief of pain? Does pain management require the informed consent of a capable patient or an authorized surrogate? Can the conflict between Carla's doctor and her parents be resolved in a way that prevents her from suffering?

More than a professional obligation, the relief of pain has traditionally been considered a moral imperative. It is also an endeavor that reflects the tension between the two fundamental ethical principles of autonomy and beneficence. As discussed in chapter 3, the notion of autonomy is expressed in the health care setting in the doctrine of informed consent. Under this doctrine, capable, knowledgeable, and voluntary consent, either by or for the patient, is required for legally and ethically valid authorization for most diagnostic and therapeutic interventions.

Yet, the requirement of informed consent is conspicuously absent from the relief of pain. The reason goes to the very core of the caring interaction and invokes the mandate to relieve pain and suffering. This imperative is so powerful that it gives rise to the presumption that, unless patients explicitly object, they would want their pain relieved. Thus, respect for autonomy requires that a capable patient's decision to refuse analgesia—either because she finds the experience of pain meaningful or she does not want to chemically compromise her awareness—must be honored.

As discussed in chapters 2 and 3, however, beneficence is elevated over autonomy in protecting and benefiting patients who are vulnerable because they cannot make decisions or advocate for themselves. Thus, an incapacitated patient who is clearly in pain must not be deprived of relief because she is unable to provide informed consent. While honoring the wishes of a capable individual shows respect for the person, withholding relief from one who cannot decide or communicate would be an indefensible abandonment. Rather, principled and compassionate caring embraces both the respect for and the protection of persons. No expressed informed consent is required precisely because relieving pain is central to the very notion of healing, and, for that reason alone, it requires no additional justifications.

Accordingly, adequate relief of Carla's pain may not be impeded by her parents' well-meaning but misguided rejection of morphine. Every effort should be made to help them understand the considerable benefits and minimal risks of opioid use in managing her severe pain, and the distinction between increasing tolerance and addiction. Including the palliative care service in this discussion would be helpful in educating and reassuring her parents about the care plan. The care team should be supportive of their desire to be responsible guardians and the focus should be on the shared goal of promoting Carla's best interest and protecting her from harm. Ultimately, however, her parents must know that, with or without their consent, Carla's pain will be managed according to the standard of care and the ethical requirements of professional practice.

Mrs. Heller, the nursing home resident with multiple medical problems, is experiencing pain severe and persistent enough to interfere with her activities and her sleep. Despite her best efforts, pain has become the focus of her attention and has profoundly impaired her quality of life. Far from rejecting pain medication, she is clearly asking for relief. Her care team has both a clinical and ethical mandate to assess her pain carefully, discuss with her the benefits, burdens, and risks of the analgesic options, and provide her with sufficient medication to relieve her suffering. The team should also identify and address the barriers to adequate pain relief that have prevented her symptoms from being recognized and managed appropriately. Her nephew's request for an ethics consultation can facilitate this process by highlighting Mrs. Heller's needs and goals, and reassuring the care team that the benefits of palliation outweigh the possible risks. Recommending a palliative care consultation should be helpful in achieving these objectives.

PHYSICIAN-ASSISTED SUICIDE

‖ The lab results of Diane's blood tests confirmed Dr. Timothy Quill's worst fears—she did indeed have leukemia. His distress reflected the disappointment common to physicians whose patients contract life-threatening illnesses as well as the special concern he had for someone who had been his patient for many years and with whom he had developed a close and trusting relationship. In addition, he greatly admired the strength and determination with which she had overcome significant physical and emotional difficulties. In the process, she had strengthened her relationships with her husband, son, and friends, and reinvigorated her business and artistic work.

Now they faced this devastating news together, going through the confirmatory tests and discussing with her husband the various options, including chemotherapy, followed by radiation and possible bone marrow transplants. Even with the most aggressive treatment regimen, the chances for long-term survival were 25 percent; the certain outcome of no treatment was death within a few months. After considerable discussion, Diane decided not to undergo chemotherapy because she was convinced that the quality of whatever time she had left was more important than the unlikely benefits of treatment. Despite Dr. Quill's misgivings and her family's attempts to persuade her to change her mind, she remained steadfast in her determination to make the most of her time at home. Ultimately, her family and physician reluctantly supported her decision.

Dr. Quill had known throughout their relationship that, for Diane, regaining and maintaining control of her life was a central value. Now he realized that being in control of her dying was just as important to her as she faced the end of her life. She became preoccupied with deteriorating, lingering, being helpless and in pain. Her anxiety about the prospect of a protracted death became so severe that it threatened to undermine the quality end of life she had as her goal. She asked Dr. Quill to help her avoid the painful, debilitating, and dehumanizing ravages in store by providing drugs that she could take to end her life when she chose. She was convinced that having the ability to control her death would give her the dignity and peace of mind that she needed.

After extensive discussion and psychiatric consultation, Dr. Quill acceded to Diane's unwavering determination, prescribed the barbiturates, and provided the information necessary for her to take her own life. She was able to spend the next several months focusing on the people, relationships, and activities that were most important to her. She received aggressive palliative treatment but, eventually, she determined that the benefits of life no longer outweighed its burdens. Her death was on her own terms, at the time and in the manner of her choosing. Yet, concerns about potential legal liability prevented her from having her family or physician with her at the end, and she died alone. (Quill, 1991)

Distinguishing Forgoing Life-sustaining Treatment, Euthanasia, and Assisted Suicide

Discussions about end-of-life issues inevitably refer to behaviors that promote, permit, or hasten death. Because these concepts are highly charged with medical, legal, ethical, and emotional significance, it is critical that we begin by distinguishing their definitions.

- Assisted suicide is clinician facilitation of a patient's death by providing the means and/or information (prescription, medication, instructions) that enable the patient to perform an act that results in self-inflicted death. The clinician's actions are taken with the knowledge that the patient intends to use the provided drugs and information to end her life, but the agent of death is the *patient*. Assisted suicide is illegal in all states except Oregon, which has adopted a formal, multistep protocol for its limited use.

- Euthanasia is clinician administration of a lethal agent with the intent of relieving the patient's untreatable suffering and/or pain. Whether the act is performed at the request of the patient (*voluntary euthanasia*) or without the patient's request (*nonvoluntary euthanasia*), the agent of death is the *clinician*. Euthanasia of either kind is illegal in all fifty states.

- Forgoing life-sustaining treatment is the withholding or withdrawing of interventions that maintain one or more organ system functions necessary to keep the patient alive. When these interventions are discontinued, the patient's death is considered to be the result of the underlying disease(s). Patients with decisional capacity, health care proxy agents, and, in some states, other surrogates acting on behalf of patients without capacity have the right to refuse unwanted life-sustaining treatments. Even when that refusal leads to or hastens death, the action is not considered suicide, assisted suicide, or euthanasia.

- Aggressive palliation is the provision of therapeutic interventions, including narcotic medications, to relieve pain and manage other symptoms effectively, especially at the end of life. While these interventions may have two possible effects, one positive (e.g., pain relief) and one negative (e.g., depression of respirations), when the intent is palliation, the action is considered medically, ethically, and legally justified under the doctrine of double effect. Therefore, although aggressive palliation at the end of life may hasten the patient's death, the action is not considered suicide, assisted suicide, or euthanasia.

Ethical Issues

It is beyond the scope of this handbook to discuss adequately the multiple and complex aspects of assisted suicide. For our purposes, it is enough to raise some of the ethical issues, including caregiver obligations, individual autonomy, public policy, and the moral imperative to relieve suffering. Some argue that respecting patient autonomy includes respecting the wish of the terminally ill to control when and how death occurs. Consistent with the principle of nonmaleficence, however, the concept of facilitating patient death is counterintuitive to those who devote themselves to promoting and protecting life. Yet, many have come to see assisting the rational suicide of a capable person as the last act in a compassionate continuum of care and forcing the patient to take that final step alone as abandonment. Some suggest that, in vulnerable and disempowered populations, such as the poor and elderly, the right to die may become the obligation to die as a way of relieving family or society of the unwanted burden of their care. Yet others counter that these same marginalized populations, which often lack access to health care and providers, may be deprived of the opportunity to end their suffering under physician care. Ultimately, there is concern that the individual, morally justified act of assisted suicide could become the generalized policy of euthanasia (e.g., Shalowitz and Emanuel, 2004; Bascom and Tolle, 2002; Emanuel et al., 2000; Salem, 1999; Thomasma, 1996).

In June 1997, the U.S. Supreme Court ruled in two cases, *Washington v. Glucksberg* and *Vacco v. Quill,* that sought to turn the right to refuse treatment into a constitutionally protected right to assisted suicide. The cases are discussed in part VI, but it is important to note here that these two rulings are more significant for what they say about palliative care than assisted suicide. Repeatedly, the Court reaffirms the doctrine of double effect, saying that it is both legally and ethically appropriate to give terminally ill patients as much medication as necessary to relieve pain, even if the effect is to hasten death. The Court also strongly reaffirms the distinction between forgoing life-sustaining treatment and assisted suicide. The critical take-away message is that providing sufficient medication to manage pain effectively at the end of life is a clinical and ethical imperative, not to be confused with assisted suicide or euthanasia. The importance of these rulings to compassionate end-of-life care cannot be overstated.

While assisted suicide is not a legal option in forty-nine states, it highlights issues that demand attention in all care settings. Both the public and professionals are troubled by the reality of overtreated disease and undertreated pain, especially at the end of life. Considerable research demonstrates that the medical profession does an inadequate job of pain management and that many people who request assistance in killing themselves are actually asking for the assurance of pain relief. It is a matter of concern when the debate centers on the questionable constitutional right of terminally ill patients to receive physician assistance in *ending* rather than *easing* their lives.

Among health care's most pressing challenges, then, is the need to improve palliation along the entire therapeutic continuum, especially as death approaches. Encouraging clinicians to collaborate with palliative care specialists can be a valuable contribution of clinical ethics consultation.

REFERENCES

American Board of Internal Medicine. 1996. Committee on Evaluation of Clinical Competence. *Caring for the Dying: Identification and Promotion of Physician Competency.* Philadelphia: American Board of Internal Medicine.

Bascom PB, Tolle SW. 2002. Responding to requests for physician-assisted suicide: "These are uncharted waters for both of us . . ." *Journal of the American Medical Association* 288(1):91–98.

Blackhall LJ, Frank G, Murphy ST, Michel V, Palmer JM, Azen SP. 1999. Ethnicity and attitudes towards life sustaining technology. *Social Science & Medicine* 48(12):1779–89.

Brock DW. 1997. Death and dying. In Veatch, RM, ed. *Medical Ethics.* 2nd ed. Sudbury, MA: Jones and Barlett Publishers, pp. 363–94.

Cassel CK, Vladeck BC. 1996. ICD-9 code for palliative or terminal care. *New England Journal of Medicine* 335(16):1232–34.

Cassell EJ. 1982. The nature of suffering and the goals of medicine. *New England Journal of Medicine* 306(11):639–45.

Dworkin R. 2003. Assisted suicide: The philosophers' brief. In Steinbock B, Arras JD, London AJ, eds. *Ethical Issues in Modern Medicine.* 6th ed. Boston: McGraw-Hill, pp. 382–85.

Dworkin R, Nagel T, Nozick R, Rawls J, Scanlon T, Thomson JJ. 2003. The philosophers' brief. In Steinbock B, Arras JD, London AJ, eds. *Ethical Issues in Modern Medicine.* 6th ed. Boston: McGraw-Hill, pp. 386–94.

Emanuel EJ, Fairclough DL, Emanuel LL. 2000. Attitudes and desires related to euthanasia and physician-assisted suicide among terminally ill patients and their caregivers. *Journal of the American Medical Association* 284(19):2460–68.

Emanuel LL. 1998. Facing requests for physician-assisted suicide: Toward a practical and principled clinical skill set. *Journal of the American Medical Association* 280(7):643–47.

Fischberg D, Meier DE. 2004. Palliative care in hospitals. *Clinics in Geriatric Medicine* 20(4):735–51.

Furrow BR. 2001. Pain management and provider liability: No more excuses. *Journal of Law, Medicine & Ethics* 29(1):28–51.

Johnson JA. 2004. Withdrawal of medically administered nutrition and hydration: The role of benefits and burdens, and of parents and ethics committees. *Journal of Clinical Ethics* 15(3):307–11.

Johnson SH. 1996. Disciplinary actions and pain relief: Analysis of the pain relief act. *Journal of Law, Medicine & Ethics* 24(4):319–27.

Joranson DE, Gilson AM. 1996. Improving pain management through policy making and education for medical regulators. *Journal of Law, Medicine & Ethics* 24(4):344–47.

Hyman CS. 1996. Pain management and disciplinary action: How state medical boards can remove barriers to effective treatment. *Journal of Law, Medicine & Ethics* 24(4):338–43.

Lisson EL 1987. Ethical issues related to pain control. *Nursing Clinics of North America* 22:649–59.

Lo B. 2000. *Resolving Ethical Dilemmas: A Guide for Clinicians.* 2nd ed. Philadelphia: Lippincott Williams & Wilkins.

Lopez SR. 1989. Patient variable biases in clinical judgment: Conceptual overview and methodological considerations. *Psychological Bulletin* 106(2):184-203.

Morrison, RS, Meier, DE, Cassel, CK. 1996. When too much is too little. *New England Journal of Medicine* 335(23):1755–59.

Post LF 2007 (forthcoming). Ethics and the delivery of palliative care. In O'Mahony S, Blank AE, eds. *Choices in Palliative Care.* New York: Kluwer Academic/Plenum Publishers.

Post LF, Blustein J, Gordon E, Dubler NN. 1996. Pain: Ethics, culture and informed consent to relief. *Journal of Law, Medicine & Ethics* 24(4):348–59.

Post LF, Dubler NN. 1997. Palliative care: A bioethical definition, principles and clinical guidelines. *Bioethics Forum* 13(3):17–24.

Quill TE. 1991. Death and dignity: A case of individualized decision making. *New England Journal of Medicine* 324(10):691–94.

Quill TE, Lo B, Brock DW. 1997. Palliative options of last resort: A comparison of voluntarily stopping eating and drinking, terminal sedation, physician-assisted suicide, and voluntary active euthanasia. *Journal of the American Medical Association* 278(23):2099–2104.

Quill TE, Meier DE. 2006. The big chill: Inserting the DEA into end-of-life care. *New England Journal of Medicine* 354(1):1–3.

Salem T. 1999. Physician-assisted suicide: Promoting autonomy—or medicalizing suicide? *Hastings Center Report* 29(3):30–36.

Shalowitz D, Emanuel E. 2004. Euthanasia and physician-assisted suicide: Implications for physicians. *Journal of Clinical Ethics* 15(3):232–36.

Steinbock B, Arras JD, London AJ. 2003. Moral reasoning in the medical context. In Steinbock B, Arras JD, London AJ, eds. *Ethical Issues in Modern Medicine.* 6th ed. Boston: McGraw-Hill, pp. 1–41.

The SUPPORT Principal Investigators. 1995. A controlled trial to improve care for seriously ill hospitalized patients. The Study to Understand Prognoses and Preferences for Outcomes and Risks of Treatments (SUPPORT). *Journal of the American Medical Association* 274(20):1591–98.

Thomasma DC. 1996. When physicians choose to participate in the death of their patients: Ethics and physician-assisted suicide. *Journal of Law, Medicine & Ethics* 24(3):183–97.

Vacco v. Quill, 521 U.S. 793 (1997).

Washington v. Glucksberg, 521 U.S. 702 (1997).

Weissman DE, Block SD, Blank L, Cain J, Cassem N, Danoff D, Foley K, Meier D, Schyve P, Theige D, Wheeler HB. 1999. Recommendations for incorporating palliative care education into the acute care hospital setting. *Academic Medicine* 74(8):871–77.

8

Justice, Access to Health Care, and Organizational Ethics

⦀ Mrs. Gomez is an undocumented person from Colombia. Since coming to this country in 1976, she has been employed as a housekeeper. Because she has no health care coverage, she has received all of her care in the emergency rooms of various local hospitals.

Last week Mrs. Gomez came to General Medical Center quite ill and was admitted to the medical unit, where she was found to be in kidney failure. She was begun on dialysis and remained in the hospital for three days, until she had been dialyzed twice. When she was ready for discharge, the medical resident in charge of her care inquired whether she would be eligible for Medicare support for her future dialysis under the end-stage renal disease program. He was told that, although Mrs. Gomez's in-patient costs might be covered by Medicaid—something that still needed to be determined—she was clearly not eligible for Medicare.

The medical resident, not to be defeated in his pursuit of care for his patient, asked the ER staff what is usually done when a patient in kidney failure who needs dialysis comes to the ER. He was told that, under an arrangement between the ER and the dialysis unit, these patients are transferred directly to the unit for emergency dialysis treatment. The medical resident told Mrs. Gomez to come to the ER three times a week so she could have the dialysis she needs. When this plan was discovered, the director of the ER exploded and said that this could break the budget for his service. He also pointed out that a nearby city hospital with a dialysis unit is designed to take care of poor people with no insurance.

If the topics in this chapter—access to health care, justice, resource allocation, organizational ethics—seem abstract and unrelated to your committee's function, stay tuned. From its beginnings, the scope of bioethical inquiry has encompassed both clinical matters and the therapeutic relationship *and* the broader questions of social justice and the distribution of health care. While the preceding chapters have focused on the former issues, this chapter takes up the latter.

Let's begin by acknowledging a difficult truth: the ethical principles and concepts that we have been discussing can seem almost impossible to apply in an environment that makes health care available in an unjust manner. "But wait," you say. "Even if the nation's health care delivery system needs work, we can't be expected to take on those huge problems. We have enough to worry about right here in our own health care facility." Precisely. As the local arbiter of moral reasoning and ethical practice, your committee's responsibilities include monitoring and guiding the way organizational decisions are made and how they affect the delivery of health care in your institution. So, let's look at the big picture as background and then see how it applies to what you do.

ACCESS TO HEALTH CARE IN THE UNITED STATES

Any discussion of health care entitlement should begin by distinguishing between a *moral* right and a *legal* right: a moral right might exist even if it is not recognized by law. Health care in the United States, with some exceptions, is not a legal right. If, however, it is a moral right, then disparities in access to care that exist in our society may be criticized as unjust.

The following overview examines the extent to which there is a *legal* right to health care in the United States. Since World War II, most health insurance in this country has been private, a fringe benefit of employment. Employers provided health insurance, often for the individual employee and his dependents; later, the employee contributed as well. Such a system of providing health insurance is extremely vulnerable to fluctuations in the economy and job market. Those who are not wealthy enough to either purchase outright all the health care they want or buy enough insurance to cover their needs depend on their employers for coverage. In periods of economic downturn, unemployment rises and many employers cut back on the benefits they provide their employees.

The two main public insurance programs in the United States are Medicaid (a joint federal and state program, mainly for the poor) and Medicare (a federal program mainly for the elderly, but also for persons with end-stage renal disease and some disabilities). Enormous variation exists in the percentage of poor people covered by state-run Medicaid programs, and states are free to restrict the range of "optional" services and the number of allowable hospital days for Medicaid patients. Moreover, Medicaid is often an entitlement in name only. Physicians often refuse to treat Medicaid patients because of low reimbursements, and hospitals that treat a predominantly Medicaid population are sorely understaffed and undersupplied.

Medicare, by contrast, has been an enormously successful program. It provides universal access to generally high-quality health care for those over 65 and has also reduced poverty in that population. Concerns have been raised, however, about the adequacy of coverage. For example, despite the passage of legislation that provides modest drug coverage under Medicare, the high cost of medication places an increasingly large financial burden on the elderly. In addition, in recent years Medicare reimbursements for care have been cut back. Larger premiums and co-payments have meant that affluent Medicare patients experience fewer problems when they need medical care than do the less prosperous elderly, who find the required out-of-pocket expenditures, especially for increasingly expensive drugs, very burdensome. The new Medicare Part D prescription drug benefit, which went into effect in 2006, covers cumulative drug expenses up to $2,250, but not between $2,251 and $5,100. The result is a $2,850 "doughnut hole" in coverage where it is likely that beneficiaries will have to cut back on even essential medications.

Despite widespread coverage, existing forms of health insurance do not reach many people. The estimate usually cited by year is that more than 44 million people in this country are without any form of health insurance coverage, either public or private. This figure, however, reflects the number of uninsured during a twelve-month period. According to some estimates, far more people are without coverage for at least some portion of the year (Rhoades, 2005). During the two-year period 2001–2, almost one-third of people under 65 (79.8 million) were without insurance for at least one month (Nichols, 2004). The uninsured population includes those who are not poor enough to qualify for Medicaid and yet are unable to afford private health insurance. They are the working poor, as well as many in the middle class and self-employed persons who cannot pay high health insurance premiums. In addition, there are many more millions in our society who are underinsured.

Private hospitals and academic medical centers have long assumed some of the responsibility for providing uncompensated care to the poor and indigent, but their budgets are steadily shrinking. This trend is due largely to the extension of prospective payment, spurred by the adoption of diagnosis-related groups (DRGs) for hospitalized Medicare patients. Likewise, preferred provider arrangements have eliminated cross-subsidies through which hospitals have covered the costs of providing uncompensated "charity" care by increasing charges for insured patients and those who pay directly out of pocket. Most managed care plans negotiate payment to the lowest level, making such cross-subsidies difficult.

Public hospitals continue to provide access to health care for those who cannot otherwise afford it but, under the pressure of fiscal crises, local and state governments have found such institutions burdensome to maintain. Both because of the resources available to them and the insurance status of their clientele, these institutions may be inferior to hospitals in the voluntary, not-for-profit sector.

Two other pockets in our health care system guarantee access to care in specific circumstances. Under the federal "antidumping" law, the Emergency Medical Treatment and Active Labor Act (EMTALA), patients who arrive at an emergency room must be assessed and stabilized before they can be transferred. Prisoners also have guaranteed rights to health care under rulings of the U.S. Supreme Court, although the quality of that care is regularly challenged in federal courts.

Mrs. Gomez's case illustrates the issues raised in a system that denies some people access to health care that it makes available to others. Health care institutions, especially those in poor or minority communities, are often considered to have a special obligation to provide health care to residents. When patients are uninsured or underinsured, staff sometimes feel the need to get around the rules by "gaming the system" in order to provide necessary care. In this case, the solution blurs the distinction between two types of care. Emergency care is limited to traumatic, unanticipated, often life-threatening injuries and illnesses that require immediate treatment. In contrast, clinic care is planned, routine primary care, including the monitoring and treatment of chronic conditions. Because emergency care is episodic, it does not provide the continuity, comprehensiveness, and multidisciplinary resources so important in the ongoing treatment of chronic illnesses, such as renal disease.

Mrs. Gomez clearly needs care that the institution can and would provide under other circumstances. Because her renal failure has been corrected in the hospital, she no longer requires emergency care. Her condition could be managed on an outpatient basis as long as she receives regular dialysis. Without it, her condition will again become unstable and she will eventually need urgent care. Her undocumented status, however, means that she is uninsured, making her ineligible for clinic care. Given this set of circumstances, the staff feels compelled to search for creative ways to ensure that she continues to receive needed treatment.

Gaming the system in this way heightens the tension between the organization's ethical obligation to benefit one patient and the obligation to steward resources responsibly to benefit all patients. Undocumented persons who require sustained treatment, such as dialysis, should not be denied care because they are unable to pay. Nevertheless, the fiscal realities prevent institutions like General Medical Center from providing all services to all those who need them, regardless of cost. However well intended the staff's motives, it is reasonable to question whether the *predictable need* for emergency care justifies a practice of using the resource *preventively.* The routine proactive use of emergency resources may well impair the hospital's ability to provide care for true emergencies. Because the public hospitals have historically covered care for the uninsured, the doctors can refer Mrs. Gomez to a city hospital for treatment. Given the increasing financial drain, however, even the municipal system may not be able to continue providing uncompensated care indefinitely.

The literature also reveals racial and ethnic disparities in health care, including diagnostic, curative, life-sustaining, and palliative care interventions (Post, forthcoming; Wolf, 2004; Epstein and Ayania, 2001; Phillips et al., 1996). These reports are of special concern because of what they reveal about both effect and cause. The health consequences of disparate care are reflected in the reported underuse among nonwhite patients of diagnostic and therapeutic interventions projected to improve clinical outcomes. Moreover, these disparities have remained relatively unchanged for decades in the United States, as has the average life expectancy of blacks, which is six years shorter than that of whites (Epstein and Ayania, 2001; Freeman and Payne, 2000). According to one estimate, compared to the vast sums dedicated to improving medical technology in an effort to save lives, five times as many deaths could be averted if the disparities in health care were corrected (Woolf, 2004).

Racial disparities in medical services suggest possible discrimination or bias, either deliberate or unintentional, by health care providers, including physicians and institutions. It is argued that the causes of the inequities implicate health care systems rather than just individual providers, and will need to be addressed systemically (Epstein and Ayania, 2001; Freeman and Payne, 2000). Although the disparities in health care tend to fall along racial and ethnic lines, commentators caution against viewing the problem as stemming only from patients' cultural values and provider discrimination. Rather, it has been suggested that the overarching problems are the socioeconomic conditions of marginalized populations and the societal priorities that do not have as a goal a "common standard of wellness." What is lacking, then, may not be the national resources to create a just health care system, but the national resolve (Woolf, 2004, p. 54).

As this brief review makes clear, there is no universal legally protected right to health care in the United States. Everyone in this country is legally free to seek health care and, when the proper arrangements are made, to receive it. But, with the noted exceptions, there is no recognized societal *obligation* to provide it. Instead, our society permits access to health care to depend on one's ability to pay or the source of one's health insurance. As a result, health care is not equally available to all those who need it. This is an especially serious problem for the many uninsured in our nation, because health status is to a large extent dependent on access to health care. The socially sanctioned inequality of opportunity that deprives some people of the health required to realize their potential fully is a moral abdication that rises to the level of true injustice.

A RIGHT TO HEALTH CARE?

Given the limited legal right to health care in this country, is there at least a moral claim that can be supported? The President's Commission for the Study of Ethical Problems in

Medicine and Biomedical and Behavioral Research confronted this issue in its influential 1983 report entitled *An Ethical Framework for Access to Health Care*. According to the commissioners, health care is different from other consumer goods, such as televisions and automobiles, because it is crucially related to the length and quality of life. Moreover, like education, health care is necessary to achieve equal opportunity in society. Without decent access to care, health status is likely to suffer and poor health status prevents people from enjoying the range of opportunities that would otherwise be available.

Because the nation's health care needs are vast, sometimes unpredictable, and extremely costly, the President's Commission concluded that the free market alone cannot meet them adequately and society has an obligation to assume part of the burden. The commissioners cautioned, however, that this societal obligation is not unlimited; it must be constrained by the balance of costs and benefits to the population. Moreover, they argued, the fact that society is morally obligated to provide *some* care does not mean that everyone is entitled to an equal amount or quality of health care. In other words, not all *inequalities* in access to health care amount to *inequities* in access, and it is only the latter that justice requires us to eliminate. As long as everyone is guaranteed access to an *acceptable* or *decent* level of health care, the report maintains, society will have fulfilled its moral obligation.

It is worth noting that the President's Commission self-consciously chose not to use the language of "rights" to frame its notion of a social duty. Yet many bioethicists, using the same arguments presented in the commission's report, have concluded that each citizen has a moral right, as distinguished from a legal right, against the government to a decent level of health care.

THEORIES OF JUSTICE

Answers to questions about allocation and access presuppose some views on the nature of individual rights, social obligations, and notions of fairness, even if they are not articulated. If there is a *moral* right to health care, it must be grounded in and justified by some more general theory about the nature of social justice. Generally speaking, a person is treated justly if he is treated according to what is fair, due, or owed. The specific term *distributive justice* refers to fair, equitable, and appropriate distribution of the benefits and burdens of social cooperation. Here we refer to the equitable distribution of the benefits and burdens of health care resources. Three theories of distributive justice—libertarian, utilitarian, and egalitarian—dominate current thinking, and each has very different implications for the right to health care.

In the libertarian theory of justice, espoused most prominently by Robert Nozick and Tristam Engelhardt, individuals have moral rights to life, liberty, and property, which a just society must recognize and respect. In this view, the sole function of government is to prevent these rights from being interfered with and to protect the individual's life, liberty, and property against force and fraud. Everything else in society is a matter of individual, not societal or governmental, responsibility. For the libertarian, there is no moral right to health care and no societal obligation to provide it.

The utilitarian theory of justice, articulated by John Stuart Mill and Jeremy Bentham, is committed to maximizing the common good. Acts, practices, and rules are to be judged better or worse, right or wrong, according to how effectively they promote this goal. Whereas libertarians stress freedom from government interference, utilitarians are more disposed to government welfare programs because these may be necessary to promote the good of society as a whole. For utilitarians, there is a moral right to health care insofar as its provision contributes to the overall good of society's members.

The egalitarian theories of justice reject libertarianism because it fails to include what egalitarians perceive as a fundamental moral concern: those who have more than enough should help those in need. Egalitarians reject utilitarianism because it fails to provide sufficiently strong support for individual moral rights. A leading twentieth-century egalitarian theorist, John Rawls, maintained that inequalities in the distribution of "primary social goods" (e.g., income, opportunities) are justified only if they benefit the least-well-off members of society. Egalitarians, such as Norman Daniels, generally embrace some notion of a moral right to health care.

RATIONING

It is hard to deny that individuals in this country are not equal with respect to the availability of health care. Beyond concerns about the costliness and inefficiency of the nation's health care system, disparities in access to care raise fundamental questions about whether the system is fair and just. Given the number of competing goods that require the investment of societal resources, such as housing, jobs, education, and defense, it appears that guaranteeing all citizens access to health care is not in the immediate future. Accordingly, it is necessary to confront the challenge of health care rationing and recognize that, while some forms of rationing are morally justifiable, others are not.

Rationing Defined

In the ongoing debate about health care, *rationing* has become a highly charged term with moral overtones. The basic ethical problem is how to structure our health care system so that it *fairly* distributes limited resources and provides *equitable* access to health care at *manageable cost*. To accomplish these various and sometimes conflicting tasks, many now call for the adoption of some explicit form of societal rationing or limit setting. As noted earlier, much of the U.S. health care system already involves a kind of implicit or covert rationing—that is, rationing by ability to pay and level of personal resources. Rationing on this basis is objectionable because of the special nature and importance of the good of health care, making its deprivation an injustice. The notion of rationing has several meanings, according to Daniel Wikler:

- Trimming: "cutting back on services that few people want and no one needs" (e.g., targeting inefficient and ineffective care)
- Cutting: "refusing genuinely needed and wanted care on the grounds that the cost is 'too high'" (e.g., a provider's decision not to provide a nonexperimental organ transplant to a medically suitable candidate based on a payer's refusal to reimburse for it)
- Tailoring: "eliminates care which is (1) of questionable effectiveness, even though it may be popular or even standard, or which has marginal effectiveness relative to risk; or (2) care which prolongs conditions which are marginally endurable" (e.g., using expensive medical technology to sustain patients who are in a persistent vegetative state or have an extremely poor quality of life) (Wikler, 1992, p. 399).

Cutting, that is, withholding care expected to be of net benefit to the patient, is the most ethically troubling form of rationing and the one that both proponents and opponents of rationing chiefly have in mind. Commentators disagree about whether cutting is really necessary, except in special circumstances. Trimming and tailoring, some optimistically argue, will for the most part eliminate the need for this more problematic form of rationing. Others disagree, arguing that the aging of the population, the onward march of medical progress, and the limits of societal resources make the more extreme form of rationing imperative.

Societal versus Bedside Rationing

Rationing health care can be done on a societal or community level, through a process of public deliberation leading to general guidelines for limit setting as a means of cost containment. This approach is known as macroallocating resources. Alternatively, it can be done "at the bedside," by individual physicians making decisions to deny particular interventions to particular patients as a means of controlling health care costs. This process is known as microallocating.

An example of macroallocating, or societal rationing, is the Oregon Health Plan, officially enacted in February 1994. The Oregon plan originated in a choice faced by the state legislature in 1987, when it decided to invest its limited health care dollars in prenatal care for thousands of uninsured poor women rather than fund organ transplants of questionable efficacy for a relatively small handful of patients. The Oregon program involves the following elements: an attempt to guarantee universal access to health care through the expansion of the state Medicaid program to include everyone officially defined as poor; recognition of the necessity of limits in the care that is provided to everyone on Medicaid, these limits to be determined by how much money the state can afford to spend on health care in any given year; and an open and democratic process for making these difficult decisions about limit setting.

The Oregon plan has been criticized on the grounds that it achieves the goal of cost control solely at the expense of those who are already disadvantaged, namely, poor women and children. The plan has been praised for making a social commitment to guaranteeing some level of health care for all poor people in the state and for relying on an open and publicly accountable system for making rationing decisions.

Microallocating is highly controversial. On the one hand, it is argued that bedside rationing is inevitable and that it is the responsibility of physicians to participate in cost containment in morally credible ways. Physicians, in this view, are the stewards of health care resources at the site of use and in the best position to assess both clinical and cost effectiveness. On the other hand, bedside rationing is criticized on several grounds: physicians may allow their personal biases to influence their decisions about which interventions are not worth the cost; variability from physician to physician means that there will be no uniform standards for limit setting; and physicians cannot be both agents of cost containment and advocates for the best interests of their patients. A middle ground would see some modest form of rationing as appropriate, and possibly obligatory, for physicians.

HEALTH CARE ORGANIZATIONAL ETHICS

||| The asthma control program at Gotham Medical Center was started by the group physician practice (GPP) in 2000. The GPP is an example of a mixed economic model. Rather than a fully capitated practice, it participates in a health maintenance organization (HMO), but also provides care on a fee-for-service basis.

The asthma program was directed by a nurse administrator who was hired by the GPP and to whom referrals were made by physicians in the group. Her role was to work with patients to enhance their understanding and management of their medical conditions. Information was provided by phone and in person to both children and adults about symptoms, appropriate medications and when to take them, and how to manage asthma attacks without having to go to the emergency room for care. The asthma program seemed to have been clinically effective, based on the decreased number of ER visits for asthma treatment and the reports of improved patient and family satisfaction. The program had also been an important health care resource for the community.

Despite its benefits, however, controversy had arisen about the asthma program's financial implications. On one hand, the program's administrative costs had been borne by the GPP. In addition, the program's clinical success had resulted in fewer patient visits to physicians' offices and less frequent hospital admissions, decreases that had cut into the GPP's revenues. From the standpoint of the HMO, however, reducing physician and ER visits and hospital admissions had kept medical costs down, which was one of the HMO's primary missions. In 2002, the GPP decided to terminate the asthma program, based on the increased administrative costs and the decreased revenues.

What interests are in tension when organizations consider which health care services to provide? Do health care organizations have ethical, as well as financial and business, obligations that inform their decisions? What role can ethics committees play in organizational matters?

From Bioethics to Health Care Organizational Ethics

In the ever-widening scope of concerns addressed by health care ethics committees, organizational ethics is a relatively new consideration. Until a few years ago, the study of ethical issues in health care focused on the moral conflicts in the clinical setting that have been addressed in the preceding chapters of this handbook. Increasingly, however, clinicians and administrators have come to recognize that how a health care organization makes decisions directly affects the quality of the care it delivers. For your ethics committee to address both organizational and clinical issues, it is important to appreciate the relationship between the two areas of concern.

Largely as a result of efforts to limit the rapid and uncontrolled rise in health care costs, the care delivery system has changed radically during the past twenty-five years. New and often competing scientific, economic, and political imperatives demand attention. The physician-patient relationship no longer controls the clinical dynamic; managers and administrators make and enforce policies that restrict the available options and the ability of physicians and patients to make choices about them. New analytic frameworks are necessary to meet current challenges in allocating health care resources and decision-making authority.

The response to skyrocketing health care costs has been a new environment in which medical practice is managed by organizations that impose economic discipline on clinical decision making. While fiscal concerns remain significant in the changing health care system, other factors, including heightened interest in the quality of care, have also promoted greater organizational control of clinical decision making. As a result, the increasingly prominent mechanisms of quality assurance and measures of clinical effectiveness have been motivated by both economic considerations and concern to improve clinical practice.

Organizational ethics introduces an *intermediate* level of analysis between the narrower set of clinical concerns and the broader societal policy issues. Health care organizations—hospitals, nursing homes, visiting nurse agencies—make daily decisions about resource allocation, clinical priorities, conflicting interests, and community responsibilities, all of which have ethical implications. In this analytic perspective, the organization as health care provider assumes ethical rights and responsibilities similar to but distinct from those of individual health care professionals. Of central importance in distinguishing clinical from organizational ethics is the notion of moral agency. Traditionally, bioethics has examined the actions of *individual* agents—clinicians, patients, family members—and has held them accountable in light of ethical principles, norms, and obligations. In the intermediate analysis, the locus of moral agency differs from that of clinical ethics and the *organization* itself is seen as having obligations to adhere to certain norms of ethical behavior.

This perspective has particular relevance to ethics committees, which have traditionally functioned as their health care institutions' analytic and consultative resource on moral issues and conflicts. This handbook argues that the committee's role should not be limited to considering the ethical aspects of individual clinical interactions, but should encompass scrutiny of how the organization creates an environment in which quality care is provided because ethically sound decisions are made.

Moral Responsibilities of Health Care Organizations

⫿⫿⫿ Central Hospital is considering some innovations in an effort to make its operation more efficient. In the process, it is confronting a conflict between its role as a health care delivery system and its role as a risk-bearing entity. For example, one of the suggestions under consideration is the establishment of an observation suite in or near the ER. Sometimes when patients come to the ER, their presenting symptoms (chest pain, shortness of breath, abdominal pain, asthma) do not make it clinically apparent whether they need to be hospitalized. An observation suite would provide a place where they could be observed closely for up to twenty-four hours while their condition either stabilizes or changes and their medical needs become clearer.

From the risk perspective, the advantage is the opportunity for twenty-four hours of monitoring, which is much less expensive than a hospitalization. From the hospital's viewpoint, however, such a resource may not be economically advantageous because it would drive up the cost of an ER visit without generating additional revenue to offset the cost. Because most patients are not in the risk category, the hospital would only be entitled to reimbursement for an ER visit.

Organizational ethics draws its core notions from the disciplines of both business and health care ethics. Traditional bioethics views organizations merely as settings for encounters between individual patients and individual clinicians. Its focus on the ethics of professions, including medicine, nursing, psychology, and social work, neglects the organizational climate that promotes or impedes the ethical delivery of health care. Business ethics recognizes medicine as a business enterprise but fails to appreciate the distinctive nature of health care as a good and the special quality of the provider-patient relationship. What distinguishes organizational ethics is the notion that organizations are more than aggregates of individuals with their own roles and responsibilities. As we have argued at greater length elsewhere (Blustein et al., 2004; Blustein et al., 2001), organizations can usefully be thought of as moral agents with interests, values, and obligations that inform their goals and the means they use to achieve them.

How these matters are considered not only has philosophical significance, but enormous practical significance as well, especially for health care ethics committees. If organizations are moral agents, they should be expected to develop a sense of what is morally acceptable and unacceptable practice and to manifest that sense in their policies and procedures. If they are only powerful economic entities, they cannot be expected to exercise moral responsibility and society would be well advised not to trust them to be self-regulating.

It would be naïve to suggest that health care organizations can be guided only by their moral codes. Like other business entities, they have a parallel and often competing responsibility to remain fiscally sound to meet their obligations to patients, employees, and the communities they serve. Central Hospital's decision about establishing an observation suite, for example, pits the benefits of risk reduction and improved clinical care against the economic burden of creating an expensive and under-reimbursed service. Because hospitals have fixed budgets, the analysis will require a balancing of goods, considering the worth of this unit in relation to other programs that may have to be delayed, downsized, or eliminated altogether.

In an analogy to the clinical setting, it might be asked whether organizations have the *capacity* for morally responsible conduct or whether, like individuals who lack this capacity, they can only be kept in line by external regulation, such as compliance requirements. We argue that organizations can be motivated not only by economic self-interest, but by a capacity to regulate their actions according to a set of moral imperatives. This position has important implications for ethics committees in determining the scope of their involvement in the goals, policies, and procedures of the institutions they advise.

Health care organizations can act in morally responsible ways only if they have a clear sense of their core values in relation to other organizational goals. These values, typically articulated in the organizational mission statement and code of ethics, become an essential part of an organization's identity. As an example of how an institution might express its governing moral philosophy, part V offers a sample code of organizational and clinical ethics. This code was developed by the Montefiore Medical Center Bioethics Committee, endorsed by the administration, and formally adopted by the board of trustees.

But neither a mission statement nor a code of ethics is worth much if executives do not appreciate the need for monitoring and evaluating performance to determine the organization's effectiveness in light of its values and goals. The organization can only act as a moral agent through individuals who use the mission of the organization as a benchmark for assessing organizational behaviors. Although the mission should be taken seriously at all levels of the organization, executives play a special leadership role in ensuring that organizational activities reflect its stated goals and values.

Organizational Ethics and Compliance

Recognizing that the transformation from fee-for-service to managed care presents ethical problems in addition to those that arise in clinical care, in 1995 the Joint Commission on Accreditation of Healthcare Organizations (JCAHO) changed the name of its standards chapter from Patient Rights to Patient Rights and Organization Ethics. The new standards require health care organizations to develop and operate according to a code of ethical behavior that addresses "marketing, admission, transfer and discharge, and billing practices" and "the relationship of the hospital and its staff to other health care providers, educational institutions, and payers" (Joint Commission on Accreditation of Healthcare Organizations 1998a:55–56, Standards RI.4.1 and RI.4.2).

Although JCAHO refers to its new standards as "organizational ethics," we use the term to distinguish a normative reach beyond the minimum required for adherence to laws and regulations. A separate but related area of organizational scrutiny, compliance, focuses on those obligations whose nonfulfillment amounts to fraud and abuse, while organizational ethics is concerned with obligations whose nonfulfillment provokes specifically moral condemnation. Organizational ethics recognizes that organizations confront many ethical problems for which no applicable laws and regulations exist; in other words, unethical conduct may not be illegal. Moreover, because ethical problems often resist neat and easy solutions, they may demand a more nuanced analysis than the determination of whether compliance has or has not occurred.

Hospitals and other health care organizations have responded to legal and regulatory requirements by appointing people whose responsibility is monitoring institutional compliance. Working with the offices of risk management and legal counsel, compliance officers are charged with ensuring that institutional policies and procedures meet or exceed specified governmental standards. Your institution likely has an office of compliance, dedicated to this effort. In contrast, your ethics committee's function is to provide the principled analyses and recommendations that will promote ethically sound organizational decisions and actions.

Ethics and the Allocation of Resources

III   City Hospital has a fifteen-bed intensive care unit and, as usual, tonight the unit is fully occupied. When the ICU is full and the ER has also reached its limit, this hospital, like others in the region, typically closes its ER to ambulances because it cannot accommodate additional patients. Ambulances that would normally bring patients to this hospital are diverted to the nearest hospital with an open ER. On this night, all area hospitals have closed their ERs because they are filled to capacity. Patients picked up by the emergency medical service (EMS) must be taken somewhere, however, so City Hospital must admit a patient despite its saturation.

The last patient admitted to the ICU is a 45-year-old chronic schizophrenic man with a high fever and overwhelming infections who has been brought in from one of the city's state-operated psychiatric facilities. Another bed is already occupied by a 96-year-old woman brought to the ER from a nursing home, where she had been found unresponsive. Efforts to restore her to consciousness have so far been unsuccessful.

A third patient in the unit is a 23-year-old woman, an IV drug user with two children, who presented in the ER with symptoms of *Pneumocystis carinii* pneumonia (PCP). Because of her pulmonary disease, she is in respiratory distress and needs to be stabilized before starting antiretroviral therapy. The remaining ICU beds are occupied by patients whose average age is 75 and for whom continued ICU treatment has been deemed essential.

The patient who has just been brought to the ER is a 63-year-old professor of internal medicine who has just had a heart attack. The university where the professor teaches recently endowed a new wing of the hospital.

Which patient, if any, should be removed from the ICU to make room for the professor? What criteria should be used in determining eligibility for ICU care? In what way do decisions about allocating ICU beds involve issues of justice?

Questions about resource allocation are among the most common and important in organizational ethics. Allocation decisions are trade-offs, necessitated by the fact that health care resources and the economic assets needed for their provision are limited. Sometimes the trade-offs involve hard choices between doing things that would improve the health of a population in serious need and doing what is necessary to preserve the fiscal integrity of the organization and, thereby, its long-term ability to continue serving the needs of the community. More commonly, the trade-off is not between some needed program and institutional survival, but between a new program and those that are already in place meeting other needs.

Resource allocation decisions often have to balance and rank a number of competing considerations. For example, resources devoted to very costly cutting edge treatments and technologies that might benefit a few patients diminish what is available for less expensive care that can benefit a larger number. Investing in large-scale marketing campaigns to attract more patients may result in less being spent on providing care to those who are already patients. A growing problem for organizations is determining how to budget for the care of undocumented persons, as well as citizens who are uninsured or underinsured.

In these and similar cases, the central questions are: who wins, who loses, and what alternatives do the losers have for getting their needs met? Because resource allocation decisions confer benefits on some (the winners) at the cost of not conferring benefits on others (the losers), they raise issues of distributive justice. The distribution of the benefits and burdens inherent in resource allocation decisions should be done in a way that is fair to all concerned and does not discriminate against any group or individuals.

One distinction is between expensive and scarce resources. For example, in City Hospital, ICU beds are an *expensive* resource that is made into a *scarce* resource by an organizational decision limiting the number of beds. If the institutional budget permitted ICU expansion, more beds could be made available. In contrast, solid organs, such as hearts, are from the outset a scarce resource because of their finite supply. Because ICU beds are expensive and limited, not all persons who could potentially benefit from critical care can receive it in the ICU.

Another useful distinction is between rationing and triage. Rationing, discussed above, is setting limits on spending to allocate limited resources among competing care and treatment needs, thereby denying beneficial care to some. Triage, the approach used in most ERs and ICUs, is determining the order in which care is provided, using as criteria the urgency of the care needs and the likelihood of benefit. Generally accepted medical criteria exclude from the ICU patients considered unlikely to benefit from critical care because it would be physiologically futile, patients who are in PVS, or those who have met the criteria for brain death. Priorities are established and patients with a greater likelihood of benefiting from ICU care are given preference over those who are less likely to benefit from care in that setting. The alternative to this approach is to increase the ICU census by admitting more patients and potentially decrease the quality of care.

Decisions regarding the allocation of limited resources in City Hospital should be based on sound medical and ethical criteria. It is reasonable to question whether giving the ICU bed to the professor, simply because his university has endowed a new wing of the hospital, is fair to the other patients who are already benefiting from ICU care. This might well be seen as an unjustified form of favoritism that has little to do with medical criteria, clinical benefit, or distributive justice. The ethics committee role in reviewing institutional policies would contribute a principled analysis to the guidelines for ICU admission, focusing on the just and clinically indicated allocation of a limited resource.

Ethics Committees and Organizational Issues

III The Atlas Hospital medical director has brought the following issue to the Atlas Bioethics Committee for consideration. Especially during protracted hospitalizations, patients' conditions and, therefore, their medical needs change. Often patients who were admitted to one medical or surgical service subsequently need to be transferred one or more times to a different service for continued care. In each instance, the process requires the medical team on the first service to communicate with the medical team on the second service, explaining why the patient would benefit from the transfer. Depending on its evaluation of the patient's condition and its own clinical burdens, the second service has the option of accepting or rejecting the transfer. It has come to the medical director's attention that clinical services are avoiding accepting transfers for reasons other than clinical indication.

Atlas Hospital is also working to promote clinical efficiency and discourage unnecessarily long hospitalizations. Accordingly, when a patient either leaves the hospital or dies, the length of stay (the number of hospital days) is credited to the discharge service, not the admitting or transferring service. That means that, if a patient spends sixty days on a surgical service and is transferred to a medicine service for two days prior to discharge, the entire sixty-two-day length of stay will be credited to the medicine service. Because the costs incurred during a hospitalization are applied to the clinical service caring for the patient, it is in each service's interest to minimize lengths of stay. Under this system, it is also unsurprising that services are not eager to accept patients who have or are likely to have long lengths of stay.

The organization's ethics committee serves a vital function by monitoring the consistency of the institutional mission and goals with the policies and procedures that guide them, and the administrative decisions that realize them. Its effectiveness requires the recognition that ethical issues arising in health care cannot be neatly compartmentalized and addressed separately from other institutional matters. Because clinical and business concerns are interrelated, decisions about them must be grounded in or consistent with the ethical principles and values that inform the institutional mission. The committee's composition and agenda should be expanded to reflect this broader scope. The membership should include both clinicians and administrators, and the issues it considers should include clinical and organizational priorities and decisions.

The interservice transfer issue is a good example of how ethics committees can influence organizational decision making and, thereby, promote better clinical decision making. The Atlas committee analyzed the situation in terms of the conflict between the obligation to promote patient best interest and the obligation to be responsible stewards of institutional resources. Patients are benefited by transfer if their treatment needs can be met more effectively in another clinical setting. Transfer burdens them if they are deprived of the clinical judgment, skill, and continuity of care on which they rely. The committee also recognized that even physicians who intend to act in their patients' best interests will be reluctant to make medically appropriate decisions that appear to disadvantage their clinical services. Organizational involvement and support are essential to developing solutions that are medically and ethically sound. The committee's ethical principles and suggested guidelines for interservice transfer appear in part III.

Your ethics committee's utility as an analytic and advisory resource, however, is only as good as its access to and active involvement in organizational planning and decision making. Genuine integration of the ethics perspective in the formulation and execution of institutional activities requires a fundamental and often difficult culture change. The significant differences between the clinical and organizational cultures challenge both ethics committees and institutional leadership seeking meaningful collaboration. Transparent and inclusive decision making, which is central to ethical process, may be seen by financial and business management as intrusive and inhibiting. Administrators may need the reassurance of sustained demonstration that ethical analysis and recommendation can enhance the efficacy and validity of organizational decision making without compromising its efficiency or security. These issues, as well as strategies for addressing them, are discussed at considerably greater length in *Ethics for Health Care Organizations: Theory, Case Studies, and Tools* (Blustein, Post, and Dubler, 2002).

REFERENCES

Blustein J, Post LF, Dubler NN. 2004. Holding healthcare organizations morally accountable. *Keynotes on Health Care* 35(3):1–8.

Blustein J, Post LF, Dubler NN. 2002. *Ethics for Health Care Organizations: Theory, Case Studies, and Tools.* New York: United Hospital Fund.

Daniels N. 1985. *Just Health Care.* New York: Cambridge University Press.

Daniels N. 1991. Is the Oregon rationing plan fair? *Journal of the American Medical Association* 265(17):2232–35.

Emanuel EL.1991. *The Ends of Medicine: Medical Ethics in a Liberal Polity.* Cambridge, MA: Harvard University Press.

Emergency Medical Treatment and Active Labor Act (EMTALA), 42 U.S.C. §1395dd et seq.

Engelhardt T. 1991. *Bioethics and Secular Humanism: The Search for a Common Morality.* Philadelphia: Trinity Press International.

Epstein AM, Ayanian JZ. 2001. Racial disparities in medical care. *New England Journal of Medicine* 334(19):1471–73.

Freeman HP, Payne R. 2000. Racial injustice in health care. *New England Journal of Medicine* 342(14):1045–48.

Hall RT. 2000. *An Introduction to Healthcare Organizational Ethics.* New York: Oxford University Press.

Joint Commission on Accreditation of Healthcare Organizations. 1998. *Comprehensive Accreditation Manual for Hospitals.* Oakbrook Terrace, IL: Joint Commission on Accreditation of Healthcare Organizations.

Lo B. 2000. Conflicts of interest. In *Resolving Ethical Dilemmas: A Guide for Clinicians.* 2nd ed. Philadelphia: Lippincott Williams & Wilkins, pp. 231-82.

Mill JS. 1957. *Utilitarianism.* New York: Liberal Arts Press.

Morreim EH. 1989. Fiscal scarcity and the inevitability of bedside budget balancing. *Archives of Internal Medicine* 149(5):1012–15.

Nichols LM. Myths about the uninsured. Taken from a Hearing on the Uninsured before the U.S. House of Representatives Committee on Ways and Means Health Subcommittee, March 9, 2004.

Nozick R. 1977. *Anarchy, State, and Utopia.* New York: Basic Books.

Pearson SD, Sabin JE, Emanuel EJ. 2003. *No Margin, No Mission: Health-Care Organizations and the Quest for Ethical Excellence.* New York: Oxford University Press.

Phillips RS, Hamel MB, Teno JM, Bellamy P, Broste SK, Califf RM, Vidaillet H, Davis RB, Muhlbaier LH, Connors AF, Lynn J, Goldman L—for the SUPPORT investigators. 1996. Race, resource use, and survival in seriously ill hospitalized adults. *Journal of General Internal Medicine* 11:387–96.

Post LF. 2007 (forthcoming). Ethics and the delivery of palliative care. In O'Mahony S, Blank AE, eds. *Choices in Palliative Care.* New York: Kluwer Academic/Plenum Publishers.

President's Commission for the Study of Ethical Problems in Medicine and Biomedical and Behavioral Research. 1983. *Securing Access to Health Care.* Washington, DC: U.S. Government Printing Office.

Rawls J. 1971. *A Theory of Justice.* Cambridge, MA: Harvard University Press.

Rhoades JA. 2005. The long-term uninsured in America, 2001–2002: Estimates for the U.S. population under age 65. *Agency for Healthcare Research and Quality, Statistical Brief #67.*

Spencer EM, Mills AE, Rorty MV, Werhane PH. 2000. *Organization Ethics in Health Care.* New York: Oxford University Press.

Wikler D. 1992. Ethics and rationing: "Whether," "how," or "how much"? *Journal of the American Geriatrics Society* 40:398–403.

Woolf SH. 2004. Society's choice: The tradeoff between efficacy and equity and the lives at stake. *American Journal of Preventive Medicine* 27(1):49–56.

PART II

Clinical Ethics Consultation

This is the part that you've been waiting for—where ethical theory meets clinical reality. A key function of ethics committees is providing clinicians with an analytic framework for identifying and resolving ethical dilemmas that arise in the clinical setting. As discussed in part I, these challenges usually reflect the inherent tensions between and among the ethical obligations incumbent upon health care professionals. Sometimes the situations are matters of life and death, with elements of high drama. More often, they concern the rights and responsibilities of patients, families, and caregivers as they struggle to make decisions that are clinically, ethically, and legally valid. In that process, the perspective of the ethics committee is an invaluable resource.

Whether ethics committees assume responsibility for conducting clinical consultations on an ad hoc or rotating basis or periodically review the work done by a dedicated consultation service, members need a foundation in ethical analysis and a sense of why similar cases invoke certain reasoning. While consultation considers each case individually, the ethical concepts and principles that inform the process, presented in part I, provide analytic clarity and consistency. Part II begins with a discussion of the fundamentals of clinical ethics consultation, including the goals and descriptions of two different approaches that committees might adopt. Committees also may find it useful to compile a library of cases that can serve as analytic models. So, in addition to the case examples in part I, this section includes sample cases with the type of analyses they might receive in clinical ethics consultations.

Approaches to Ethics Consultation

KENNETH A. BERKOWITZ, M.D., AND

NANCY NEVELOFF DUBLER, LL.B.

Our goal in this chapter is to provide an introduction to health care ethics consultation, including a conceptual overview followed by descriptions of two very different consultation approaches. The CASES approach was developed by the Veterans Health Administration's National Center for Ethics in Health Care to set explicit standards for performing ethics consultation at nearly 160 Veterans Health Administration (VHA) medical centers nationwide. The second approach, bioethics mediation, reflects the work done during the past twenty-five years by the Bioethics Consultation Service at Montefiore Medical Center, Bronx, New York.

Ethics consultation is one way to help patients, care professionals, and other parties resolve ethical concerns in a health care setting and is now widely recognized as an essential part of health care delivery. The vast majority of U.S. hospitals have active ethics consultation services, usually a function of the institutional ethics committee, but these services vary widely in their approach, intensity, and effectiveness (Fox, 2002). In some places, such as Montefiore Medical Center, for idiosyncratic historical reasons, the ethics consultation service developed separately from the ethics committee.

Ethics consultation has been endorsed by numerous governmental and professional bodies, and is legally mandated under specific circumstances in several states (Tulsky and Fox, 1996). By providing a forum for discussion and a method of careful analysis, effective ethics consultation promotes health care practices consistent with high ethical standards, helps to foster consensus and resolve conflict in an atmosphere of respect, honors participants' authority while respecting their values and preferences in the decision-making process, educates providers to approach current and future cases according to agreed-upon principles, and fosters the notion of justice by ensuring that like cases will be treated in similar ways. Ethics consultation has also been shown to save health care institutions money by reducing the provision of nonbeneficial treatments, as well as certain hospital lengths of stay (Schneiderman et al., 2003; Schneiderman, Gilmer, and Teetzel, 2000; Dowdy, Robertson, and Bander, 1998; Heilicser, Meltzer, and Siegler, 2000). But these instrumental uses of bioethics consultation are welcome by-products of the intervention rather than the primary goal, which is to promote sound health care decision making, with respect for clinicians, patients, and families, and support for caregiver concerns.

As discussed in the introduction to this book, the three goals of most ethics programs and ethics committees are education, policy development, and case consultation. At the beginning of ethics committee development, most case consultation was retrospective, and that often remains the approach today for committees just starting to do consultation. Increasingly, as committee members gain experience with each other and with the ethical norms in their institution, and as the committee becomes comfortable with reflective analysis, real-time consultation becomes more customary. Thus, ethics committees and consultation services, to one degree or another, are involved in:

- retrospective review either of a case on which the consultation service consulted or a case handled without ethics participation
- prospective case consultation that involves members of the ethics consultation service intervening to affect the outcome of an active case

This chapter focuses on the latter of these tasks, prospective consultation on active patient cases.

THREE MODELS OF ETHICS CONSULTATION

Health care ethics consultations are typically performed by an individual ethics consultant, an ethics committee, or an ethics consultation team. As discussed below, each of these models has advantages and disadvantages. Although some ethics consultation services might rely exclusively on one of these three models, we generally recommend against this because each has its effective application under different circumstances. Instead, consultation services should determine which model is most appropriate for each consultation, depending on the ethical and clinical issues raised, the parties involved, the consultation skills required, and the staff available.

That said, it is important to note that a given institution may prefer one or another consultation model and be structured to facilitate that mode most easily. For example, at Montefiore, the bioethics mediation approach typically utilizes an individual consultant on each case. Whenever possible, however, the consultants prefer to work together so that they can co-mediate, a process that maximizes skills.

In this model, one person—either an independent "solo" consultant or a member of an ethics consultation team or committee—is assigned to perform a consultation alone. The advantages of the individual ethics consultant model are that it provides fewer logistical hurdles (e.g., scheduling meetings) and facilitates quick response to urgent consultation requests. The disadvantages are that the consultant must possess all required knowledge and skills to perform the consultation, and there are fewer checks and balances to protect against the intrusion of the consultant's own values and biases. One way to counter this problem is suggested by the Montefiore approach, in which the consultant's initial meeting is with the entire involved health care team, making the collective knowledge and skills of the team available as the baseline for the consultation.

It is incumbent on the individual ethics consultant to recognize her strengths and limitations, and to get help when needed. The successful ethics consultant builds a web of strong, collegial relationships within the health care facility and network, and calls on others for assistance with particular clinical, ethical, legal, cultural, or religious concerns. Even the most highly trained and experienced ethics consultant benefits from confidentially discussing complex cases with other experts.

In addition, individual consultants should engage in systematic review of their consultations with colleagues. In the Montefiore approach, difficult cases are shared with the other ethics consultants on the service and retrospectively with the ethics committee. Another check on the process comes from entering a note in the patient's chart, where it can be read by clinicians, administrators, lawyers, and risk managers, alerting them to a developing problem. At Montefiore, the note is placed in the chart before perspectives are solicited from other persons who have different roles in the institution and may provide useful information and feedback to the consultant.

In the second model, a standing interdisciplinary committee—that is, a relatively stable group of typically between six and twenty people—jointly performs the consultation. The advantages of this model are that it facilitates collective proficiency and includes ready access to diverse perspectives and multidisciplinary expertise. Its disadvantages are that it requires a great deal of staff time, is not well suited to situations that require a rapid response, and diffuses responsibility among committee members, which can contribute to "groupthink." Most important, the potential for patients and family members to feel intimidated by a large group of white-coated professionals makes this model the opposite of a mediation approach, which seeks to "level the playing field." Using a small subset of the committee as the link between the committee and the patient or family can help to minimize this power imbalance.

The committee model may be especially useful for ensuring broad organizational input into difficult consultations, including those that might establish institutional precedent or end up in the media or the courts. This notion of consultation has less to do with solving the immediate problem and more to do with structuring the situation if the problem gets magnified or blows up. This model may also be useful to facilities that are relatively new to ethics consultation, handle a low volume of consultations, and/or lack specialized ethics expertise. Most committees are good at talking; some are proficient in analysis; and some, with experience, can bring perspective and wisdom to the enterprise.

In the team model, responsibility for the ethics consultation is shared by a small group of people selected from a pool of qualified consultants based on the knowledge and skills required by the circumstances of the case. The advantages of the consultation team model are that it lends itself to rapid responses and ensures diverse perspectives and expertise because the members of the team can vary to meet the situation. Small groups can be less intimidating for patients and families, and the team itself provides a natural forum for support and reflection. Conversely, the team model is less efficient than the individual consultant model and provides fewer checks and balances than the committee model.

The team model allows tasks to be divided among members of the team, accommodates a wide range of situations and levels of consultant expertise, and is in some ways a compromise between the individual and committee models. It is the most common consultation model, used by more than two-thirds of hospitals in the United States (Fox, 2002).

CRITICAL SUCCESS FACTORS FOR ETHICS CONSULTATION SERVICES

Regardless of the consultation model(s) used, certain factors are critical for an ethics consultation service to achieve its goals and, for this reason, they should be formally incorporated into institutional policy. Ethics consultation services need to have integration, leadership support, expertise, staff time, and other resources. Access, accountability, organizational learning, and evaluation are also essential. These critical success factors are described below and, in greater detail, in the VHA primer *Ethics Consultation: Responding to Ethics Concerns in Health Care* (Fox et al., 2005).

The successful ethics consultation service must develop and maintain positive relationships with the various individuals and programs that shape the health care organization's ethics environment and practices. In this way, it serves the entire institution, not just a particular category of staff (e.g., physicians), a particular setting (e.g., intensive care), or a particular clinical service (e.g., surgery). A fully integrated ethics consultation service responds to the entire range of ethics concerns faced by the organization.

The ethics consultation service should look for opportunities to forge strong connections with other departments and services within the organization, share activities and skills, and identify and work toward achieving mutual goals. The integrated service can develop ongoing working relationships with programs and departments that commonly encounter ethics-related issues (e.g., pastoral care, patient advocacy, legal counsel, risk management, research, compliance, human resources). Collaborating with different services and programs will enhance staff understanding of each other's skills and roles and contribute to the overall organizational efficiency.

One critical element in the notion of integration is access to the consultation service. If the service is to be available to all staff and patients, it is useful to have a policy that encourages any member of the staff—subinterns to senior attendings, nurses and social workers—to request a consultation. Under such a policy, if the person calling for a consultation is not the attending of record, a call informing that physician about the consultation is an important early step in the process.

Explicit organizational leadership support is essential if the goals of ethics consultation are to be realized. Ultimately, leaders are responsible for the success of all programs, and health care ethics consultation is no exception. Organizational leaders establish institutional priorities and allocate the resources to implement those priorities. Unless leaders support—and are perceived to support—the facility's ethics consultation service, its function cannot succeed.

Health care facility leaders should ensure that ethics consultation services have the requisite expertise, including the knowledge, skills, and character traits necessary to perform competent and effective ethics consultation. Regardless of the consultation model used, the proficiencies outlined in *Core Competencies for Health Care Ethics Consultation* (American Society for Bioethics and Humanities, 1998) must be represented on the ethics consultation service.

Ethics consultants need adequate dedicated time to perform consultation activities, the requirements of which will vary depending on the types of consultations handled. Even a straightforward ethics case consultation typically takes several hours, while more complex cases—especially those that are novel or precedent setting—may continue for more than a week, requiring twenty or more hours of effort by multiple individuals. In addition, consultation services, often supported by their ethics committees, handle a variety of other activities, including requests for general information or education, clarification of policy, review of documents, ethical analysis of hypothetical or historical ("nonactive") cases or organizational ethics questions, or ethics teaching. Consultants should have a clear understanding with their supervisors that ethics consultation is not an optional or voluntary activity, but an assigned part of their jobs that requires dedicated time.

Ethics consultants need ready access to other resources, such as library materials, clerical support, training, and continuing education. Because many facility libraries lack a good selection of health care ethics references, a consultation service often needs its own core set of books and journals. A variety of useful ethics resources is also available online, making access to the Internet essential as well. Finally, ethics consultants need training and regular continuing education to develop, maintain, and improve their knowledge and skills.

As indicated earlier, an effective ethics consultation service must be readily accessible to all patients, families, and staff. The service should be available not only in acute care hospitals, but in all care settings. Ethics consultation services should take steps to ensure that patients, families, and staff in the various sites of health care delivery are aware of the ethics consultation service, what it does, and how to access it.

Like any other important health care function, ethics consultation must have a clear system of accountability to organizational leadership and be plainly situated within the reporting hierarchy. To ensure accountability, responsibilities relating to ethics consultation should be explicitly described in the performance plans of everyone involved, from senior leaders to frontline staff.

Ethics consultants should contribute to organizational learning by sharing their knowledge and experience. Group discussion of actual cases (appropriately modified to protect the identities of participants) is an excellent way to engage and educate clinical staff. With relatively little effort, a consultation service note can be reworked into a newsletter article that summarizes an important ethics topic. Policy questions handled by the service can be turned into Frequently Asked Questions and posted on a website. Efforts such as these not only increase staff knowledge, they also enhance the visibility, credibility, and relevance of the ethics consultation service.

The success of the ethics consultation service requires ongoing evaluation, defined as the systematic assessment of the operation and/or outcomes of a program compared to a set of explicit or implicit standards, as a means of contributing to the continuous improvement of the program (Weiss, 1998). Evaluation efforts need not be elaborate or costly. Experts within the facility, such as quality managers, can assist in developing appropriate ways to assess these factors, ensuring that the measures used are valid and that data are collected and analyzed in a minimally burdensome fashion.

POLICY

The structure, function, and processes of ethics consultation should be formalized in institutional policy that addresses the following topics:

- the goals of ethics consultation
- who may perform ethics consultation
- who may request ethics consultations
- what requests are appropriate for the ethics consultation service
- what requests are appropriate for ethics case consultation
- which consultation model(s) may be used and when
- who must be notified when an ethics case consultation has been requested
- how the confidentiality of participants will be protected
- how ethics consultations will be performed
- how ethics consultations will be documented
- who is accountable for the ethics consultation service
- how the quality of ethics consultation will be assessed and assured

TWO APPROACHES TO CLINICAL ETHICS CONSULTATION

The following two approaches to ethics consultation reflect the quite different natures of the institutions that use them, as well the perceptions of the professionals involved regarding their expertise, authority, and responsibility. In the CASES approach, developed for use throughout the VHA system, ethics consultants are systematically guided through the process and practice of ethics consultations involving active patient cases. Bioethics mediation, the approach developed and used at Montefiore Medical Center, is based on the consult team's experience that calls for ethics consultations are generally requests for help in resolving or managing conflict. Thus, it may be that the CASES approach will be very useful for certain medical centers or health systems, while the mediation approach may be more suited to others. Alternatively, some combination of these approaches or one of the several others not discussed here might prove useful, depending on the circumstances of a particular consultation.

The CASES Approach

The National Center for Ethics in Health Care is the primary office of the VHA for addressing the complex ethical issues that arise in patient care, health care manage-ment, and research. The mission of the National Center for Ethics in Health Care is to clarify and promote ethical health care practices within VHA, the country's largest integrated health care delivery system. Toward this end, the National Center for Ethics in Health Care developed the CASES approach to health care ethics case consultation, a systematic step-by-step approach to providing consistent and effective ethics case con-sultation at VHA facilities. Ethics consultants or committees wishing to learn more about the CASES approach and consider its applicability are encouraged to consult the comprehensive discussion, including tools, templates, sample cases, and other re-sources, presented in *Ethics Consultation: Responding to Ethics Concerns in Health Care* (Fox et al., 2005).

The CASES approach involves five steps:

Clarify the consultation request.
Assemble the relevant information.
Synthesize the information.
Explain the synthesis.
Support the consultation process.

These steps were designed to guide ethics consultants through the complex critical thinking needed to perform ethics case consultation effectively. They are intended to be used in much the same way clinicians use a standard format for taking a patient's history, performing a physical exam, or documenting a clinical case. Even when spe-cific, observable action is not required, each step should be considered systematically as part of every ethics case consultation. Although the steps are presented in a linear fashion, *ethics consultation is a fluid process and the distinction between steps may blur in the context of a specific case.* At times, it may be necessary to repeat steps or perform them in a different order than presented here.

Clarify the Consultation Request

The first step requires the consultant to gather information from the requester to form a preliminary understanding of the circumstances and reasoning that prompted an ethics consultation request. Two initial questions should help the consultant confirm whether the request is appropriate for ethics consultation:

Question 1: Does the requester want help resolving an ethics concern, that is, uncertainty or conflict over which decisions or actions are ethically justifiable? *If the answer is "no," and there is no uncertainty or conflict over which decisions or actions are ethically justifiable, the request is probably not appropriate for ethics consultation.* Requests that do not pertain to ethics concerns should be referred to other offices within the organization. *If the answer is "yes, there is an ethics concern," consider the second question.*

Question 2: Does the request pertain to an active patient case? *If the answer is "no," the request may still be appropriate for the ethics consultation service but not necessarily the CASES approach, which was specifically designed to address active cases.* Many ethics-related requests are for information or education, policy clarification, document review, or ethical analysis of issues or historical cases. Many of the CASES steps may also be relevant to other types of ethics consultation but, in noncase situations, the consultant should tailor the approach to the nature of the request. *If the answers to both Questions 1 and 2 are "yes, there is an ethical concern about an active patient case," the request should be handled through the CASES approach.*

Occasionally, a case-related question may appear so simple or the consultant may be so pressed for time that a formal consultation may not seem necessary. The temptation to cut corners should be resisted lest it undermine the quality of the consultation process. Ethics cases are often more complex than their initial presentation or perception, and each case deserves to be addressed systematically and comprehensively rather than handled through an "informal" or "curbside" approach. *If and when ethics consultants do comment informally on a clinical ethics question, they should be clear that they can only respond in general terms, and absolutely cannot give recommendations about a specific patient case without completing the CASES approach.*

After verifying that the request is appropriate for the CASES approach, basic information should be obtained, including the requester's demographics, role in the case, and understanding of the circumstances; the steps already taken to resolve the ethics concern; and the type of assistance sought. The consultant should establish with the requester realistic expectations about the consultation process and begin a preliminary determination of the personnel best suited to address the specific concern(s).

Next, the consultant should formulate the ethics question, a sometimes difficult but essential part of ethics case consultation. Clarity about the ethics question allows all participants to focus on the same concerns and work efficiently toward resolution, while an imprecisely formulated question can sidetrack or derail the consultation process. Accordingly, the consultant should formulate the ethics question early in the consultation process and examine it again once all the relevant information is assembled.

In a case consultation, *an ethics question asks what should be done in the face of an ethics concern, that is, in the face of uncertainty or conflict about values.* The initial formulation should not emphasize abstract concepts, but should state the question in a way that will focus and assist those who will participate in resolving the case. At the risk of reducing important issues to a formula, the ethics question might be constructed in one of the following two ways, with the consultant providing the case-specific information called for in the parentheses:

1. *Given (the ethical concern/uncertainty or conflict about values), what decisions or actions are ethically justifiable?* or
2. *Given (the ethical concern/uncertainty or conflict about values), is it ethically justifiable to (decision or action)?*

Assemble the Relevant Information

Next, the consultant assembles the information necessary to develop a comprehensive picture of the circumstances and work through the case to facilitate an answer to the ethics question. The CASES approach builds on the work of Jonsen, Siegler, and Winslade (2002) in defining topics that should be reviewed in every ethics consultation, but reframes relevant information into four categories (medical facts, patient's preferences and interests, other people's preferences and interests, and ethics knowledge).

Some cases can be resolved merely by clearing up factual misunderstandings among patients, families, and the health care team. In addition to examining the patient's medical record, ethics consultants should speak directly to involved health care providers and seek out other relevant documents, including advance directives, court papers, and health records from other providers. Consultants with advanced clinical training have an advantage over their nonclinical colleagues, who generally require more effort to identify, collect, and understand the salient medical facts.

Eliciting the patient's preferences and interests is critical because they are central to the consultation. Whenever possible, they should be obtained directly from the patient in face-to-face interaction, even if the patient is said to lack decisional capacity, as well as from advance directives or authorized surrogates. Other parties and medical record notes can also add important insights that put the patient's perspectives in context.

Consultants should collect information about the interests of family, friends, and other stakeholders who may be affected by the outcome of the case. Appreciating these diverse and potentially competing perspectives enriches the consultant's grasp of the situation's complexities and often leads to new insights and ideas.

Considering the ethics question requires a review of the relevant ethics knowledge, which might include codes of ethics, ethical standards and guidelines, consensus statements, scholarly publications, precedent cases, applicable institutional policy, and law. The ethics consultant will be helped by familiarity with ethics-related journals and texts and an ability to perform computer-assisted information searches. Depending on the consultant's expertise, preparation may include selected readings or a literature review and sometimes discussion with a more experienced consultant.

Synthesize the Information

The consultant next analyzes and synthesizes the assembled relevant information into practical terms, applying the ethics knowledge to the other case-specific information and the ethics question. This difficult yet important proficiency requires a foundation of strong analytic skills, drawing on different approaches to moral reasoning and augmented by reading, study, and supervised practical experience.

Based on the circumstances of the case, the consultant should determine whether synthesis would be promoted by a formal meeting of the parties, separate face-to-face discussions, or, in simple situations, telephone or deidentified electronic communication. Formal meetings, conducted skillfully and professionally, require that the consultant set ground rules about respectful and fair interaction, and try to develop a common goal of answering the ethics question. During synthesis, the consultant should identify and guide the ethically appropriate decision maker in reaching decisions within an ethically justifiable range (American Society for Bioethics and Humanities, 1998). In the case of unresolved conflict, bioethics mediation or other conflict resolution techniques should be considered (Dubler and Liebman, 2004).

Explain the Synthesis

The completed synthesis should be made clear to others involved in the case through direct communication to key participants and documentation in both the medical record and consultation service records. The medical record note communicates important information to involved staff, promotes accountability and transparency, and serves an educational purpose. In consultation service records, consultants can record additional observations on power dynamics, workload data, performance improvement ideas, or comments on the ethics consultation process.

Support the Consultation Process

The consultant's final step is to support the overall process of ethics case consultation by following up with participants and learning what was done; completing a critical self-review after each case; soliciting feedback from peers; and assessing how the ethics consultation service is perceived by systematically surveying the participants in the case. Ethical issues that need to be addressed at the systems level should be brought to the attention of the appropriate individual or body.

Effective ethics consultation rests in part on sound consultation practices. The CASES approach is intended to help facilities respond appropriately to ethics concerns. By working systematically through the activities of clarifying consultation requests, assembling relevant information, synthesizing that information to identify morally acceptable solutions, explaining the synthesis to involved parties, and supporting the overall consultation process through follow-up and evaluation to refine its practices, the CASES approach helps the consultation service to ensure that ethics concerns are addressed consistently throughout the health care facility.

The Montefiore Medical Center Model: Bioethics Mediation

The following brief description is intended only to introduce bioethics mediation as one model for consultation services prepared to engage in the necessary training. Ethics committees wishing to learn more about bioethics mediation and consider its applicability are encouraged to consult the comprehensive discussion, including case analyses and role plays, presented in *Bioethics Mediation: A Guide to Shaping Shared Solutions* (Dubler and Liebman, 2004). (Much of this material appeared in an earlier form there.)

■

All bioethics consultation services, including yours, have creation narratives that describe their origins. The Montefiore Medical Center (MMC) Bioethics Consultation Service was established in 1978 and, by the mid-1980s, the original bioethics consultants (one lawyer and one philosopher) were responding to increasing requests for clinical ethics consultation. Over time they noted that the team's arrival at a consultation brought a particular value-added, which they came to think of as "neutral turf." The consultants had not previously been involved in the case, had not issued the care orders that, however wise and well-intentioned, might have contributed to the problem, had not been at odds with anyone on the care team, and had not antagonized either the patient or the family members. In addition, the consult team came fresh to the presentation of the case history and problems, and could ask the questions that had already been asked and answered, but this time eliciting different and more revealing responses.

The team's makeup also accounted for the way it developed and functioned. It was clear that one lawyer and one philosopher were not about to tell medical staff what needed to be done in the clinical setting. Therefore, the "facilitation" aspect of the discussion became both the method and the model, encouraging the consultation staff to think precisely about the dynamic of the discussion and the structure of the decision.

Initial discussion often revealed that some care team members had opposing notions of the patient's prognosis and different arguments for what should be the appropriate care plan. Often these conflicting opinions had been communicated either explicitly or implicitly to the patient and family. As you well know, different staff telling the patient and family different things is a sure recipe for confusion and discord. Sometimes the opportunity that the consultation service provided for all opinions to be presented, clarified, and discussed was, in itself, the beginning of conflict resolution. Once the staff was communicating the same information about diagnosis and prognosis, much of the conflict about the care plan disappeared. Often, although the staff may have reached consensus on the medical facts and the diagnosis, differing opinions about the prognosis remained. In those instances, the value added by mediation would be identifying and clarifying the areas of agreement and disagreement. Over the years, we came to realize that, rather than providing ethics directives or even analysis, what we were doing was some form of alternative dispute resolution or mediation.

As we became more knowledgeable about and more trained in mediation, we realized that another huge benefit emerged from a mediation model for consultation—facilitation skills that could be taught. In addition to a mastery of the rights, interests, and agreed-upon principles of bioethics—an indispensable knowledge base—mediation adds techniques for managing and resolving conflict. Constructing a working hypothesis, framing and reframing issues, identifying underlying interests, concerns, and available options, supporting and stroking the parties, caucusing, and reaching incremental points of agreement are all skills that can be conveyed by training. It is all very well to say that a bioethics consultant mediator needs to be able to facilitate discussion and decision making, but the necessary skill set must be learned.

Fortunately, as mediation is increasingly valued for its effectiveness in resolving conflicts in many fields, its techniques are being taught in many forums around the country. Courses are given by mediation centers, as well as local and state bar associations, universities, and corporations trying to enhance employee productivity. The Internet provides an extensive array of options.

To further clarify this brief introduction to ethics mediation, consider the following questions:

1. Why mediation?

Mediation is a technique that is particularly well suited to conflict resolution in the health care setting. Bioethics mediation combines the clinical substance and perspective of bioethics consultation with the techniques of mediation and dispute resolution to:

- identify the parties to the conflict (although disagreements between family and care providers are common, most conflicts have more than two sides)
- understand the stated (presented) and latent interests of the participants
- level the playing field to minimize disparities of power, knowledge, skill, and experience (to the degree possible) that separate medical professional, patient, and family
- help the parties define their interests
- help maximize options for a resolution of the conflict
- search for common ground or areas of consensus
- ensure that the consensus can be justified as a 'principled resolution,' compatible with the principles of bioethics and the legal rights of patients and families
- help to implement the agreement
- conduct follow-up (Dubler and Liebman, 2004, p. 10).

Bioethics mediation is different from bioethics consultation. *Bioethics consultation* refers to a directed substantive process. The consultant listens to the parties and helps move them toward a principled resolution of the dispute by explaining ethical principles and legal rules, applying them to the facts, and presenting the social consensus on the permissibility of different practices. *Bioethics mediation* refers to the use of classical mediation techniques to identify, understand, and resolve conflicts. Bioethics mediation and bioethics consultation may both be employed in a particular case at different points in the process. Mediation is more inclusive and empowering, and consultation is more authoritarian and hierarchical; either or both may be required in any complex case, even within a single meeting. (Dubler and Liebman 2004, p. 14)

2. Why is bioethics mediation well suited to the resolution of conflicts in the health care setting?

In difficult cases, the real question is, which is the "least bad" process for drawing out and resolving the issues? Conflict must and will be resolved because the delivery of care demands that physicians, nurses, and other care providers be guided by a coherent plan. If necessary, that plan can be imposed by the medical or the administrative staff.

But the bioethics mediator, in contrast to an authoritarian decider, will more often be able to ensure that the options are based on respect for the interests and rights of patients and families, regard for the parties' differences, and awareness of cultural and religious imperatives, within the framework of bioethics theory. Because of its focus on "leveling the playing field," it is more likely that a meditative process will be just and will ensure that similar cases are treated in like ways. Ideally, mediation can produce a solution agreed to by all parties who feel a sense of ownership in and responsibility for the plan.

One of the greatest advantages of using the mediation process in bioethics disputes is its flexibility. The general structure of mediation can be altered and adapted to fit the needs of the participants and the clinical realities. But the starting point is always the same: respect for the patient, the family, and the care providers, and an impartial stance regarding what should be the outcome in any particular case.

One exception to the extended flexibility is the need to reach a "principled resolution." This requires that the rights of the parties, as distinct from their interests, be protected. Thus, it would not be possible to agree that a decisionally capable and adequately informed patient should be excluded from a decision about discontinuing life-sustaining treatment. It might, however, be possible to postpone that decision, until one or more of her family members has had time to adjust to the inevitable outcome. It is key to this intervention to remember that the process is a part of the product.

3. What are the limitations of bioethics mediation?

Bioethics mediation is not for every situation. Parties to a mediation must want to reach agreement. In some cases, the patient or family members may not have the emotional strength to face difficult facts or make hard choices. They may need to have some decisions *made for them*. But most often there are three reasons that mediation fails:

- Sometimes the conflict is out of control before it comes to the attention of the mediator.
- In many cases, some psychological problem or psychiatric diagnosis affects one of the parties and is at the heart of the disagreement. In such cases, reason and argument will be ineffective because of illness and distortion.
- Outsiders may have an interest in augmenting conflict. This is especially evident in prominent end-of-life cases, such as the tragedy of Terri Schiavo, where the use of legal process and the press to make political points dooms private reconsideration and resolution.

4. Why should bioethics consultants try techniques of mediation?

In the experience of the Montefiore Medical Center Bioethics Consultation Service, mediation often works for the reasons discussed above. Even when it does not work, it often helps to define and delineate the conflict. Finally, after the consultation service is experienced and has integrated mediation into practice, its collegial process may mean that medical staff will be more willing to call for help. This is especially the case when experience indicates that the bioethics consultant "doesn't generally make it worse and sometime makes it better."

REFERENCES

American Society for Bioethics and Humanities, Task Force on Standards for Bioethics and Humanities. 1998. *Core Competencies for Health Care Ethics Consultation: The Report of the American Society for Bioethics and Humanities*. Glenview, IL: American Society for Bioethics and Humanities.

American Society for Bioethics and Humanities, Clinical Ethics Task Force. 2007. *Improving Competence in Ethics Consultation: A Learner's Guide*. Glenview, IL: American Society for Bioethics and Humanities.

Dowdy MD, Robertson C, Bander JA. 1998. A study of proactive ethics consultation for critically and terminally ill patients with extended lengths of stay. *Critical Care Medicine* 26(2):252–59.

Dubler NN, Liebman CB. 2004. *Bioethics Mediation: A Guide to Shaping Shared Solutions*. New York: United Hospital Fund.

Fox E. 2002. Ethics consultation in U.S. hospitals: A national study and its implications. Annual Meeting of the American Society for Bioethics and Humanities. October 24, Baltimore, MD.

Fox E, Berkowitz KA, Chanko BL, Powell T. 2005. *Ethics Consultation: Responding to Ethics Concerns in Health Care*. Washington, DC: Veterans Health Administration. [On-line] www1.va.gov/integratedethics/download/EthicsConsultationPrimer.pdf; last accessed May 1, 2006.

Heilicser BJ, Meltzer D, Siegler M. 2000. The effect of clinical medical ethics consultation on health-care costs. *Journal of Clinical Ethics* 11(1):31-38.

Jonsen AR, Siegler M, Winslade WJ. 2002. *Clinical Ethics: A Practical Approach to Ethical Decisions in Clinical Medicine*. 5th ed. Columbus, OH: McGraw-Hill Medical.

Schneiderman LJ, Gilmer T, Teetzel HD. 2000. Impact of ethics consultations in the intensive care setting: A randomized, controlled trial. *Critical Care Medicine* 28(12):3920–24.

Schneiderman LJ, Gilmer T, Teetzel HD, Dugan DO, Blustein J, Cranford R, Briggs KB, Komatsu GI, Goodman-Crews P, Cohn F, Young EWD. 2003. Effect of ethics consultations on nonbeneficial life-sustaining treatments in the intensive care setting: A randomized controlled trial. *Journal of the American Medical Association* 290(9):1166–72.

Tulsky JA, Fox E. 1996. Evaluating ethics consultation: Framing the questions. *Journal of Clinical Ethics* 7(2):109–15.

Weiss CH. 1998. *Evaluation Methods for Studying Programs and Policies*. 2nd ed. Upper Saddle River, NJ: Prentice Hall.

10 Sample Clinical Cases

The following sample cases are representative, but not exhaustive, of the kind likely to come before an ethics committee or consultation service. They appear as they would be presented for consideration, with a description of the clinical situation and an overview of the key ethical issues that would receive attention in an ethics consultation or case review. Three cases are supplemented by sample chart notes that illustrate how the ethics consultation might be documented in the medical record. To enhance their accessibility and utility, we have categorized the cases according to the issues they illustrate. Each category contains one detailed case with analysis, in some instances followed by a similar case that presents variations or raises additional issues. Further information about the concepts and principles discussed in the analyses, as well as other case examples, can be found in the relevant chapters in part I.

- Advance Directives
- Autonomy in Tension with Best Interest
- Confidentiality
- Decisional Capacity
- Disclosure and Truth Telling
- End-of-life Care
- Forgoing Life-sustaining Treatment
- Goals of Care
- Informed Consent and Refusal
- Medical Futility
- Parental Decision Making
- Surrogate Decision Making

ADVANCE DIRECTIVES

||| Mrs. Dunn is a 94-year-old woman who was admitted to the hospital from a nursing home for surgical repair of a hip fracture. Her baseline mental status was described by the nursing home as "moderate dementia with intermittent confusion and inattentiveness." The nursing staff says that she is usually vocal in refusing treatments and medications, and that coaxing is often required to obtain her cooperation for therapy.

According to the living will that Mrs. Dunn signed in 1992 when she was admitted to the nursing home, she has been a devout Jehovah's Witness for over thirty years. The living will directs that "no transfusions of blood or blood products be given to me under any circumstances, even if physicians deem such necessary to preserve my life or health." At the same time she executed the living will, she also appointed her son, Tom, to be her health care proxy agent.

Although her health has been reasonably good, Mrs. Dunn has been hospitalized several times during these years, for pneumonia, kidney stones, and appendicitis. When she provided consent for the 1988 appendectomy, it was with the clear understanding that no blood transfusions would be given, and, fortunately, none was needed.

On admission to the hospital for hip surgery, Mrs. Dunn was evaluated and found to lack the capacity to make decisions about her treatment. She appears very uncomfortable, confused, and frightened. When attempts are made to examine her, she responds by pulling away and saying, "No, no!" Now that surgery is being considered, her son, Tom, has been contacted to assume the decisional authority of her health care agent. When the clinical situation is explained, he says, "Do the surgery and give her blood if she needs it. At this point, she's too out of it to understand or object. The important thing is to give her the best chance to come through this safely and comfortably."

Dr. Lewis, the orthopedic surgeon, has requested a bioethics consult because of his expectation that she will need blood transfusions either during or after the surgical hip repair. If she needs blood and does not receive it, life-threatening complications (e.g., hemorrhage, heart attack) could result. If she does not have the surgery and the fracture is treated with bed rest, other complications (e.g., thrombophlebitis, pulmonary emboli, pneumonia, pressure ulcers) could develop.

Dr. Lewis is troubled because he believes that surgery, with blood if necessary, is clearly the preferred option and that it is his professional responsibility to advocate for that approach. Yet, he also knows that Mrs. Dunn's living will is a legally enforceable expression of her preferences. He questions whether a surgeon can be asked to undertake this type of surgery without giving blood if it becomes necessary during or after the operation. He also questions whether a surgeon may refuse to operate under those circumstances and, if so, what happens to the patient.

This is a case that cries out for a clinical ethics consultation. It invokes the principles of autonomy, beneficence, and nonmaleficence, and raises issues of decisional capacity, informed consent and refusal, advance care planning, and surrogate decision making. It involves the interests of a vulnerable patient, concerned family, conscientious physician, and responsible institution. It's practically a mini-course in bioethics all by itself.

Because the consult request comes from Dr. Lewis, his perspective is the ethics consultant's introduction to the case. His concern is that he may be asked to compromise his professional judgment and obligations by withholding clinically indicated care, thereby putting the patient at risk. Knowing the likely complications of orthopedic surgery without blood transfusion, he is worried about Mrs. Dunn's well-being. He is also understandably nervous about his reputation and possible legal liability if foreseeable adverse events occur. How can he, as a responsible doctor, not protect his patient from likely harm? On the other hand, how can he abandon his patient by refusing to operate? Not surprisingly, the similar interests of the institution, represented by the offices of legal counsel and risk management, also reflect the organizational responsibilities to promote the patient's well-being and protect her from harm.

But the ethics consultant understands that this case presents multiple, sometimes competing, interests that need to be considered during the consultation meeting. While the concerns of the care professional and the institution are important, the central figures in this or any ethics conflict are the patient, the family, and, if available, the health care proxy agent.

Ideally, the capable patient is able to articulate her own goals and wishes in explaining her choice of a particular course of action. Clarity and consistency are especially important when the decision is to refuse potentially life-saving treatment. In this case, however, Mrs. Dunn is no longer able to advocate for herself and her wishes will have to be communicated through other means. Of course, this is where advance directives are critical in making sure that the voice of the now-incapacitated patient is still heard in the care planning. Perhaps anticipating that her religious beliefs would conflict with her medical needs, Mrs. Dunn's living will explicitly and unambiguously rejected blood and blood products under any and all circumstances, including the preservation of her life and health. The authenticity of this statement is bolstered by over thirty years as a devout Jehovah's Witness, indicating a firm and settled adherence to the tenets of the religion. Her refusal of blood transfusions when she had the appendectomy suggests that she understood and accepted the risks of bloodless surgery, including possible death, making it likely that she would make the same decision now. Indeed, the theory underlying advance care planning is that respect for autonomy is demonstrated by continuing to honor the value-based wishes articulated and demonstrated by the patient when capable.

Her son, Tom, presents yet another perspective. His expressed goal is to protect his mother from what he perceives as foolish decisions that put her health and life in jeopardy. Because he does not share her religious beliefs, he sees them as a dispensable barrier to her well-being. He insists that his appointment as her health care agent empowers him to make decisions that respond to her current medical condition, even if they depart from her living will.

Tom is in a somewhat conflicted position because his two roles present competing interests and responsibilities. As a concerned son, his somewhat paternalistic approach is that advancing his mother's health and safety justifies overriding what he considers her self-destructive wishes. As a health care agent, however, his obligation is to represent what he knows of her wishes and values, unless they do not apply to her current situation. Unless he can demonstrate a reasonable likelihood that she would have changed her mind and accepted transfusions during the proposed surgery, her unambiguous living will and prior decision history argue forcefully for treatment that does not involve blood or blood products.

A clinical ethics consultation should surface these issues, explore the ethical reasoning, and help develop an appropriate care plan. Goals should include helping Tom to appreciate the importance of honoring his mother's long-held values. Skillful intervention should assist him in accepting that, while this would not be the decision he would want for himself or his mother, the refusal of blood is one of her core values, an essential part of who she is. His responsibility as her trusted agent includes being her voice and making the decisions that are authentic for *her*. He should be supported in making this very difficult decision and reassured that aggressive attention will be given to her medical needs, focusing on her comfort.

The consultation should also support Dr. Lewis's decision about whether he or another doctor should assume responsibility for Mrs. Dunn's care. He should be helped to understand that, if he cannot provide what he believes to be high-quality care within the limitations of the patient's wishes, he can meet his professional obligations by exploring alternatives. Considerations will include the potential for surgery without blood in this institution or transfer to a hospital that specializes in bloodless surgery. Because symptom management and end-of-life care will be important, a member of the palliative care service would be a helpful addition to the consultation. Additional guidance and support for Dr. Lewis might come from the institution's offices of legal counsel and risk management.

⫶ Mrs. Barnes is a 77-year-old woman who suffers from chronic obstructive pulmonary disease, peripheral vascular disease, and early dementia. During the six years that she has lived in the nursing home, her medical condition has remained fairly stable, although her cognitive status has gradually declined. Nevertheless, she is still able to interact with her family, care providers, and other residents, as well as make simple decisions about her daily activities. When she entered the nursing home, Mrs. Barnes completed a health care proxy, appointing her daughter, Carol, as her primary agent and her son, Philip, as the alternate agent. A living will executed at the same time contains care instructions, including a statement that she would not want dialysis if she were terminally ill or permanently unconscious.

Recently, Mrs. Barnes complained of chest pain and shortness of breath, and exhibited a change in her mental status, becoming more confused and agitated. She was admitted to the hospital, where tests revealed that she had suffered a mild heart attack and was in acute renal failure. Her attending and a renal consultant have recommended a few dialysis treatments to improve her kidney function and possibly clear her mental status while the extent of her heart damage is assessed. When her care team determined that she was unable to make care decisions or provide informed consent to treatment, the clinicians turned to her appointed health care agent and alternate. Carol has consented to the recommended dialysis, but Philip argues that such a course would violate their mother's living will. Carol responds, "If Mom had known that temporary dialysis might improve her condition, especially while we are waiting to see about her heart, she certainly would have agreed to that. What she never wanted was to be dependent on long-term dialysis or to have it just prolong her dying."

An ethics consult has been requested to help resolve the conflict.

This case also presents an inconsistency between a patient's living will and the decision of the appointed proxy agent. Two critical differences, however, should be appreciated and highlighted by a skilled ethics consultation. First, the provisions of the living will may not apply to the patient's current clinical condition. Until further clinical assessments are completed, it is not possible to know whether Mrs. Barnes is in an irreversible or terminal condition that she would find unacceptably prolonged by dialysis. Until that determination is made, dialysis may enhance the possibility of a successful outcome.

Second, the statements in the living will may not accurately or fully express the patient's wishes. Carol's knowledge of her mother provides insights that are not available in the written instructions. As a result, she is able to interact with the care team, respond to a clinical situation the patient did not anticipate, and interpret what her mother would want in current or future circumstances. Ethics consultation can provide the explanation and support that will reassure all parties that the proxy agent's authority and knowledge and the patient's trust enable her to make the decision that the patient would make if she could.

AUTONOMY IN TENSION WITH BEST INTEREST

III Mrs. Miller is an 88-year-old woman with obstructive and restrictive lung disease and severe chronically undertreated hypothyroidism. She was admitted to the hospital in respiratory distress, hypothermia, and hypotension and intubated in the ER. She has had several other admissions over the last six months for similar symptoms. She was extubated easily and is improving with treatment. She should be ready for discharge within the next week.

The staff is concerned about how Mrs. Miller's home situation has contributed to her medical condition. She lives at home with her 91-year-old husband, who has moderate dementia, and her 40-year-old son, Terry, who has psychiatric problems. Both Mr. Miller and Terry appear disheveled when they visit Mrs. Miller in the hospital.

Mrs. Miller appears to be neglected at home and is continually readmitted to the hospital in critical condition. Her colostomy has been poorly maintained, and it is uncertain whether the bruises on her arms are from senile purpura or physical abuse. She has some dementia even when she is receiving medication to keep her thyroid functioning normally and she seems unable to manage her care without help. After prior discharges, Terry has dismissed the visiting nurse service (VNS) or other help sent to the home.

Mrs. Miller's younger son, Larry, is her legally appointed health care proxy agent, but he does not visit and has been unwilling to be involved in her care. Attempted interventions by social service have been rebuffed. The family has been reported to adult protective services, but the results of that investigation are not known. In the past, when Mrs. Miller was treated and improved, she has stated consistently that she does not want to go to a nursing home. The care team is concerned about how to provide a safe discharge for her while respecting her wishes.

This case is a graphic illustration of the tension between honoring the patient's wishes and promoting her best interest. Arranging a safe discharge is the professional and legal duty of the health care team and the institution. Mrs. Miller's multiple and escalating care needs plus her limited ability to meet them mean that she should be in an environment, either her home or a skilled care facility, that provides assistance and support. Yet, she has clearly and consistently rejected the option of nursing home placement, choosing to return to a situation where her needs are not met and she is in jeopardy. In addition, the risk of elder neglect and abuse is substantial in this case, heightening the obligation to protect this vulnerable patient.

Capable patients have the right to make decisions about discharge, even decisions that appear to put them at risk. As the risk of harm increases, the level of capacity needed to understand the implications and accept the consequences is increased. Mrs. Miller's past decisions to remain at home, despite the apparent neglect that impairs her health and safety, require heightened scrutiny of her capacity to understand her risks and options. Because she was not receiving medication regularly, her thyroid malfunction resulted in periodic cognitive impairment. Her diminished or fluctuating capacity increases concern about her ability to assume responsibility for an unsafe living situation.

If Mrs. Miller is shown to lack sufficient capacity to make discharge decisions, that responsibility will fall to her health care proxy agent. The fact that Mrs. Miller appointed her son, Larry, indicates that she considered him the most reliable person to speak on her behalf. This trust should not be readily overridden unless the agent is shown to be incompetent, unwilling to make decisions, or acting clearly against the best interests of the patient. It would be important to encourage Larry's participation in the decision making. His lack of involvement may be the result of family dynamics, anger toward the patient, an estranged relationship, or incomplete understanding of his role as the proxy agent. He may need education and support so that he does not feel abandoned to make critical decisions alone.

Without an able and willing proxy agent, decision making for the incapacitated patient is challenging. One option is a court-appointed guardian. Drawbacks include the six to nine months the appointment process typically takes, during which she would be in an unsafe environment, and the guardian's lack of familiarity with her values and wishes.

The health care team's primary responsibility is to the patient, promoting her best interest and, if possible, respecting her wishes. While the team's function is not to do family therapy, minimizing the barriers to consensus can facilitate care planning. In cases like this one, bioethics consultation can perform a valuable mediation function by helping all involved parties to reach consensus on a discharge solution for the patient. Even if Mrs. Miller lacks the capacity to make discharge decisions, her assent to the plan would be critical to its success and to her feelings of self-determination. She considers nursing home placement unacceptable and, in attempting to balance her wishes with her safety, it would be important to explore with her the reasons she objects to residential care facilities and perhaps arrange for her to visit a few.

Social service involvement is necessary to discharge planning, which can touch upon very intimate family matters, as well as resource issues. Psychiatric counseling may be useful as well. Without assurance that necessary care services will be available and accepted at home, however, nursing facility placement may be the only responsible option.

III Ms. Powell is a 35-year-old woman who has been HIV-positive for ten years, presumably due to her history of IV drug use. She lives alone in a single-room occupancy (SRO) building, but she has been incarcerated in the past. She has been in and out of detoxification programs ten times and reports that her sister died of an overdose. She has not adhered to her anti-retroviral regimen, but details of her HIV care were not available. At her last methadone clinic appointment, she was noted to have anemia and increasing renal failure, and she presented to the ER with cough, fever, and flank pain. She was admitted and, because there was also a question of tuberculosis, she was placed in isolation.

In the ER, Ms. Powell was initially noted to be agitated and showing signs of opiate withdrawal but, when the physician returned to complete the exam, she appeared lethargic. This pattern has continued in the hospital and appears to coincide with the appearance of certain visitors. The house staff suspects that she is actively using heroin in the hospital and, because she was also receiving methadone, they are concerned for her safety. When asked, she denies drug use in the hospital.

The case has been discussed twice at staff rounds and several issues were raised. The initial concern was how to deal with Ms. Powell's apparent active drug use while in the hospital. The staff believes that, if all visitors are barred, she will probably sign out against medical advice. Questions included whether staff could legally search her belongings and how to guard against a fatal overdose if she is using heroin at the same time she is receiving methadone. At the second meeting, the focus was on whether to place a shunt for hemodialysis when the patient is believed to be an active heroin user, knowing that the shunt could easily be used to administer drugs. Another question was whether staff could refuse to continue caring for a patient who would not adhere to a treatment plan and puts herself at risk.

This is another instance in which clinicians' obligation to respect the patient's autonomy by honoring her wishes is in tension with their obligation to promote her best interest and protect her from harm. While no one is questioning Ms. Powell's capacity to understand the risks of her behavior, it might be suggested that her addiction makes her unable to control her behavior. In the continuum of capacity, the compulsion of an addict may become an impediment to understanding the risks and benefits of a proposed treatment or course of action. If a person can comprehend the risks intellectually but cannot behave in a way that demonstrates appreciation of the risks, the argument can be made that decisional capacity is lacking. Addicts are often well aware of the danger of their behavior and some genuinely do want to stop drug use. But the addictive nature of drugs prevents them from controlling their self-destructive impulses. Their capacity to understand is not translated into the behavior that would promote adherence to treatment or avoidance of risk.

The conflicts here concern both the patient's behavior and the care team's responses to it, and an ethics consultation can be useful in unpacking and analyzing the issues. While the clinical interaction is always a critical element, some situations are especially difficult for professionals. Here, the team faces the problems of substance abuse, institutional policies, and the obligation to promote the best interests of a difficult patient who is resisting help.

Drug rehabilitation treatment is often associated with temporary success and frequent relapses. Detoxification efforts require patience and persistence. The expertise of specialists who deal with active drug users is needed in this situation. The house staff was expending time and energy attempting to deal with the problem in a logical fashion, while lacking the experience and resources to do so. Their frustration stems from their inability to implement a beneficial plan of care or protect the patient from self-inflicted harm.

Establishing a good and trusting clinical relationship may be especially difficult with some patients. They may not be candid about their medical history or adhere to appointments and treatments; they may engage in disruptive and self-destructive behavior. While it is important to be empathic, patient, and persistent, doing so can be frustrating. Often a contract approach can be effective in setting limits. If the contract is reasonable and fair, and all parties can agree to it, this approach may facilitate the treatment program.

Placing a shunt sets up a therapeutic dilemma. Used for its intended purpose, the shunt would allow regular dialysis to improve Ms. Powell's renal function. Providing her with venous access, however, greatly increases the possibility of drug abuse and possibly overdose, as well as bacterial infection. In dealing with a capable patient, staff should initiate a thorough discussion of the risks and benefits of the procedure and hope that the patient makes the prudent decision. If the staff believes that the shunt will place the patient at significant risk, alternatives should be explored.

Health care professionals have a well-established duty to treat patients in need of medical care and not abandon them. Withholding dialysis, which has a clear benefit to Ms. Powell, because of a highly foreseeable risk of nonadherence, misuse, and infection may be considered paternalistic. The obligation to protect the patient from likely harm justifies staff concern, however, and this is best addressed candidly with Ms. Powell to see if she wants to take the risk of the dialysis shunt.

Transferring the patient's care to another professional because the clinician's values conflict with those of the patient may be justified if the conflict poses a significant barrier to communication or care. This can be done when the reason is explained to the patient and accepting clinicians are available. Transferring the treatment responsibility because the patient is difficult and frustrating may be less easily justified and should be carefully considered.

CONFIDENTIALITY

III Laura Chase is a 40-year-old woman who has been a source of anxiety to the MICU staff for thirty-six days, ever since she was admitted in severe sepsis and respiratory failure. According to the medical team, her condition is the result of a rare and virulent multi-drug-resistant infection that she developed in response to the multiple medications she takes for her HIV infection. Despite aggressive treatment, her condition has continued to deteriorate. In a relatively short time, she has gone from an active and healthy-looking woman to a patient who is intubated, sedated, and only intermittently aware of her surroundings. Her prognosis is very poor.

Mrs. Chase's unusual syndrome, young age, and rapid decline have made her the focus of considerable attention by the care team. Attending physicians, nurses, medical students, and house officers meet regularly outside her room to consider modifications in her treatment plan. Dr. Ewing, chief of the MICU, and Marianne Haber, clinical care coordinator, are particularly involved in managing her care and interacting with her family.

Laura's family consists of her husband, Frank, and her two sisters, Phyllis and Rita. Frank has been a constant and devoted presence at his wife's bedside. As her legally appointed health care proxy agent, he has taken an active role in learning about her condition and making decisions on her behalf. He and Dr. Ewing meet regularly to discuss Laura's prognosis and various treatment options. He has advocated using whatever drugs or other therapies might help her and give her a chance to beat this illness. Within the past week, however, especially as her condition has deteriorated, his daily visits have been getting shorter.

During one of their early meetings, Frank told Dr. Ewing that Laura's sisters are very worried about her and very angry with him. "They don't know that she's HIV-positive, so they cannot understand what is wrong with her. Laura never wanted them to know about her diagnosis and she has hidden it from them ever since she found out. She believes they would think she was worthless and she made me promise that they not be told. They know I'm not telling them everything and they think the worst."

Phyllis and Rita are very concerned about their sister and, as Frank indicated, very angry about what they perceive as people being less than candid with them. They suggest that Frank should be removed as the health care proxy because they believe he is a threat to Laura's safety.

Within the past few days, the care team has determined that the endotracheal tube should be replaced with a tracheostomy, which will be more comfortable and also lessen the risk of additional infection and bleeding. In this way, the intervention would both be palliative and potentially promote cure. When the recommendation was presented to Frank, he concurred with the reasoning but refused to consent to the procedure without the agreement of his sisters-in-law. Marianne has spoken at length with Phyllis and Rita, who appear to understand and even agree with the proposed trach but are adamantly opposed to anything that Frank approves.

Here, respecting the patient's autonomy by protecting her confidentiality has exacerbated a strained family dynamic and threatens to impede her treatment by interfering with decision making. The benefits of confidentiality include a respectful and trusting relationship between clinician and patient, and the patient's willingness to be candid about sensitive issues so that accurate diagnosis and effective care management can be achieved. Health care professionals have a duty to keep confidential any patient information learned in the course of the clinical relationship. Exceptions are usually related to situations that place others at imminent and significant risk of harm.

The capable patient can determine who should receive confidential information and under what circumstances. Laura has made it clear that she does not want her diagnosis shared with others, none of whom are placed at risk by her request. The proxy agent or surrogate is bound by the patient's wishes regarding health information. In this case, Laura has instructed her husband, who is her health care agent, that her HIV diagnosis not be disclosed to others and, unless others are placed at direct risk, her wishes should be honored.

Frank agrees to the recommended tracheostomy and feeding tube, but he wants the concurrence and support of Phyllis and Rita. His ability to act as Laura's decision maker is inhibited by the lack of consensus generated by their hostility. This intrafamilial conflict threatens to prevent or at least delay care that would clearly benefit the patient. While consensus among family members is a worthy goal, the primary responsibility of the health care team remains the patient. As Laura's appointed proxy agent, Frank is the person she chose and trusted to make decisions in case of her incapacity. Her wishes and values are to be expressed and implemented through him, although his job is made considerably more difficult by the constraints she has placed on what he can disclose. So long as he can competently and responsively function in this capacity, he should be supported by the team. The sisters' concern for the patient is also legitimate and should be acknowledged, but it cannot be allowed to interfere with care planning. In the event that consensus is not achievable, Frank may need support in consenting to the recommended treatment even without the concurrence of his sisters-in-law.

Bioethics mediation may be helpful in arriving at an appropriate plan of care and perhaps enhanced communication. The consult would seek to help Frank, Phyllis, and Rita focus on their shared concern for Laura and their mutual goal of identifying a care plan that promotes her best interest. Recognition that the care team supports Frank's decisions as responsible and beneficial may diminish some of the sisters' anxiety. Working to achieve these goals should not be confused with attempts to help the family resolve long-standing resentments and conflicts. Bioethics consultation is not family therapy and the focus should remain firmly on resolving the patient's care issues.

||| Mrs. Cole is a 32-year-old woman admitted to the MICU with bilateral pulmonary infiltrates and impending respiratory failure. Her hospital course has included treatment for AIDS-related opportunistic infections. While her clinical picture and past history are suggestive of AIDS, she has not been tested and has consistently refused to address AIDS as a possible diagnosis. She has required mechanical ventilatory support since admission. Prior to intubation, she told her mother, the nurse, and the social worker, "Don't let them label me with AIDS. I know they are thinking that and you can't let them do it."

Mrs. Cole's mother, Mrs. Davis, and her seven siblings have held a constant vigil during her forty-three-day hospitalization. Mrs. Cole's children, ages 7 and 14, appear to be in good health and visit often. Her husband of more than five years has been incarcerated for the past six months. Although Mrs. Cole is being treated for AIDS-related complications, her family has not been directly told her diagnosis because of her expressed wishes. Mrs. Davis, without asking the name of her daughter's illness, acknowledges that her immune system has been compromised. She has agreed to the use of AIDS-related medications if they are potentially beneficial to her daughter and, yesterday, consented to a DNR order. Mrs. Cole's death appears imminent.

Here, the confidentiality issue is complicated by the patient's fear and denial, and the threat posed to other parties at risk. Not only does Mrs. Cole not want her possible AIDS diagnosis revealed to others, she does not want to confront it herself. She is saying, "Don't tell my diagnosis to me *or* anyone else."

The duty of confidentiality precludes professionals from disclosing anything learned in the clinical interaction, whether from the patient or from diagnostic work-up. Based on patients' expectation of confidentiality, they are likely to feel safer seeking care and more comfortable discussing sensitive issues. Although she did not want to acknowledge her likely AIDS, on some level Mrs. Cole obviously recognized it as a possibility. Despite her anxiety, she sought treatment with the understanding that, if the dreaded diagnosis were confirmed, it would not be revealed to her or others. In other words, "Treat me for whatever I have, just don't say that it's AIDS."

Patients have the right not to know about their conditions if they request non-disclosure and treatment does not require an explicit label. Certainly, patients have the right to determine who has access to their personal information. Breaching confidentiality is justified only when withholding information places third parties at significant and imminent risk. The laws in many states include this exception to the confidentiality obligation to require notification of identified sexual or needle-sharing partners of patients with HIV/AIDS. The threshold at which confidentiality may be breached must be set fairly high to avoid casual disclosure of sensitive information.

Mrs. Davis, acting on behalf of her daughter, would likely have difficulty understanding the clinical situation or making sound decisions without complete medical information. Ordinarily, this would set up a conflict between the professional obligations of confidentiality and beneficence to the patient. Because she appears to recognize that her daughter has AIDS, however, she is providing consent without asking that confidentiality be breached. The implicit message is, "You don't have to tell me she has AIDS, just treat her for it."

Mrs. Cole's children, husband, and any other sexual or needle-sharing partners, however, are another matter because they are all at risk. Warning them (or, in the case of the children, those responsible for them) may afford timely diagnosis and treatment if they are infected and may also prevent further spread of HIV infection to unidentified third parties. The significant consequences justify breaching confidentiality and discussing with Mrs. Davis the need to test and potentially treat her grandchildren for HIV. How these sensitive issues are considered and handled will benefit from bioethics involvement.

In some instances, patients will discuss their medical conditions with their care professionals but insist that their diagnoses not be disclosed to their health care agents. These restrictions most commonly occur with stigmatizing conditions, such as HIV/AIDS. In such situations, every effort should be made to help the patient appreciate that the agent's ability to interact with the care team and make appropriate surrogate decisions will depend on his or her having the same clinical information that the patient would have in making decisions. Emphasis should be placed on the relationship of trust that underlies the proxy appointment and the agent's commitment to act in the patient's best interest.

Sometimes patients are more concerned about how the information will affect their relationship with the agent than they are with having it disclosed. Often the most distressing prospect is having to face the agent with information the patient may consider shameful. One approach is to ask, "Is there a time when you would feel comfortable having us tell your agent about your condition?" One patient with end-stage AIDS, whose mother was her health care agent, replied to this question, "When I'm too sick to see the disappointment in her eyes, then you can tell her."

DECISIONAL CAPACITY

⫼ Mrs. Andrews is a 77-year-old widow living in the community who was admitted via the emergency room encrusted with feces and covered with maggots. Her nutritional status was poor, and she was both malnourished and dehydrated. On medical examination she was found to have an umbilical hernia, bilateral knee contractures, urinary incontinence, multiple neurological impairments, and marked dementia. After surgery and physical and occupational therapy, her ambulation was improved but she remained incontinent.

In the hospital, Mrs. Andrews was noisy and disruptive and required a single room. When engaged one-on-one, however, she was charming and articulate. She was soon able to feed herself and after two weeks she is neither malnourished nor dehydrated.

Prior to her hospitalization, Mrs. Andrews had lived alone in an apartment in the same building as her son, his wife, and their three children. Her social security check is over $1,200 per month. Her son has no apparent source of support, other than a $500 check every other month from social security disability. It is not clear whether he has been misappropriating her funds, but staff suspect that might be the case. What is clear is that Mrs. Andrews cannot care for herself and her family does not seem willing or able to provide the support that she needs to keep herself clean, well-fed, and ambulatory.

The care team believes that Mrs. Andrews needs to be placed in a nursing home where she will receive consistent care. She has regularly refused this placement and said that she wants to return home. "What else does an old lady have in the world besides her children and grandchildren?" On other days she says, "I don't know what to do. Whatever my son says is fine with me." A liaison psychiatry consultation has concluded that "the patient has significantly impaired ability to form a judgment about her discharge plan."

Decisional capacity refers to the ability to process information, make decisions, appreciate their implications, and assume responsibility for their consequences. This ability is decision-specific because most people have the ability to make some but not all decisions. Capacity can be constant, diminished, or fluctuating. It can be exercised entirely by the patient, supported by others, or delegated by the patient to trusted surrogates.

Mrs. Andrews is a good example of a person with fluctuating capacity. Her ability to understand her situation and make decisions in her best interest appears to be affected by her medical condition, her dementia, and her anxieties about being in unfamiliar surroundings. She seems to benefit physically, emotionally, and cognitively from being in a setting where her care needs are met and she has regular interpersonal contact. Yet, she expresses the desire to return to her home and family, a situation that does not seem to promote her best interest and may put her at significant risk.

Discharge planning for Mrs. Andrews would require a benefit-risk assessment. If she goes home, she may not live as long as she could if she were to go to a nursing home, where she would receive the care she needs. Nevertheless, many elderly patients choose to return home, knowing that they may compromise the extent or the quality of their lives. The notion of "home" is powerful, encompassing one's possessions, memories, comfort, and sense of self. Even if the nursing home represents "better care," it can also be regimented, unfamiliar, and impersonal.

Yet, some patients who initially refuse placement eventually adjust to the nursing facility and do very well, especially in contrast to an unsafe home environment. Care providers need to advocate for the solution that they think is best for each particular patient and accept that, in some cases, patients will choose unwisely. Clearly, capable patients who make risky decisions are a source of concern to staff, even though their choices usually should be honored. The personal intellectual and emotional calculus of each patient is unique and not necessarily consistent with the rational, professional judgments of caregivers.

For many elderly patients, like Mrs. Andrews, however, there are moments of confusion or periods of diminished capacity. In these instances, consistency over time may be a substitute for total clarity. If every time the patient is clear, she answers the same way, this pattern of choice has weight in those times of some cognitive compromise. This is especially persuasive if her choices are consistent with her prior history of capacitated decision making.

The principles in tension are autonomy, beneficence, and nonmaleficence. Care providers have an ethical obligation to support the capable patient's exercise of autonomy. That obligation may, as in this case, come into direct conflict with the obligation to promote the patient's best interest and protect the patient from harm, especially if she is vulnerable because of diminished or uncertain capacity.

Finally, there is a difference between autonomously consenting to or refusing a medical intervention and choosing a home care plan. In the latter instance, the rights and interests of others besides those of the patient are at issue. In the home care context, the principle at issue is *accommodation,* that is, how the patient's wishes and desires can be met or modified by the ability or willingness of those whose cooperation is needed to carry out the plan. In this instance, the degree to which Mrs. Andrews' family can or will provide needed assistance is very uncertain. With the help of social service, it may be possible for her to return home if a home care agency and adult protective services can monitor her progress. If she is unable to safely remain at home, the nursing facility option can be revisited.

||| Mr. Jeffers is a 58-year-old man with a history of diabetes, hypertension, coronary artery disease, peripheral vascular disease, and cocaine use. He is divorced and his family consists of his mother, with whom he lives, his sister, and three adult children with whom he has limited or no contact.

Mr. Jeffers has undergone several toe amputations and a femoral-popliteal bypass operation to stem the vascular damage related to his diabetes. He has consistently refused recommended coronary artery bypass surgery and left the hospital last time against medical advice. He was admitted this time with shortness of breath and right foot cellulitis. Because of the worsening peripheral vascular disease, a below-the-knee amputation (BKA) may not heal adequately and an above-the-knee amputation (AKA) might be required. He has refused amputation and all diagnostic measures. His sister can sometimes convince him to cooperate for an examination or test.

Mr. Jeffers' capacity has been difficult to assess because he refuses to complete an interview. During the most recent evaluation, he said that his "foot is very sick" and that he does not want to die; however, he terminated the interview after a brief time. Although he signed consent for the BKA, he refused testing necessary to plan the surgery and said that his foot "will get better by itself." His capacity to weigh the risks and benefits of the care plan is unclear. Moreover, these benefits and risks cannot be identified or assessed without the additional tests that he is refusing. A successful outcome will require his cooperation over a long multistep recuperative period; the care plan is complex and the prognosis, even under optimal circumstances, is guarded. The amputation is not considered to be an emergency at this time, but will likely become one in the near future.

In this case, the consequences of decision making by a patient without capacity are more immediate and serious. Unlike Mrs. Andrews, Mr. Jeffers does not have the opportunity for leisurely decisions or timed trials. Refusing amputation may lead to death, while having the amputation should greatly improve the length and quality of his life.

It is important to assess Mr. Jeffers' capacity to make two decisions in light of his interests and values. The highly difficult decision about amputation has significant negatives, whichever course is chosen. To make an informed decision, he needs to understand fully the benefits and risks of both amputation and nonamputation. If he cannot make this potentially life-saving decision, he may still be capable of appointing someone, such as his sister, to be his health care proxy agent, with the authority to make the decision on his behalf.

Even if Mr. Jeffers lacks decisional capacity, he deserves care that demonstrates respect for him as a person. Forcing treatment, especially something as invasive as amputation, against his will poses serious threat to his dignity. Treatment over the objections of a patient, even one without capacity, can generally be justified only if there is a clear benefit to imposing the interventions. The less clear the benefit, the less acceptable the infringement of his right to noninterference. Here, the amputation may be the only thing that will preserve the patient's life.

Even if Mr. Jeffers is incapable of making informed decisions, he can and should be given the opportunity to provide assent, which also demonstrates respect for him as a person. If his sister can convince him to assent to recommended treatment, his cooperation with the care plan will facilitate surgery and recuperation. Without either his consent or assent, surgery may not be a safe or effective plan.

DISCLOSURE AND TRUTH TELLING

||| "I didn't know what to do," said Dr. Lewis, the intern. "I was about to go into Mrs. Gold's room to get consent for the colonoscopy when suddenly they were all there in my face saying, 'Don't tell Mama if she has cancer. Tell her anything else, but not that, not even that it's a possibility. It would kill her.'"

The "they" Dr. Lewis referred to were the grown children—a son and a daughter—of the patient who had been admitted two days ago. Mrs. Gold is an 82-year-old woman who was brought to the hospital by her daughter after several weeks of fatigue, weakness, and gastrointestinal disturbance. Her history and physical strongly suggested colon cancer and a colonoscopy would be necessary to establish the diagnosis and develop a treatment plan.

"I was so startled I just kind of nodded at them and mumbled something about not having anything definite to tell anyone yet," Dr. Lewis continued. "We all trooped into Mrs. Gold's room and they stood there while I explained that we needed her consent to do some tests to see why she is not feeling well. I don't know if I sounded as evasive as I felt. When I told my resident, Carol, what had happened, she was furious. She said that patients have the legal right to know their medical information and the family has no business telling us not to disclose it. When we made rounds the next morning, the family was waiting outside the patient's room and warned the team again. Carol explained about the patient's right to information and the son said, 'Listen, I'm a lawyer and I know all about rights. If you say anything that upsets or harms my mother, you'll find out firsthand what the law has to say.' Before things got even more tense, however, the attending, Dr. Martin, stepped in and assured the family that we would not do anything to put the patient at risk."

Mrs. Gold's tests have revealed that she does, indeed, have colon cancer. Dr. Martin put a big note on the front of the chart saying, "Patient is not to know her diagnosis as per instructions of family." There is considerable difference of opinion on the team about the appropriate way to handle the situation during the time she is hospitalized for surgery and subsequent treatment. The effort to avoid talking with Mrs. Gold about her condition has been very awkward for the house and nursing staff. Several people feel that they are being dishonest and not spending as much time with her as she deserves. Others feel intimidated by the threat of a lawsuit if they disregard the family's instructions.

Because truth telling is a moral obligation, withholding the truth requires a morally compelling justification. Benefits of patients knowing their diagnoses and prognoses include adequately informed decision making, better adherence to treatment, and a more trusting clinical relationship. The burdens to the patient of disclosure (anxiety, sadness, or other types of stress) have been empirically shown to be normally outweighed by the benefits of knowing the facts. The therapeutic exception to the disclosure obligation is a rare instance in which the information is expected to pose a significant and imminent threat to a patient (such as suicide or serious destabilization of an already fragile condition).

More often, concerned and protective families, such as the Golds, wish to spare the patient distressing information. These requests usually reflect the family's sadness about the patient's condition and the belief that, while it may not be possible to protect her from illness, it may be possible to protect her from anxiety and fear. Because they see themselves as shielding her from harm, it is important to avoid the adversarial climate that would be created by focusing on the clash of "rights."

Rather, the family's devotion to and intimate knowledge of their mother should be acknowledged and supported. Efforts should be made to determine how the patient has handled bad news in the past and what approaches have been successful. In addition, the cultural norm of truth telling varies widely and the patient's background and family dynamics should be considered in determining how and to whom information is provided. Finally, they should know that, because multiple health professionals are caring for Mrs. Gold, there is no guarantee that the information can be successfully kept from her.

Mrs. Gold should be approached, independently of her family, and asked what she knows about her condition, what she wants to know, how much she wants to be involved in choices about her care, and how much she wants her family to participate in decisions. She should be reassured that she can choose to know or not to know, to make decisions or voluntarily delegate that task to her children.

A bioethics consultation can help put the focus on the goal, shared by family and care team, of doing what is in Mrs. Gold's best interest. A collaborative resolution may be achieved by explaining that the quality of care the family wants for the patient depends on a trusting therapeutic relationship that includes open communication. The family should be helped to understand that, while lying to the patient is ethically unacceptable for care professionals, if Mrs. Gold indicates that she does not want medical information, she will not be burdened with it. If she requests information, it will be provided in a way that minimizes her distress. She will not be subjected to massive amounts of painful or confusing information all at once. Rather, her questions will be answered over time as part of a process that includes adequate support.

Sample chart note

Re: Edna Gold

Reason for consultation: Family's request to withhold clinical
    information from patient.

Mrs. Gold is an 82-year-old patient who has colon cancer, as revealed by colonoscopy. She has not been told her diagnosis and her son and daughter adamantly refuse to permit the care team to discuss her diagnosis with her. As they put it, if she were to find out she has cancer, or even to suspect that she may have cancer, "it would kill her."

Cases like this are not uncommon. Family members have mixed motives for not wanting their loved ones to get bad news: it may be partly to protect the patient and partly to protect themselves. Family wishes regarding disclosure should certainly not be disregarded or discounted, but they need to be carefully and critically examined.

First, we must determine whether Mrs. Gold possesses or lacks decisional capacity. Decisional capacity is decision specific, so we have to inquire whether Mrs. Gold is able to make specific decisions about her illness—about whether and how it should be diagnosed and treated. There is no indication that Mrs. Gold is incapable of doing this. Ethically and legally, a capable patient normally has the right to receive information about his or her diagnosis and prognosis, and to provide informed consent to tests and treatment. Though Mrs. Gold was not told why the tests were being done, it is open to question whether the doctors were required at that point to inform her of their suspicions. But once the tests revealed colon cancer, the moral situation changed significantly. The patient should have the opportunity to decide what, if anything, she wants to do about her illness. There is also a practical concern: if the patient undergoes chemotherapy and/or radiation, how will the nature of her illness be kept from her?

When family members say the truth would kill their loved one, this is the start of series of questions. What evidence do they have for saying this? How has she responded to bad news in the past? Are they afraid that she will kill herself and give up the will to live, or just that she will be depressed? Depression is normal when bad news is disclosed, but depression itself is not life-ending. An important part of the discussion should also address whether the patient herself has any suspicions about the nature of her illness. If she suspects something serious is wrong, but is not told, studies have shown that this only increases patient anxiety and sense of isolation.

I would explain to the family that, while we respect their viewpoint, we need to assure ourselves that the patient herself does not want to know her diagnosis. This is a matter of professional ethics. Questions, such as "How much would you like to know about why you are here?" can be asked without the family being present and may reveal the patient's true preferences without inadvertently disclosing the nature of her disease. If the patient lets us know that she does not want to be involved or wants to be involved only marginally, this should be respected. To lessen the family's anxiety, they can be told that the word *cancer* does not have to be used with the patient, since the word itself is frightening to many people.

III Mr. Wernick is a 30-year-old recently married man with metastatic testicular cancer. In a patient this young, the cancer, although very aggressive, should respond well to treatment. The recommended plan would be an orchiectomy (removal of the testis), followed by a course of systemic chemotherapy, giving him an excellent prognosis. Dr. Bond also knows that this regimen carries a significant risk of impotence and infertility.

Mr. Wernick has told Dr. Bond that he and his wife plan to begin a family as soon as possible. In fact, their shared love of children is one of the first things that attracted them to each other. Dr. Bond believes that knowledge of the likely side effects might well discourage the patient from undergoing the recommended therapy. His concerns are echoed by Mrs. Wernick, who stops him in the hall and says, "Just don't tell him about the possibility that he'll be infertile. We can always adopt. The important thing is to get him well."

In this case, the justification for disclosure is far more compelling. As a capable adult who has not waived his right to information, Mr. Wernick needs to assess what is in his best interest and make this important decision with full knowledge of the risks and benefits involved. Surviving cancer with a loss of function (impotence and infertility) may be an acceptable trade-off for some people but not for others. Armed with an understanding of the consequences, he may refuse potentially life-saving chemotherapy to avoid infertility, thereby increasing his risk of dying or he may choose life-saving therapy and alternative strategies for becoming a father. Manipulating information to influence his decision is unethical, preventing him from making an informed and autonomous decision.

Mrs. Wernick is deeply troubled by her husband's cancer diagnosis and what she fears will be his preference—to forgo life-saving treatment. Wanting him to accept chemotherapy and survive, she can encourage, persuade, and even pressure him. Although Dr. Bond has a primary duty to his patient, which includes disclosing information material to his decision, the wife's concerns should be addressed, even if her request to withhold information cannot be honored. Dr. Bond can offer support and counseling, including advice on the issues she might raise with her husband.

END-OF-LIFE CARE

III Lucy Ajuba is a 17-year-old from Kenya, who was diagnosed in January with a cancer that had invaded one kidney and metastasized to her bones, lungs, liver, and aorta. Given the extent of the metastases, her prognosis was determined to be poor. Lucy underwent surgery in June to remove the diseased kidney and began a nonexperimental course of chemotherapy, but she showed no improvement. She was placed on an experimental chemotherapy protocol, but a scan done in July showed new metastases in her bones. By the fall, Lucy was experiencing significant abdominal pain, but the use of a fentanyl patch brought her some relief.

Shortly after her increased pain problems, Lucy was admitted to the pediatric critical care unit (PCCU) in renal failure. She continued to experience significant pain and, despite the fentanyl patch, she was often very restless and unable to lie still, although every movement was painful. She was also terrified because she was clearly getting worse instead of better. For example, her abdomen had become quite distended and she repeatedly asked "why my belly is so big?" After a few days in the PCCU, she was stabilized and transferred back to the floor, but her remaining kidney was found to be heavily infiltrated with cancer.

Lucy is emotionally immature for her age and unusually dependent upon her parents, especially her mother. Before moving to this country, Mr. and Mrs. Ajuba had lost their only other child to malaria and they are very protective of Lucy. From the time of her diagnosis, they have insisted that she be told nothing about her medical status or prognosis. In spite of this, Lucy has indicated her awareness that her disease is serious and, more recently, that she is terminally ill. Both Mr. and Mrs. Ajuba are very religious and repeatedly express their faith that God will cure their child from what her father describes as a "white man's disease." They also insist that all aggressive measures be used to keep Lucy alive, although Mrs. Ajuba appears to be more realistic about her daughter's condition and prognosis.

Shortly after Lucy was transferred out of the PCCU, her oncologist recommended that, in light of her irreversible deterioration, a DNR order would be appropriate and that curative treatment should be replaced by aggressive palliation. After considerable resistance, her parents reluctantly agreed to the DNR, but the next day, her father rescinded the order. A few days later, Lucy's condition worsened and she was readmitted to the PCCU and intubated. Within the past twenty-four hours she has experienced four hypotensive episodes, each of which has been treated aggressively. She is receiving escalating support to maintain respiration, blood pressure, and other vital signs. In addition, she requires increasingly heavy sedation to manage her pain and agitation.

The treating team is concerned about continuing aggressive curative treatment that appears increasingly ineffective. Her oncologist has requested a bioethics consultation to engage the team and the family in considering appropriate end-of-life care.

Parents have discretion in making decisions about their children's health care because they customarily act in ways that promote the children's best interests. Their decisions usually are based on their own preferences and values because children are not mature enough to have developed long-range interests and goals. How best interest is defined depends on how the benefits, burdens, and risks are perceived and valued. In this case, the notion of best interest is disputed, with Lucy's parents arguing for continued life-sustaining treatment and the care team advocating a palliative approach.

Lucy's parents' wish to continue aggressive life-sustaining treatment may be multifactorial, including misunderstanding of the clinical facts and unrealistic expectations that must be addressed. They may not be getting the information necessary to understand Lucy's clinical condition or they may be unable to understand the information because of their educational level, their cultural background, their fears and suspicions, or the emotional stress of caring for a critically ill child. An additional barrier may be their understandable inability to face the possible loss of another child. Care professionals are expected to be sensitive to the importance of cultural values and traditions in decisions about health, life, and death, and should provide information, especially bad news, in a supportive and accessible manner.

Here, the key parties include the patient, even though she is a minor. Lucy clearly has indicated awareness of the gravity of her illness and a sense of isolation and fear because she has been excluded from discussion about her condition. Involving the adolescent in information sharing and decision making in the face of likely death is both extremely important and challenging. Paternalism may be justified if an adolescent is (1) not able to understand the information, or (2) too immature to act in ways that would be beneficial. As the adolescent grows and matures, these justifications progressively weaken. Even if minors are not able to exercise autonomous decision making fully, it is usually desirable to help them understand their condition and obtain their assent to the care plan.

An important goal of ethics consultation is to help the family and care team arrive at consensus on a care plan that promotes the best interest of the patient and addresses the concerns, values, and preferences of all parties. The dying child needs palliation of symptoms and reassurance. The grieving parents need clinicians to share the burden of difficult decisions and provide emotional support and access to additional resources. Barriers to consensus include family history and conflict, information imbalance, and cultural background. Through effective communication and mediation, the parties may be able to reach agreement on mutually acceptable goals and plan of care.

III Mrs. Ewing is an 86-year-old widow with dementia and severe heart disease. She lives in a nursing home, where she has been bedridden for a year. She occasionally speaks and follows some commands, but does not communicate in a consistent fashion. It is uncertain if she recognizes any of her family members or the people who care for her.

Mrs. Ewing was transferred to the local hospital, where she is being treated for congestive heart failure. Despite aggressive medical treatment, her condition has remained grave. Fluid has been removed from her lungs via a needle in the chest wall (thoracentesis), only to reaccumulate in two days. Recognizing that the prognosis is poor, her physician has addressed the treatment plan with her family. Her daughter has become extremely upset and insists that "everything should be done" for her mother. Mrs. Ewing's son, a dermatologist who does not live in town, has been in telephone contact and says, "Do whatever you have to do to keep her alive." He insists that his mother be transferred to the intensive care unit and that a second thoracentesis be performed.

The attending physician has explained that the available interventions would be painful and possibly unsafe, and would not likely alter the disease course. A permanent chest tube would need to be placed to continue withdrawing fluid, and Mrs. Ewing might require mechanical restraints to prevent her from pulling out the tube or the intravenous lines. If she has a cardiac or respiratory arrest, which is almost certain to occur soon, attempted resuscitation would likely be unsuccessful. If she were revived, she might face uncomfortable days on a respirator before her death. He advocates for a palliative care plan. The family remains adamant, however, stating that "nothing is worse than death."

Like parents of dying children, the adult children of dying parents often issue instructions to "do everything" or ask for specific interventions judged to be therapeutically ineffective or otherwise inappropriate. How these requests are handled can determine not only the effectiveness of the care plan, but also the residue of family comfort or guilt after the patient has died. If Mrs. Ewing's children believe that she was deprived of life-saving treatment because they were not good advocates, her death may be seen as their preventable failure. As an initial matter, then, ethics consultation should seek to defuse any sense of a power struggle with the family on one side demanding treatment and the professionals on the other side withholding it. The focus should begin and remain on the shared goal of identifying and promoting the patient's best interest.

Requests to "do everything" are a signal that the parties may not share the same understanding of the patient's condition and prognosis, the goals of care, the available treatment options, and the expected outcomes of the interventions being requested. The fact that Mrs. Ewing's son is a physician does not mean that he can be entirely objective in assessing the clinical situation. He may be experiencing the same unrealistic hopes for improvement as his sister and the same need to advocate for all available treatments. Indeed, as the family's in-house medical professional, he may feel additional pressure to effectively manage his mother's care.

Among the first things to determine are what "do everything" means to the family and what the interventions in question are expected to accomplish. Discussion should focus on clarifying the goals of care, the likely effectiveness of the proposed treatments in achieving those goals, the obligation to prevent suffering without benefit, and further explanation of the recommended plan of care. The family should be reassured that, while improvement is no longer feasible, comfort is an achievable priority that will receive the full attention of the team. The notion of aggressive palliative care as active intervention should be reinforced.

Ethics consultation can also reaffirm the special moral standing of the family. Mrs. Ewing's children may have intimate knowledge of her wishes that could inform the goals of care. Engaging in a benefit-burden assessment of the treatment options, including what is known about the patient's values and preferences, would be useful in decision making. If her wishes are unknown, the analysis should be based on the best interest standard. Discussion can emphasize their critical role in protecting Mrs. Ewing from interventions that will increase her suffering without providing benefit. In the event they disagree about care, the focus should be on their shared concern for their mother's well-being.

Physicians' concerns about honoring family requests may also need attention. Physicians are not obligated to follow every family demand, some of which are for medically inappropriate or futile treatment. Problematic requests should trigger discussion, clarification, and mediation where appropriate. Guided by their professional judgment and personal moral codes, physicians may legitimately refuse some requests. Their position, rationale, and commitment to the patient, as well as their offer to transfer the patient's care to another doctor, should be made clear to the family.

Limitation, either scarcity or expense, of resources introduces an additional and uncomfortable ethical element into the decision-making mix. If the decision is made to "do everything" for Mrs. Ewing, should she be given access to expensive resources, including a bed in the ICU? What if a critically ill 32-year-old also needed the bed? What makes sense clinically may not be the most appropriate course of action. Even if the decision is made to treat Mrs. Ewing aggressively, it is still ethically appropriate to weigh her medical needs against the needs of others, when resources are limited.

FORGOING LIFE-SUSTAINING TREATMENT

‖ Mrs. Martel is a 61-year-old hospital employee admitted for total abdominal hysterectomy (bilateral removal of uterine tubes and ovaries) and debulking for stage IV ovarian cancer. In the recovery room, she was without heartbeat for five minutes and suffered significant anoxic brain damage, although she retains brainstem function. She has been comatose but responsive to pain for one month and her care team believes that there is no chance for improvement.

The family has consented to a DNR order and has presented letters attesting to the fact that Mrs. Martel "would never want to live connected to tubes." Her husband and children have requested that she receive only comfort care and that artificial nutrition and hydration be stopped. Legal counsel and risk management are comfortable with the family's decisions, but the nursing staff is very troubled by this course of action. Since surgery, Mrs. Martel has been on an acute care floor where the notion of limiting life-sustaining treatment is disquieting. The nurses feel that they are doing nothing but turning the patient and, because she is receiving IM Dilantin to prevent seizures, they are causing her additional pain with the injections. They think that she is becoming congested and might be having difficulty breathing. Above all, they are distressed by the notion of discontinuing nutrition and hydration and "starving the patient to death."

In contrast to the family that wants everything done, the family that wants to forgo treatment can also present an ethical challenge for care professionals. Despite family consensus and caregiver understanding of the legal and ethical principles, limiting treatment at the end of life can be counterintuitive and disturbing to those whose mission is to preserve life. An ethics consultation can be very useful in helping care providers and families articulate their concerns and in reassuring them about the validity of the care plan.

A capable adult patient has a well-settled right to make an informed decision consenting to or refusing treatment, even if the decision leads to her death. These wishes can be expressed contemporaneously or prospectively. An appointed health care proxy agent can make these decisions on behalf of the incapacitated patient, based on wishes expressed in an advance directive, substituted judgment, or the best interest standard.

Absent an advance directive, the family is often best suited to represent the patient because of their long-standing and intimate relationship. The family is usually accorded a significant degree of discretion in making decisions for the incapacitated patient, although some states restrict the authority to limit treatment. Ethically, there should be a presumption that the family's knowledge of and concern for the patient is the best guide in making decisions about end-of-life care. While Mrs. Martel had not executed an advance directive or appointed a proxy agent, her family is agreed on what she would want in her current situation.

Legally, as well as ethically, there is no distinction between withholding and withdrawing life-sustaining treatment (LST). The key issues are (1) whether the interventions are benefiting the patient or contributing to suffering and prolonging the dying process, and (2) whether the patient or the surrogate believes they should be forgone. Yet, withdrawing artificial nutrition and hydration (ANH) feels different because of its association with nurturing. The notion that forgoing ANH at the end of life is starving the patient to death needs correction. Palliative care professionals should clarify for family and staff that withholding or withdrawing ANH from patients near death does not create hunger or thirst and, in fact, has been shown to often relieve discomfort during the dying process. Some religions and cultures stress the symbolic meaning of food and water and do not permit withdrawing or withholding ANH. Both ethical analyses and legal rulings, however, discuss ANH as a medical treatment like other interventions whose benefits and risks should be assessed in care planning.

The concerns of caregiving staff should always be considered in care planning but, in this situation, they deserve heightened attention. These acute care nurses are unaccustomed to limiting life-sustaining treatment, which they find clinically counterintuitive and ethically troubling. In addition, they are caring for a colleague with whom they cannot help but identify. The nurses need reassurance that they are doing a great deal for Mrs. Martel and her family by keeping her comfortable and treating her with professionalism, concern, and respect. The focus should be that, when cure or improvement is no longer feasible, the goals of care shift to maximizing comfort, minimizing suffering, and not prolonging the dying process. Involving the palliative care service in the planning and delivery of care should be educational and supportive for the nursing staff.

One important function of bioethics consultation is working with staff, including medicine, nursing, social work, and administration, to clarify and analyze difficult ethical issues. Sometimes, more than one meeting is indicated to address multiple sets of issues. Here, bioethics might meet with the nurses to address their concerns and meet again with the family and care team to discuss the goals and plan of care, with particular attention to the most effective clinical setting. In this case, the palliative care or hospice unit is probably better equipped to attend to the patient's end-of-life needs, including identifying alternative methods for administering Dilantin and easing respirations. A bioethics consultation that includes palliative care professionals can reassure the family that, rather than a lower or less attentive level of care, the palliative care service provides expertise in symptom management at the end of life.

GOALS OF CARE

||| Frankie Abruzzi is a 31-year-old man, currently in the ICU in grave condition. He has a history of IV drug abuse, which he stopped seven years ago when he tested positive for HIV. For the past five years he has been on antiretroviral therapy. Also significant in his medical

history is a heart valve replacement due to endocarditis contracted as a result of his drug use. According to his parents and immunologist, Dr. Stern, who has known him for several years, Frankie has coped fairly well emotionally with his condition and has been very conscientious about taking care of himself. Recently, Frankie and his wife divorced, but he has maintained contact with his young daughter.

Frankie was referred by Dr. Stern to Dr. Heiken, an oncologist, because of an elevated white blood count. He was admitted to the hospital for a bone marrow biopsy, which revealed a very early stage of leukemia. Interferon was started but discontinued shortly thereafter because Frankie continued to spike fevers, one of the side effects of interferon. According to Dr. Heiken, Frankie's leukemia is definitely treatable.

While in the hospital, Frankie developed abdominal swelling due to fluid buildup. He also developed an acute retroperitoneal bleed coming from his right kidney, which was removed. During surgery, Frankie became hypotensive for a protracted period and he has not regained consciousness. He is intubated and attempts to wean him from the ventilator have proved unsuccessful. He has developed left kidney failure, for which he has received dialysis on three occasions. Because of low blood pressure, however, dialysis has had to be discontinued, at least temporarily.

Frankie has no health care proxy or living will. His family consists of his two parents and a sister, all of whom seem genuinely concerned about doing what is best for Frankie and sparing him any unnecessary suffering. Yet their approaches to his care are very different. Mrs. Abruzzi and her daughter, who want to spare Frankie further needless suffering, have requested a DNR order and the withholding of dialysis and other cure-oriented treatment. In contrast, Mr. Abruzzi contests the DNR order and argues for continuing all other aggressive treatment because "Frankie is a fighter and he wouldn't give up." Dr. Stern advocates a palliative care plan that focuses on Frankie's comfort. Dr. Heiken explains that he cannot agree with forgoing resuscitation, dialysis, and other treatments because Frankie's condition is potentially reversible and he might be "salvageable." He says that, if the family decides to withdraw treatment, it will be difficult for him to be Frankie's physician and he will ask Dr. Stern to assume care of the patient.

The concept of autonomous decision making is based on the notion that capable patients are in the best position to make care decisions consistent with their own values and interests. The concept of surrogate decision making is based on the notion that people who know and care about the incapacitated patient will make the decisions he would make if he were able to do so. These insights into what matters to the patient inform the goals of care.

The difficulty arises when trusted and well-meaning surrogates have differing ideas of what the patient would want or what would be in his best interest. Frankie's devoted family members are advocating for the goals they each believe are best for him. His two doctors also have differing goals for Frankie based on their respective assessments of his clinical condition and prognosis. These well-intentioned but conflicting perspectives threaten to create a stalemate in care planning, interpersonal tension, and residual family conflict following Frankie's death.

Achieving consensus on a plan of care requires that the family and care professionals agree on the goals of care. A bioethics consultation would promote a review of what is known about Frankie's interests and values in light of what is known about his medical condition. Expectations of what continued treatment can accomplish should be clarified in light of Frankie's condition. Through discussion of the diagnosis, prognosis, treatment options, and patient wishes, the parties can reach a mutually acceptable plan of care with clearly defined goals (such as time-limited trial of specific critical care interventions).

The consultation should also consider Dr. Heiken's motivation to continue aggressive curative care in light of the clinical realities and his possible concerns about liability. Withdrawing life-sustaining measures, thereby allowing death, is sometimes confused with euthanasia or physician-assisted suicide. In other instances, physicians may act on strongly and deeply held convictions that prevent them from acceding to patient or family wishes. An available option, suggested by Dr. Heiken, is to transfer the patient's care to another physician.

III Mrs. Pelz is a 105-year-old woman who was admitted from home with pneumonia. She lives with her daughter, Mrs. Dean, who is her health care proxy agent. For four years prior to admission, she was alert but noncommunicative, able to go from bed to chair and eat a little.

In the ER, Mrs. Pelz was intubated with her daughter's consent. Since admission, she has suffered multiple complications, including vaginal infections, pneumothorax, infections around the chest tube, and malnourishment because of poor intake. She is receiving nutrition and hydration through a nasogastric tube and antibiotics intravenously. She is currently not responsive, although her pulmonary function is improving enough that she may be able to be weaned from the ventilator.

Mrs. Pelz's prognosis is very poor and it is almost certain that, even with aggressive measures, she will never return to baseline. Her condition and prognosis have been explained to her family, including the likelihood that continued aggressive interventions will increase her suffering without providing benefit. According to Mrs. Dean, her mother had never expressed care wishes, except to say that she never wanted to be in a nursing home.

Mrs. Dean has authorized a DNR and stipulated that, if her mother is able to be weaned from the vent, she should not be reintubated and, if the nasogastric feeding tube is removed, it should not be replaced. She has based these decisions on her mother's irreversible condition and her belief that they will promote her mother's best interest by sparing her further needless suffering. Mrs. Pelz's granddaughter and great-granddaughters strenuously object to Mrs. Dean's decisions and want all supportive and curative measures continued. Their maturity and understanding of the clinical realities appear very limited, however, creating unrealistic expectations and resistance to information that is inconsistent with what they want to hear. The situation is complicated by dysfunctional family dynamics that create a passive-aggressive pattern of interaction between them and Mrs. Dean, who seems very isolated and anxious.

Even in the best circumstances, it is difficult for families to make decisions for critically ill patients. While the Abruzzi family members differed in their goals for Frankie's care, they were mutually supportive in their search for consensus on a way to promote his best interest. In contrast, decision making for Mrs. Pelz is complicated by family anger, guilt, denial, dysfunctional history, and conflicting interests, all of which are barriers to decision making.

An ethics consultation should begin by acknowledging the difficulty of the decision process and commending the family for struggling to do the right thing for the patient. Physician clarification of the clinical situation may help them recognize that the patient is dying and that care goals must accommodate that reality. When cure or improvement is no longer feasible, the goals of care become maximizing comfort, minimizing suffering, and not prolonging the dying process.

Bioethics mediation should be attempted in an effort to help the family resolve conflicts that are impeding care planning. Mrs. Dean needs special support in advocating for her mother's best interest in the face of overwhelming resistance and antagonism from her children and grandchildren. As the appointed proxy agent, she is empowered to make care decisions without family consensus and even without the guidance of her mother's explicit wishes. While family consensus is desirable, the care team's primary duty is to the patient and her best interest.

All parties should recognize that mediation is not family therapy. This family brings long-standing conflicts that will not be resolved in the clinical setting. What bioethics consultation can do, however, is emphasize the importance of leaving their interpersonal problems aside and focusing on their shared concern for Mrs. Pelz. The objective is to help family members give themselves permission to protect the patient from the burden of interventions that are no longer benefiting her.

Sample chart note

Re: Abigail Pelz

Reason for consultation: Clarification of patient's condition, prognosis, goals, and plan of care.

Mrs. Pelz is a 105-year-old woman with multiple health problems related to a recent respiratory insult and her generally debilitated condition. Despite aggressive interventions, she continues to deteriorate and will almost certainly not return to baseline. According to her attending and consulting physicians, she is dying. Her daughter, who is her health care proxy agent, has accepted the inevitability of her mother's death and requests no further cure-oriented interventions, but her granddaughter and two great-grandchildren appear to have unrealistic expectations, are reluctant to let go, and insist on pursuing aggressive treatment.

An ethics analysis considers the goals of care in the light of the patient's diagnosis and prognosis, the treatment options, and what is known about the patient's wishes. The benefits, burdens, and risks of therapeutic options are evaluated in terms of the patient's well-being. These considerations receive heightened scrutiny when, as here, the patient's condition is grave and irreversible, her prognosis is very poor, the treatments likely to benefit her are limited, she is unable to participate in decisions, and she has not communicated her health care wishes.

Under these circumstances, the goals of care focus on providing treatment that will benefit the patient without increasing her suffering or prolonging the dying process. To prevent unrealistic family expectations, it is especially important to distinguish why interventions are contemplated and what they are likely to accomplish. These issues were addressed during a meeting that included the patient's daughter, granddaughter and her husband, two great-grandchildren, the attending physician, resident, clinical care coordinator, rabbi, and bioethics consultant.

According to the care team, this patient will almost certainly not recover, despite aggressive treatment. For this reason, it would be clinically counterproductive and ethically unsupportable to burden her with additional cure-oriented interventions that would contribute to her suffering without providing benefit. Here, it is appropriate to help the family protect the dying patient from unnecessary and ineffective treatment. Accordingly, the team encouraged the family to recognize the limits of the patient's endurance, as well as the limits of what medicine can accomplish, and to focus on the goal of promoting her comfort and peace during the dying process.

The agreed-upon plan is that the patient will remain on the vent, finish the current course of antibiotics, and continue to receive nutrition and hydration, but that no additional curative treatments will be started. All measures to enhance her comfort will be pursued. It will be important to help the granddaughter and great-grandchildren to support patient's daughter and each other by recognizing their shared concern for the patient and the importance of acting together in her best interest.

INFORMED CONSENT AND REFUSAL

||| Mrs. Daws is a 57-year-old woman presenting to the ER in respiratory distress and hypoxia. She has a history of stage IV breast cancer, diagnosed five years ago, chronic schizophrenia, and mild retardation. She was treated briefly with chemotherapy, which was discontinued because she found the side effects so distressing. The cancer has metastasized to her ovaries and, following surgery three months ago, she was transferred to the medical center's long-term care facility for palliative chemotherapy. When she experienced shortness of breath today, she was brought to the ER. She is refusing intubation.

Her appointed health care agent is her husband, who is moderately mentally retarded. He is devoted to her and wants to be involved in her care. He is unable to understand her clinical condition or accept her terminal prognosis, however, and his anxiety is steadily increasing his agitation.

Mrs. Daws' level of cognitive function appears to be adequate for participation in care discussions and decisions. She seems to understand, certainly better than her husband, that she has breast cancer and that she will not recover from it. She understands, with appropriate apprehension and sadness, that there is no treatment that will make her better. The most compelling evidence of her decisional capacity is reflected in her long, close, and trusting relationship with her primary care physician and oncologist, Dr. Meyer. According to Dr. Meyer, she and the patient have engaged in many long discussions about her condition and care. In her opinion, Mrs. Daws appreciates the gravity and irreversibility of her condition.

The professionals caring for Mrs. Daws are very uneasy about whether to honor her refusal of intubation if her respiratory distress increases. The care team, including Dr. Meyer and clinicians in the ER, critical care, and pulmonary, all agree that intubation will not benefit her in the long term and that, once intubated, she will not be weanable. In the past, Mrs. Daws has been consistent, as she is today, that she does not want to die and wants treatment continued so that she can live as long as possible. She is also consistent in her refusal of intubation but it was not initially clear whether she would agree to intubation if it were the only way to remain alive.

For several reasons, Mrs. Daws is a patient who should be considered especially vulnerable to the risks of uninformed decisions with grave consequences. Her uncertain baseline capacity (compromised cognitive function and emotional instability), plus the current lack of clarity about her wishes and possible hypoxia, raise troubling questions about her ability to assume responsibility for refusing life-sustaining treatment. Further, her only family is her husband, whose cognitive deficits prevent him from functioning as an informed surrogate or even a stable support. Indeed, his emotional distress is distracting her from focusing on her own situation. Under most circumstances, this patient would not be considered to have the ability to provide informed refusal of intubation.

Two factors alter the usual analysis. First, Mrs. Daws has a long and trusting relationship with Dr. Meyer, who has known and cared for her during the past several years. She is very familiar with the patient's level of understanding, wishes, values, and fears. She knows, for example, that Mrs. Daws is afraid of suffering and does not want to subject her husband to watching her distress. She has consistently asked Dr. Meyer to promise that she will not be in pain. Second, Dr. Meyer and the rest of the care team are convinced that intubation would contribute to the patient's suffering without benefiting her. A considerably higher degree of capacity would likely have been required for the patient to refuse life-sustaining interventions that the team considered to be in her best interest.

Dr. Meyers thus provides a combination of supported autonomy, substituted judgment, and best interest analysis. Her personal and medical knowledge enables her to support the patient and her husband, and refocus the goals of care toward the palliation that is needed.

MEDICAL FUTILITY

‖ Bobby, a 6-month-old boy, was brought to the ER in full cardiac arrest by Ms. Clark, his 18-year-old mother. While bathing the infant, Ms. Clark had told her 2-year-old to watch the baby while she went to the kitchen for a moment. When she returned, Bobby was face down in the bathtub and not breathing. In the ER, he was successfully resuscitated and then transferred to the Pediatric Critical Care Unit (PCCU). At first, although he required oxygen support, he was able to breathe on his own. He also demonstrated reflexive responses to noxious stimuli. Within about twelve hours, however, he experienced respiratory failure and was intubated. At that time, all other outward indications of brainstem activity ceased. Although repeated neurological tests failed to confirm brain death, the consensus was that the baby would not regain responsiveness or any other meaningful brain function.

In conversations with Ms. Clark, the PCCU attending has attempted to explain Bobby's condition and prognosis, but she is unwilling or unable to entertain the possibility that her child will not recover. She has great trouble understanding and remembering what the physicians have told her and has some very unrealistic ideas about possible treatments. She has asked whether a brain transplant would be possible using her own brain and wanted to know whether the baby could be cloned. She is preoccupied with her responsibility for Bobby's near drowning and is unable to focus on discussions about end-of-life care, a DNR order, or transfer to a long-term care facility. She visits daily and, despite occasional glimmers of understanding, she continues to insist that her baby will make a full recovery. Although several tests now have confirmed brain death, she adamantly refuses to accept the determination or consider removal of mechanical supports.

The definition of medical futility has physiologic, qualitative, and quantitative components. The concept may be unhelpful except for the narrowest definition—failure of an intervention to achieve its therapeutic goal—which was applicable in this situation. Given Bobby's profound and irreversible neurological condition, interventions aimed at cure or improvement would be futile. Measures aimed at keeping him alive, however, might have been effective, although they would never lead to reversal of his brain damage. Now that brain death has been confirmed, mechanical supports are merely perfusing his organs, but will not return him to life. Helping his mother accept the reality of these distinctions is an essential but difficult part of the therapeutic interaction.

Ms. Clark's insistence on continued aggressive curative treatment is based on her poor understanding of medical information, compounded by her denial, guilt, and anger. The unimaginable pain of a parent unable to rescue her child is infinitely worse when she is responsible for the harm. The result is unrealistic expectations of and demands on staff, as well inability to begin the grieving process. These factors need to be addressed by the care team, including psychosocial support and counseling.

The controversial nature of futility, including where to draw lines limiting care, is inherently value-laden and subject to dispute. A critical judgment is who should make these assessments and decisions. While clinicians should not be the sole decision makers, it is unfair to ask families desperate for signs of improvement to recognize on their own when those hopes are unrealistic. Acknowledging the limits of medicine can begin the process of shared planning for what *can* be done in the patient's best interest.

Although the death of a child is always a tragedy, the determination of brain death is appropriate when supported by clinical and laboratory findings. Determination of brain death in a young child, especially one under a year old, is clinically and emotionally challenging for the care team and the family. Bobby's mother needs to be reassured that he is not suffering and that the care team will attend to his needs in a compassionate and dignified manner. Given her emotional fragility and protective denial, reasonable accommodations, discussed in chapter 6, are certainly appropriate for a specified time before mechanical supports are removed.

A final issue raised by this case is the relationship between futility and resource allocation. ICU care and life-sustaining treatment are scarce and/or expensive. The health care organization has a duty to be a judicious steward of community resources. A challenging question for the institution is whether parents' inability to accept their child's brain death because of psychological, philosophical, or religious barriers justifies continuing expensive medical care that ultimately drains community resources. Futility—the failure of an intervention to be physiologically effective—must be distinguished from misapplication of a scarce resource. Application of a scarce resource may work, but may be ruled out by the competing need of other patients. Grappling with this issue is the ongoing obligation of responsible health care organizations as they craft ethically principled policies and procedures.

PARENTAL DECISION MAKING

||| Luke is a 14-year-old boy and a long-term survivor of congenitally acquired HIV infection. His father, Mr. Bradley, is a physician's assistant, and makes all decisions regarding family medical care. Luke's mother died of AIDS and was cared for by Mr. Bradley during her illness. Nevertheless, Luke was not tested for HIV infection until he was 12 years old, at which time he tested positive. His father has been very resistant to the notion of telling Luke his diagnosis.

The medical center became involved in Luke's care shortly after his diagnosis. At that time, PCP prophylaxis and antiretroviral therapy were recommended. Mr. Bradley initially refused both, but finally was persuaded to start PCP prophylaxis with Bactrim. After his son had been on Bactrim for three weeks, Mr. Bradley discontinued medication without notifying the care professionals. The interruption in treatment was discovered during the next clinic visit, at which time Mr. Bradley explained that Luke had developed a fever and headaches, potential side effects of Bactrim. PCP prophylaxis was reinitiated with Dapsone instead of Bactrim. Again, he developed a fever and headaches and his father discontinued both the antibiotic and PCP prophylaxis.

During the summer, Luke developed neurological symptoms, including sleepiness, acting out, hypersexuality, and gait problems. In the fall, the cause of the symptoms was identified as HIV-related encephalopathy, an incurable condition that is AIDS-defining. Luke's symptoms currently are causing him a great deal of suffering. He is aware of what is happening to him, although the consensus is that he does not have decision-making capacity. He cries out that he is dying and believes that he is crazy. He is difficult to control and care for, creating disruption and distress at home. His 10-year-old sister has threatened to run away from home because of his behavior and its effects on family life. Psychotropic medications have been used to treat the effects of the encephalopathy but, because of adverse side effects, his father has discontinued all medications other than Ativan.

Care professionals have recommended that Luke receive D4T, an antiretroviral drug that will not produce a cure, but could ease his dementia and other neurological symptoms. Mr. Bradley has been considering this course of treatment, but has not made a decision to reinitiate antiretroviral treatment. Currently, Luke is (1) suffering severe symptoms caused by his encephalopathy; (2) receiving only Ativan, which is not providing significant symptom relief; and (3) not receiving medication, namely D4T, that might improve his symptoms.

Parents are typically accorded the responsibility for making health care decisions for their minor children, based on their presumed knowledge of and concern for them. The theory is that parents' mature judgment will enable them to act in ways that promote their children's best interest. Especially when the child's life is at stake, parents are usually not permitted to withhold beneficial treatment.

In this case, Mr. Bradley is indecisive about the treatment plan for many possible reasons. He may be experiencing some or all of the following emotions: denial that his child is dying, fear of losing his child, emotional stress of caring for a critically ill child, and a desire to protect his child from the distressing side effects of treatment. These barriers will have to be addressed by the care professionals in order to promote an effective care plan for Luke. Psychosocial support for the father may include involving additional support persons (other family members, friends, spiritual advisors), providing information in a comprehensible way, and allowing time for him to grasp the information and reach a comfortable decision.

Palliation of suffering must be the focus of the care plan. The effort should be to encourage Mr. Bradley to support the provision of medication that, while not curing Luke, will manage his symptoms. He should know, however, that his son's palliative needs will be met, even over his objections, and that clinicians will not withhold appropriate treatment because of his indecisiveness, beliefs, or values, however well intended. The crucial task is to empower the father and collaborate with him in ensuring that his child's best interests can be met.

Every medical intervention comes with potential benefits and side effects, some predictable, some unpredictable. The benefits of antiretroviral therapy are uncertain, as is the exact trajectory of Luke's disease. Decision making in the face of uncertainty is difficult, for patients, families, and clinicians. It is especially painful for the parents of sick and dying children, who feel powerless to make them better. Parents need consistent help from the care team, including regular consultation, counseling, and support.

Whether and how to involve the adolescent in the decision making is an individualized judgment that depends on numerous factors. The timing, manner, and content of the disclosure about his condition depends on what he knows, what he wants to know, the level of his maturity, and his ability to grasp and process the information and appreciate its implications. Here, although Luke has not been told explicitly that he has HIV/AIDS, his recollections of his mother's illness and his awareness of other sources of information make it likely that he suspects his diagnosis. The fear and isolation that he may be experiencing should be explained to his father in an effort to help him understand why Luke needs more open communication about his disease and treatment, and support and comfort during the dying process.

SURROGATE DECISION MAKING

▌▌▌ Mrs. Charles is a 47-year-old woman without significant medical history. She is employed as a watch and clock repairer, and came to the ER with a swollen right thumb several days after sustaining an injury to that thumb at work. She was admitted and underwent surgical incision, drainage, and evacuation of suspected compartment syndrome. Following surgery, her condition deteriorated and she developed overwhelming sepsis and multiorgan system failure. The following day she underwent repeat surgery for necrotizing faciitis. Her condition continued to decline and, despite aggressive treatment, she remained dependent on ventilatory support, pressors, and hemodialysis. She required heavy sedation to manage her agitation. Several days after admission, she exhibited peripheral vascular compromise and developed dry gangrene of all extremities. Orthopedic evaluation established that bilateral amputation of both hands and both feet would be necessary to preserve her life.

The care team met with Mrs. Charles' family to explain her grave condition and the fatal prognosis without amputation. Although the patient had not appointed a health care proxy agent or executed a living will, her family was certain about what her decision would be under the circumstances. Her husband, father, and two siblings were united in their opinion that Mrs. Charles would not want to live without her hands and feet. They related numerous examples of her fierce independence. In addition to the delicate nature of her work, they cited her hobbies, which include playing guitar, skiing, and sailing. They repeated that, even if her life could be saved, the loss of her hands and feet would deprive her of the ability to do the things that bring her pleasure and the self-sufficiency so important to her. Knowing her preferences and values, they agreed that she would reject the surgery, even if death were the result.

The gravity of the decision's consequences prompted the care team to attempt lightening Mrs. Charles' sedation in an effort to engage her in a discussion of her options. When the sedation was decreased, however, the patient became very agitated and hypertensive, and the plan was abandoned. It looked as though the decision about amputation would have to be made by her family, and the consensus was that she would not be able to tolerate life as a multiple amputee.

The next day, as plans were being made for surgery, the care team tried once more to lighten the sedation and, this time, Mrs. Charles responded well. When she was alert and interactive, the care team and her family engaged her in discussion about her condition and options. To everyone's surprise, she insisted vehemently and repeatedly, "If the only way to keep me alive is to take off my hands and feet, then go ahead. Do whatever you have to do, just don't let me die."

Decision making on behalf of patients without capacity uses the following standards in order of preference: the patient's wishes as expressed directly through discussions with others or in advance directives; substituted judgment when the patient's wishes are known or can be inferred; or, absent information about what the patient would choose, what is determined by others to be in the patient's best interest.

All states permit decisions about care, including end-of-life care, to be made by surrogates, based on the patient's explicitly expressed or documented wishes. Depending on the laws in the state where the patient is receiving treatment, these decisions may also be based on substituted judgment or the best interest standard.

An advance directive would have provided clear information about Mrs. Charles' wishes regarding some circumstances but perhaps not a situation as unanticipated as her current condition. Even without explicit instructions, however, her family had the benefit of knowing her values, preferences, decision-making history, and reaction to disability and dependence. Ideally, those insights could be confirmed contemporaneously by lightening her sedation enough to engage her in a discussion of her condition, prognosis, and options. Because that strategy did not appear to be feasible and time was running out, the decision fell to those who know her best. They were prepared to make the decision they genuinely believed she would make if she knew what they knew about her situation.

Given the gravity of the decision, the care team has a heightened obligation to ensure that the family clearly understands all the options, alternatives, and their implications. Efforts should also be made to confirm that the surrogate decision is grounded in promoting the patient's wishes and interests, rather than other considerations. In short, the team's obligation is to build in as many safeguards as possible to prevent a life-threatening mistake.

The unexpected twist to this case—Mrs. Charles' decision to proceed with the amputations—provides a cautionary postscript. Even when family or other surrogates are well-intended, convinced, and unanimous about what they believe the patient would choose, they may still be wrong. Like Mrs. Charles, patients who are suddenly faced with their own mortality may surprise even themselves by making choices they would not have anticipated. A critical take-away message is that, whenever possible, all efforts should be made to elicit and act on the patient's current wishes about current circumstances.

||| Mr. Feder is a 79-year-old man with end-stage dementia who was transferred to the hospital from the nursing home for treatment of pneumonia. He also has advanced metastatic prostate cancer. In the course of the diagnostic work-up, he was found to be suffering from a leaking aortic aneurysm, bilateral muscle abscesses, and an impacted bowel. The abscesses were drained and the impaction was relieved. He was started on a course of antibiotics and given a blood transfusion. The only remaining clinical issue is the aneurysm and the question is whether to perform a surgical repair.

This patient's profound dementia has left him with little responsiveness to his surroundings. He does not interact verbally, although he sometimes responds to simple commands and indicates discomfort by withdrawing from painful stimuli. His attending, Dr. Allen, says that Mr. Feder usually appears comfortable, although his recent medical problems caused him discomfort, which was evident in his behavior and reactions to clinical interventions.

According to Dr. Allen and the consultants from neurology and vascular surgery, repairing Mr. Feder's aneurysm will reduce the likelihood of a fatal rupture, but it will not improve his cognition or responsiveness. His pain will be increased postoperatively and the surgical mortality can be as high as 30 percent. Mr. Feder cannot understand his medical condition or the treatment options, and he is unable to participate in discussions or decisions about his care. He has no family or friends who might be involved in treatment planning.

Mr. Feder is an example of what has been described as the patient alone—an individual without decisional capacity, family, or other surrogates to participate in decisions about care. Patients alone are especially vulnerable because neither they nor anyone else who knows them can advocate for their interests. Without explicit information about Mr. Feder's wishes from recollected statements or advance directives, or inferences about his preferences based on knowledge of his values and decision patterns, the care team must rely on the best interest standard in determining the most appropriate course. This analysis requires others, in this case the care professionals, to consider what they believe will promote his best interest.

One criterion that is typically assessed, especially in the face of irreversible illness, is what effect the proposed intervention will have on the quality of the patient's remaining time. While quality-of-life judgments are usually reserved for the patient or those close to him, in this case that evaluation falls to his care providers. This analysis, assessing the relative benefits, burdens, and risks to the patient that would be expected as a result of the surgery, is reflected in the chart note following a bioethics consultation.

Sample chart note

Re: Kevin Feder

Reason for consultation: Question of the appropriateness of surgery
for this patient.

This patient is a 79-year-old deeply demented man, admitted with pneumonia, metastatic prostate cancer, bilateral muscle abscesses, and bowel impaction. The pneumonia, abscesses, and impaction have been treated. A CT scan revealed a leaking aortic aneurysm and the question is whether it should be surgically repaired. I have discussed this case with the house staff, Dr. Allen, the attending, and Dr. Owen, the vascular surgeon. Following these discussions, I reviewed the case with Dr. Masters, the director of medicine.

This is a patient with little or no responsiveness to the world. He is reported to be generally comfortable, except during his recent medical problems. His cognitive status and ability to respond or interact will not be improved by surgery and his pain and discomfort will certainly increase. He has no ability to comprehend his medical situation, consider his options, or participate in making treatment decisions. The consensus of the treating team is that surgery will not substantially improve his condition.

This is a patient for whom the goal is comfort rather than cure. The appropriate plan is palliative care to ensure that he is as comfortable as possible, while avoiding aggressive curative measures, such as a surgical intervention that will only increase his pain and will not provide him with any improved quality of life. For this reason, both Dr. Allen and Dr. Owen expressed reluctance to intervene surgically. They both expressed concerns about his pain and suffering, as well as the surgical mortality, which could be as high as 30 percent in a patient with these characteristics. They both stated that, if the patient had family to participate in medical decision making, they would be comfortable with a decision not to intervene. Because this patient is alone with no family and no friends, he should not be automatically consigned to aggressive intervention that will not benefit him.

Dr. Masters, in a bioethics consultation on this case, stated that, if both treating physicians agreed, he would concur with medical management and aggressive palliative care.

PART III

White Papers, Memoranda, Guidelines, and Protocols

Allocating critical care resources: Keeping the teeth in ICU triage
Justice and access to unreimbursed therapies
Guidelines for transferring patients between services
Decision-making protocol for the patient alone

A key function of your ethics committees is education—of your members and your institution. The quality of committee deliberations reflects the depth and breadth of knowledge members bring to the consideration of ethical issues that arise in the clinical and organizational settings. The utility of committee recommendations about institutional practices depends on the ethical analysis that supports them. Explaining all this to administrators, trustees, and clinical staff members enhances broader understanding of the issues, their significance, and their resolution.

One way in which ethics committees can prepare for these functions is by researching and writing about topics with particular relevance to their work and their institutions. Often, committees are asked to provide insights about an especially challenging issue. Sometimes, policy review or an untoward event triggers a closer look at how situations are or should be addressed. Occasionally, a topic in the news stimulates a desire to learn more about developments with ethical implications. Depending on the topic and the needs of the committee, these reports can take the form of detailed white papers or brief memoranda.

Because most committees are composed of busy health care professionals with interest but little formal training in ethics, your discussions will be more fruitful if members are armed with the background and key issues of selected topics, their significance in the clinical or organizational setting, the underlying ethical principles, and guidelines for implementing recommendations. While your committee is unlikely to need the breadth and depth of white papers on a regular basis, their time-consuming preparation can be most efficient and effective if a few members work together as a subcommittee whenever this level of attention is required. More often, an informational memorandum that states the issue, lays out a brief background and ethical analysis, and offers recommendations will provide useful structure for committee discussion.

In addition to preparing memoranda and the occasional white paper, ethics committees often develop guidelines and protocols that may eventually be formalized. These models are typically the result of clinical or organizational situations for which no plans of action or reasoning currently exist. Recognizing the likelihood that these scenarios may recur and wanting to avoid reinventing the wheel each time, committees find it useful to draft strategies for discussion and possible pilot testing.

The following are examples of materials developed by a medical center bioethics service, often with the help of one or two members of the ethics committee. To save time and enhance member familiarity with the issues, the documents were distributed to the full committee in advance of the meetings during which the topics would be addressed.

One white paper ("Allocating Critical Care Resources") and one memorandum ("Justice and Access to Unreimbursed Therapies") illustrate how selected topics can be researched and presented as useful committee resources. They served as discussion guides during deliberations and as the analytic framework for the committee's recommendations to the medical center's clinical and organizational staff. "Guidelines for Transferring Patients between Services" and "Decision-making Protocol for the Patient Alone" are examples of draft strategies to improve clinical and organizational processes. These working documents are offered as possible models for ethics committee response to selected situations that might benefit from structured appraisal and recommendation. They can also usefully inform clinical practice, ethics consultation, and inservice teaching.

ALLOCATING CRITICAL CARE RESOURCES: KEEPING THE TEETH IN ICU TRIAGE

JACK KILCULLEN, M.D., J.D.

More than almost any other clinical resource, the allocation of beds in the intensive care unit (ICU) generates controversy because it is both scarce and life-saving. Consequently, critical care physicians possess an ethical responsibility unique among their colleagues (outside the realm of organ transplantation) because they cannot advocate exclusively for any given patient, but must direct treatment in the ICU to the patients most likely to benefit. These decisions demand a thorough understanding of the complex interplay of a patient's underlying chronic illness and immediate threats to hemodynamic stability. Given the dangers of delay, these decisions must often be made quickly, knowing that there will now be one fewer bed available for the next patient seeking help.

Unlike the allocation of donated organs, the allocation of ICU beds is done without the authority of federal law, the safety of committee deliberation, or the methodical review among all competing preselected patients. It is often made only by a fellow and an attending, in the middle of the night and in the midst of other clinical pressures.

More important than the lack of a waiting list is the fact that the patient for whom the ICU physician must save a bed could be the one still racing to the hospital. As unwilling as our society is to confront the concept that health care has limits, rationing is a long-accepted, yet always vexing part of critical care medicine.

To the family stunned by a loved one so close to death, the critical care staff has a special responsibility to provide understanding and compassion and to promote acceptance of painful clinical realities as they become inevitable. Palliative care professionals when available can help moderate the emotional pain for families with the offer of clear comfort-based measures for the patient, thus underscoring the reality that death is imminent.

Yet, complicating the already challenging process of triage is the rare patient's family members who, often with the involvement of their own physicians and senior hospital staff, bring pressure on the ICU attending to accept patients who lack any clinical claim to these beds. The effect is to undermine the ICU attending whose authority is established by specialized training and experience. The individual triage process becomes exponentially time consuming, distracting him from clinical responsibilities. The result of a forced admission, beyond depriving someone who might later need the bed, is a polluting of precedents established by more evidenced-based decisions, leading to further distrust within the institution and future demands for "special treatment." For the critical care attending, who has enough pressures to bear, this loss of institutional support can cut deeply into that shallow reservoir of morale.

The bioethics committee's purpose in considering ICU triage is to establish the proper institutional commitment to a just allocation of one of its most precious resources. For patients at the end stage of life, there are specific points that the committee should address:

- When brain death is strongly suspected, this determination shall be made while the patient remains at his or her current location, be it the emergency room (ER), the general floor, or the ICU. Patients in the ER determined to be brain dead may be admitted to the general floor to accommodate the family beginning to adjust to their loss. In no instance should the patient be admitted to the ICU once brain death has been determined.
- Patients with irreversible comorbid conditions who present with a potentially reversible acute deterioration may, after stabilization in the ER, continue to receive limited aggressive intervention on the general floor with consultation by critical care medicine in a manner consistent with the limits of floor nursing. Palliative care services will be incorporated with these limited interventions to support the patient and family during this difficult and ongoing acceptance process.
- Patients unknown to the medical staff who present with strong evidence of irreversible and rapidly progressive disease may be admitted to the ICU for

stabilization and rapid confirmation of this dire diagnosis. They may, thereafter, be transferred to the general floor for palliative care.

- The ultimate authority for all ICU triage decisions by the ICU attendings rests with the director of critical care medicine.

PRINCIPLES RELATED TO CRITICAL CARE PLACEMENT

The following principles and guidelines use the term *triage* in reference to decisions about patient admission to, clinical management in, and transfer from critical or intensive care units. It is an ongoing active process integral to patient assessment that requires continual reexamination of the perceived need to be treated only in the ICU.

The Society for Critical Care Medicine published guidelines (Society of Critical Care Medicine, 1999) for the allocation of ICU beds in an attempt to ensure they be reserved for those who have a reasonable prospect of substantial recovery. The society encourages hospitals to articulate their own admission and discharge criteria in the light of their own available resources. The guidelines provide a classification system of descending priority. The highest priority is given to those requiring continuous and aggressive management in the face of ongoing instability (patients in shock or respiratory failure). The second priority goes to patients who need increased monitoring because they are at high risk for developing a life-threatening condition. The third priority is directed to unstable patients who have underlying terminal conditions that might be successfully stabilized but whose longevity is curtailed. Finally, there are those either too well to require ICU care or those who are so sick that, despite aggressive care, death is most likely imminent.

BRAIN DEATH

It would seem unnecessary to state that the threshold assessment of a patient newly arrived in the ER is whether she is alive. Yet, determining that neurological function has ceased down to below the brainstem is more involved than merely palpating for a pulse. This institution's policy requires an initial clinical assessment with subsequent confirmation by a physician credentialed by the Department of Neurology or Neurosurgery. A neurologist or neurosurgeon must then review the findings and, if necessary, specify whatever lab tests he considers necessary before attesting in the chart to the final outcome.

The state legislature, in recognizing that death can be defined as a permanent loss of brainstem function, gives considerable discretion to the hospital in how this determination will be made. As busy as the ER can become, it is still realistic to assume that its staff or others with appropriate credentialing could establish the necessary basis for a neurologist or neurosurgeon to make a determination in the vast majority of cases.

Because a patient who has likely suffered brain death is considered clinically and legally dead, *admission to the critical care setting is never appropriate*. Such an admission would ignore established criteria for ICU admission, which require that the patient be likely to benefit from the critical care setting and, therefore, would be counterproductive to the family's acceptance of the death.

If a family has moral or religious objections to brain death as a determination of death, state law allows hospital admission to reasonably accommodate the family as it begins to accept the death or makes arrangements for transfer to a facility where cardio-pulmonary support may be continued. These reasonable accommodations (e.g., not disconnecting the ventilator, continuing nutrition and hydration, continuing medications) should take place after transfer from the ER to another location in the hospital, but *not to the critical care setting*. The clinical staff should emphasize that the accommodations are for the benefit of the family, not the now-deceased patient.

LIMITED AGGRESSIVE TREATMENT OUTSIDE THE ICU

Acute Deterioration in a Patient with Irreversible Comorbid Conditions

The vast majority of terminally ill patients arriving in the ER are best described as "pre-hospice." They are stricken with profound disease, such as metastatic cancer or end-stage dementia, and often require substantial support to maintain life, including nursing home care, tube feeding, and mechanical ventilation. They come to the ER on multiple occasions with acute, often infectious, illness. Yet their families see the immediate deterioration as an isolated event and seek ICU admission, anticipating recovery sufficient to return them to their most recent setting.

On an informal basis, ICU admission rarely occurs. Critical care fellows and attendings need only invite a family member to describe the patient's previous six months in order to elicit how frequent these admissions have become. When the fellow observes that the patient appears to be at the end of life, most families see how easily this truth arises from their own words. Even though the patient in the ER has now been intubated and stabilized on vasopressors, families can appreciate that care on the general floor is more appropriate because it is more accommodating. They are explicitly told that the care plan is not to "do everything" and that floor nurses are not watching every patient at every moment. Still, they can agree that limited treatment (e.g., antibiotics) along with comfort measures can allow for the hope of recovery to be preserved while realistically letting "nature take its course." The inclusion of a professional palliative care service is invaluable in helping the family cope with whatever ensues. Nurses can turn over micromanagement of the ventilators to respiratory therapists. Any titration of infusions is handled by house staff. Thus, the general floor teams have become able to handle this limited aggressive care, knowing that the critical care physicians are always within reach.

CONFIRMATION OF A DIRE DIAGNOSIS

In unusual and compelling cases, a patient unknown to the hospital staff who is often only recently symptomatic may arrive in the ER with a subacute complaint, only to be found to have striking evidence of advanced terminal disease, usually a malignancy. Work-up may reveal multiple highly suspicious masses in both lungs or masses in the liver or scattered throughout the abdomen. For the family and patient, the news is completely unexpected and can be devastating.

When the patient is unstable and otherwise headed for the ICU, diversion to the floor because of a strongly suspected terminal diagnosis can further traumatize an already frightened family. Compassion would dictate that the patient be stabilized in the ICU and that a rapid tissue diagnosis be sought confirming the worst. Not only will the family be spared the immediate anxiety of the acute crisis, it will be possible to provide irrefutable evidence necessary to face the painful truth squarely. Transfer to the floor thereafter may be necessary for triage, especially if the patient has been stabilized hemodynamically. By that point some relationship of trust should have been established that would not otherwise have occurred had probability alone dictated the decision.

FINAL AUTHORITY FOR ICU TRIAGE SHOULD REST WITH THE DIRECTOR OF CRITICAL CARE MEDICINE

When the family of a patient at life's end stage becomes adamant in demanding ICU admission, the process risks disrupting the hospital. Often, the family's private physician may be asked to apply pressure on the ICU fellow or attending. Alternatively, the ER physician may feel targeted by the family's ire. Eventually, the case may reach the level of the medical director, who may be called on to intervene.

Ultimately, the decision ceases to be a medical one. If, over the objections of the director of critical care medicine, a patient is placed in the ICU, the decision invalidates the specialty nature of managing critically ill patients. It creates an adversarial climate and hinders the collaborative and trusting relationship essential for effective care. Most of all, it puts the patient's family in the role of physician, dictating the level and location of care.

No right exists to an ICU bed for every person whose life might be prolonged by unlimited medical care. Federal law, under the Emergency Medical Treatment and Active Labor Act (EMTALA), requires only that patients be evaluated and stabilized in the ER before the hospital transfers them elsewhere. Statutory and common law regarding malpractice requires adherence to a physician's general duty of care to a patient as physicians so define it.

Just as a heart transplant team cannot be expected to rescue every patient with a failing heart, the ICU staff cannot create beds where none exist. We risk denying a 30-

year-old woman in eclampsia ICU admission because the last bed was just given to a 90-year-old demented man septic from his third bout of aspiration pneumonia. Justifying that decision to the husband of the pregnant woman is far more difficult than explaining to the man's daughter that critical care started in the ER will continue to a limited degree on the floor and not in the ICU. The role of the hospital medical director is to support the decision of the critical care medicine staff and explain to the family how the institution can properly care for their loved one through medical and palliative services consistent with the best standards of the profession.

ETHICAL GUIDELINES

The Medical Center Code of Ethics articulates the following overarching institutional commitment: "We recognize that our primary mission is to ensure the provision of high quality, ethically based patient care."

The fundamental ethical principle of respect for patients underlies the health care institution's commitment to patient well-being and confers organizational obligations to promote clinical excellence, collaborative case management, and wise stewardship of resources. These institutional responsibilities require that patients be cared for in the most appropriate clinical setting, which, in the hospital, means the service with the most targeted skills and resources.

- Clinical decisions, including determinations of the most appropriate plan and locus of care, depend primarily on the patient's care needs, the therapeutic options, and the professional staff and technical resources available to provide the needed care. Particular attention should be given to the interventions that can and cannot be provided on each service.
- Triage criteria should be derived from evidence-based data about the clinical resources necessary to maximize therapeutic outcomes.
- Triage decisions should recognize that critical care is a resource and a set of clinical skills, not a location. Aspects of critical care can be delivered in non-ICU settings.
- The therapeutic objective is to provide only care that benefits the patient, without imposing unnecessary suffering or prolonging the dying process. When cure is no longer possible, the patient's comfort and dignity remain the focus, requiring close collaboration with the palliative care service.
- Patient requests for critical care and family or surrogate advocacy on behalf of patients should be considered but they are not dispositive in decisions about placement in ICUs. Decisions about admission to and transfer from ICUs are not to be dictated by patients or families. Care providers have an obligation to use clinical judgment, establish boundaries, and provide guidance and support in the triage process.

- Budgetary and bureaucratic concerns, while important to deliberations about resource allocation, must not impede or compromise the care of individual patients.
- Patients and families must be helped to understand the changing clinical picture and the goals, potential, and limits of critical care in order to prevent misunderstanding, unrealistic expectations, disappointment, and confrontation.

REFERENCES AND ADDITIONAL READING

Bone RC, McElwee NC, Eubanks DH., Gluck EH. 1993. Analysis of indications for intensive care unit admission: Clinical efficacy assessment project: American College of Physicians. *Chest* 104(6):1806–11.

Charlson ME, Sax FL. 1987. The therapeutic efficacy of critical care units from two perspectives: A traditional cohort approach vs. a new case-control methodology. *Journal of Chronic Disease* 40(1):31–39.

Emergency Medical Treatment and Active Labor Act (EMTALA), 42 U.S.C. §1395dd et seq. Examination and treatment for emergency medical conditions and women in labor.

Griner PF. 1972. Treatment of acute pulmonary edema: Conventional or intensive care? *Annals of Internal Medicine* 77:501–6.

Kalb PE, Miller DH. 1989. Utilization strategies for intensive care units. *Journal of the American Medical Association* 261(16):2389–95.

Kollef MH, Canfield DA, Zuckerman GR. 1995. Triage considerations for patients with acute gastrointestinal hemorrhage admitted to a medical intensive care unit. *Critical Care Medicine* 23(6):1048–54.

Kraiss LW, Kilberg L, Critch S, Johansen KH. 1995. Short-stay carotid endarterectomy is safe and cost-effective. *American Journal of Surgery* 169(5):512–15.

Manthous CA, Amoateng-Adjepong Y, Al-Kharrat T. 1997. Effects of a medical intensivist on patient care in a community teaching hospital. *Mayo Clinic Proceedings* 72:391–99.

Mulley AG. 1983. The allocation of resources for medical intensive care. In President's Commission for the Study of Ethical Problems in Medicine and Biomedical and Behavioral Research. *Securing Access to Health Care.* Washington, DC: U.S. Government Printing Office 3:285–311.

Multz AS, Chalfin DB, Samson IM, Dantzker DR, Fein AM, Steinberg HN, Niederman MS, Scharf SM. 1998. A "closed" medical intensive care unit (MICU) improves resource utilization when compared with an "open" MICU. *American Journal of Respiratory and Critical Care Medicine* 157(5):1468–73.

Oliver MF, Julian DG, Donald KW. 1967. Problems in evaluating coronary care units: Their responsibilities and their relation to the community. *American Journal of Cardiology* 20(4):465–74.

Ron A, Aronne LJ, Kalb PE, et al. 1989. The therapeutic efficacy of critical care units: Identifying subgroups of patients who benefit. *Archives of Internal Medicine* 149:338–41.

Society of Critical Care Medicine Guidelines for ICU Admission, Discharge, and Triage. 1999. *Critical Care Medicine* 27(3):633–38.

JUSTICE AND ACCESS TO UNREIMBURSED THERAPIES

The following memorandum had its origins in discussions with the Medical Center Heart Transplant Program about justice issues related to access to ventricular assist devices (VADs). In researching these issues, however, it became apparent that VADs were but one instance of the following generic problem confronting the Medical Center and other health care institutions: an expensive technology that can potentially benefit large numbers of people has recently received or is likely to receive Food and Drug Administration (FDA) approval, but reimbursement for its use will be significantly delayed. How should the lack of reimbursement enter into organizational decision making about providing the therapy? The same question arises for many new pharmaceuticals that are awaiting or have recently received FDA approval. The issues and reasoning in this memorandum, therefore, have much wider application than to VADs alone.

BACKGROUND

A recently completed study, Long-Term Use of a Left Ventricular Assist Device for End-Stage Heart Failure—dubbed the REMATCH study (Randomized Evaluation of Mechanical Assistance for the Treatment of Congestive Heart Failure)—compared the device with the latest drugs for patients with the most severe heart failure. The study found that the risk of death was 48 percent lower among patients who received the device, compared with those who received the most potent cardiac drugs. Although mortality was statistically reduced, few of the study patients who received the assist device survived longer than two years. The authors of the study conclude the following: "The use of a left ventricular assist device in patients with advanced heart failure resulted in a clinically meaningful survival benefit and an improved quality of life. A left ventricular assist device is an acceptable alternative therapy in selected patients who are not candidates for cardiac transplantation" (Rose et al., 2001, p. 1435).

Cardiac assist devices are extremely expensive. Associated costs are estimated to be about $68,000 to $71,000 for the device itself and about $160,000 for the pre- and postsurgical and medical care during the twenty-five- to thirty-day hospital stay required for left ventricular assist devices (LVADs). Balanced against the costs of the new technology are the possible savings from factors like reduced need for hospital admissions and years of life gained.

The FDA has approved the use of ventricular assist devices as a bridge to transplant and, as of November 2002, as a destination therapy as well. The important distinction is that a bridge therapy is used as a necessary support only until a more permanent or destination therapy, in this case, heart transplant, is available. Prior to its FDA approval as a destination therapy, the use of VADs for that purpose could not be reimbursed by Medicare or private insurance. Now that the FDA has approved VADs as a destination therapy, the question will be whether Medicare will pay for them. This public policy issue will likely be debated in Congress and it is unclear how long it will be before VADs are approved for Medicare payment when used as destination therapy.*

VADs are but one example of a new generation of cardiac devices that hold out the prospect of benefiting large numbers of patients. Two other recent examples are implantable cardiac defibrillators (ICDs) and drug-eluting stents.

A recent study, entitled Multicenter Automatic Defibrillator Implantation Trial II (MADIT II), found that the death rate in patients with a prior myocardial infarction and advanced left ventricular dysfunction can be reduced by over 30 percent with small devices called implantable defibrillators. The study also expanded considerably the number of patients for whom ICDs could be indicated. Estimates of the number of patients who meet the criteria of the MADIT II trial are between 400,000 and 600,000 (Moss et al., 2002). At the same time, the device itself costs about $20,000 and the surgical costs are around $10,000. With the number of new patients each year who could benefit from the device plus the three million patients who already have had serious heart attacks and could be helped, the total potential costs are enormous. FDA approval of the device for this large patient group is expected shortly and much of the cost burden is likely to fall on Medicare.†

The newest device in this area is the drug-eluting stent. Studies seem to indicate that this new type of stent is significantly better than bare-metal stents in preventing restenosis. Hospital administrators and device manufacturers are predicting that there will be a rapid conversion from bare-metal to drug-eluting stents and a slightly less rapid conversion from coronary artery by-pass graft (CABG) to the new devices. These next-generation stents are projected to cost between $3,000 and $4,000 each. FDA approval is not expected until the third or fourth quarter of 2002, with Medicare funding expected to follow.‡

THE PROBLEM OF DELAYED REIMBURSEMENT

LVADs, ICDs, and drug-eluting stents share a number of common features and raise similar ethical problems. In each case, when the number of patients appropriate for the device is multiplied by the costs of the device and the care associated with it, the total expenditure is considerable. In each case, FDA approval has either recently been obtained or has not yet been obtained but is expected in the near future.

Finally, in each case, there is a temporary issue of reimbursement because the decision

* Medicare reimbursement for LVADs as destination therapy was approved in 2003.

† In July 2002, the FDA approved the MADIT II indications for the first ICD, and, in June 2003, the Centers for Medicare and Medicaid Services (CMS) approved coverage for a select subgroup of MADIT II patients. The FDA has since approved several other ICDs, and CMS has expanded its coverage.

‡ Two drug-eluting stents received FDA approval for sale in the United States, one model in April 2003 and another in March 2004. Codes for Medicare funding became effective July 1, 2003.

by Medicare to cover the device is not expected until after FDA approval. Even after FDA approval, reimbursement is delayed because each new device is typically assigned a unique ICD-9 billing code, which is used to compile one year of cost data in order to determine appropriate coverage. As a result, hospitals must often wait a long time, sometimes years, for reimbursement that adequately compensates for the costs associated with these technological breakthroughs. This delay places hospitals in a financially precarious and ethically uncomfortable position. They must consider whether and to what extent they are prepared to take a financial hit by providing patients with FDA-approved devices before Medicare and other insurance reimburse for them.

ETHICAL PRINCIPLES

The issue raised by VADs, ICDs, and drug-eluting stents is essentially one of responsible and prudent stewardship of limited health care resources. In accordance with the principle of responsible stewardship articulated in its Code of Ethics, the Medical Center needs to consider how it should respond to these new technological breakthroughs, not just one at a time but from a broader perspective. This task is made more difficult because of the rapidity and frequency with which these new technologies become available. Discussions of this memorandum by the Medical Center Bioethics Committee generated the following guidelines:

- When there is a time lag between FDA approval of a new therapy and its coverage by public or private health insurance, the Medical Center should evaluate on a program-by-program basis how and to what extent it can absorb the cost of the new therapy.

Explanation: Every new decision involving nonreimbursable care has to be considered on its merits and not merely as an adjunct to a decision that has already been made. For example, providing VADs as a bridge to transplant does not obligate the Medical Center to provide VADs as a destination therapy, if the latter is not reimbursable.

This guideline is compatible with the following:

- The Medical Center should take a proactive stance with insurance companies to ensure speedy and adequate payment for new devices.
- The Medical Center should pursue creative strategies for making FDA-approved devices available to patients who can benefit from them without having to take a financial hit for doing so.

Finally,

- The principle of informed consent requires that patients be fully informed about which cardiac devices are available to them and the conditions under which they will be provided.

CONCLUSION

New and challenging ethical issues arise when new therapies become available but are not yet reimbursable by public or private health insurance. The Medical Center will need to decide whether and to what extent it will offer FDA-approved but not-yet-reimbursed therapies. Such decisions necessarily involve trade-offs, specifically determining what other services and programs will need to be forgone or curtailed as a result of providing these new treatments. The problem of reimbursement will become even more pressing as new or modified devices improve upon the current generation of VADs and other cardiac devices, such as ICDs and drug-eluting stents, receive FDA approval and are clinically indicated for more patients.

REFERENCES

Barold HS. 2003. Using the MADIT II criteria for implantable cardioverter defibrillators—What is the role of the Food and Drug Administration approval? *Cardiac Electrophysiology Review* 7(4):443–46.

Bigger JT. 2002. Expanding indications for implantable cardiac defibrillators. *New England Journal of Medicine* 346(12):931–33.

Centers for Medicare & Medicaid Services. 2003. Medicare announces its intention to cover ventricular assist devices as destination therapy. *Medicare News*, www.cms.hhs.gov/apps/media/press/release.asp?counter=881 (last accessed May 11, 2006).

McClellan MB, Tunis SR. 2005. Medicare coverage of ICDs. *New England Journal of Medicine* 352(3):222–24.

Moss AJ, Zareba W., Hall WJ, Klein H., Wilbur DJ, Cannom DS, Daubert JP, Higgens SL, Brown MW, Andrews ML. 2002. Prophylactic implantation of a defibrillator in patients with myocardial infarction and reduced ejection fraction. *New England Journal of Medicine* 346(12):877–83.

Rose EA, Gelijns AC, Moskowitz AJ, Heitjan DF, Stevenson LW, Dembritsky W, Long JW, Ascheim DD, Tierney AK, Levitan RG, Watson JT, Meier P. 2001. Long-term use of a left ventricular assist device for end-stage heart failure. *New England Journal of Medicine* 345(20): 1435–43.

U.S. Food and Drug Administration. 2003. FDA approves drug-eluting stent for clogged heart arteries. *FDA News* P03–31. www.fda.gov/bbs/topics/NEWS/2003/NEW00896.html (last accessed May 11, 2006).

GUIDELINES FOR TRANSFERRING PATIENTS BETWEEN SERVICES

Patients are transferred between clinical services based on where their care needs will be most effectively met. The determination of when, how, and where transfers take place has been the subject of controversy in some instances when services have refused to accept transfers that the original treating services considered to be in the patient's best interest. This type of dispute may result in compromised patient care.

Because interservice transfer has both clinical and organizational ethical implications, the Bioethics Committee was asked to consider the issues, identify the relevant principles, and propose a set of guidelines as a way to preempt disputes over patient transfers and resolve conflicts if they occur.

ETHICAL PRINCIPLES

The Medical Center Code of Ethics articulates the following overarching institutional commitment: "Medical Center recognizes that its primary mission is to ensure the provision of high quality, ethically based patient care." The code expressly articulates this commitment by recognizing that the institution's responsibilities include:

- "promoting continuity of care by coordinating services among providers . . .
- promoting collaborative clinical management and supporting the authority of specific multidisciplinary teams
- supporting attending physicians' professional judgment and authority, while requiring institutional oversight and joint clinical management and implementing a plan of care that reflects the patient's best interest, regardless of financial compensation
- promoting cost-effective care through cooperative clinical decision making that uses resources wisely . . .
- supporting a principled dispute resolution system that addresses treatment and interpersonal conflicts, strives for consensus and is based on ethical, medical and legal principles."

The fundamental ethical principle of respect for patients underlies the health care institution's commitment to patient well-being and confers organizational obligations to promote clinical excellence, collaborative case management, and wise stewardship of resources. These institutional responsibilities require that patients be cared for in the most appropriate clinical setting, which, in the hospital, means the service with the most targeted skills and resources. Because the delivery of high-quality patient care requires institutional direction and support, the organization must take ownership of facilitating appropriate interservice transfers.

- Clinical decisions, including determinations of the most appropriate plan and locus of care, depend primarily on the care needs of the patient, the therapeutic options, and the professional staff and technical resources available to provide the needed care. Particular attention should be given to the interventions that can and cannot be provided on each service.
- Transfer decisions should recognize that relocation between services or even units within services may not be in the patient's best interest and should not be considered without compelling clinical reason(s).

- Transfer criteria should be derived from evidence-based data about the clinical resources necessary to maximize therapeutic outcomes.
- Budgetary and bureaucratic concerns, while important to deliberations about resource allocation, must not impede or compromise the care of individual patients.
- Physicians have a responsibility for the care of their hospitalized patients that transcends financial considerations or length-of-stay imperatives.
- Plans of care that respond to patients' treatment needs may require that individual physician case management be replaced by collaborative case management. This may require transfer to services that provide different types of care.

INTERSERVICE TRANSFER GUIDELINES—DRAFT POLICY

Clinical Guidelines

- Transfers should be initiated with a request by the patient's attending or house staff for consultation by the service that is being asked to accept the patient. The request should specify the patient's clinical condition, diagnostic and/or treatment needs, and the reasons why transfer is considered necessary, including the resources and interventions that may be provided more effectively on the receiving service (e.g., wound debridement, psychiatric treatment).
- Within twenty-four hours, the consultation request should be answered by a physician who evaluates the patient for transfer, communicates with the requesting physician, and enters a note in the chart reflecting the transfer decision. If the clinical situation is urgent, the request should be answered within one hour. Both the discussion and the note should address the patient's care needs, the transfer criteria, and the available resources. The note should clearly explain why the patient will or will not benefit from transfer to a different service.
- Upon transfer, further care of the patient becomes the responsibility of the accepting service, including the determination of type, level, and location of care.
- If, after discussion, there is disagreement about whether the patient should be transferred—if the patient's current service believes that transfer is appropriate and the consulting service refuses to accept the patient—the matter should be escalated to senior physicians on each service. The lines of communication should be resident–resident, service attending–service attending, and service chief–service chief. In this way, the matter is escalated to physicians of comparable experience, expertise, and authority on each service.
- Additional consultations from other services should be requested at any point if the deliberations would benefit from different perspectives and expertise.

- If disagreement remains, the matter should be referred to the medical director for resolution. If the clinical situation is urgent, the medical director's decision will be binding.
- The entire process of consultation, escalating discussion, and appeal should be expedited as much as possible.
  —If the situation is urgent, the question of transfer should be resolved within two hours.
  —If the situation is not urgent, the question of transfer should be resolved within forty-eight hours.

Organizational Guidelines

- Institutional policy should recognize that interservice transfer decisions should be based on (1) the patient's best interest, and (2) whether specific services have the clinical resources and skills to meet the patient's health care needs.
- The institution should take steps to promote efficient and effective transfer decisions, and to minimize administrative barriers, including length-of-stay consideration and attribution.
- Institutional policy should articulate and support conflict resolution mechanisms that address the care needs of patients and the resource needs of clinical services.

DECISION-MAKING PROTOCOL FOR THE PATIENT ALONE

Adult patients are presumed to have the capacity to make decisions about their health care. In the clinical setting, decisional capacity consists of the ability to:

- understand the basic facts of one's medical situation, including current condition and prognosis
- weigh the benefits, burdens, and risks of the presented treatment options, including the option of no treatment
- apply a set of personal values
- arrive at a decision that is consistent over time
- communicate the decision

Patients determined to lack decisional capacity need treatment decisions made for them to promote their health and protect their rights of bodily integrity. Under most circumstances, guidance in making decisions for the incapacitated patient may come from an advance directive, expressing the wishes of the patient before losing capacity, or from family or even close friends with knowledge of what the patient would want or what would be in the patient's best interest. The notion of patient best interest is specific to the individual, but it is considered to include pain and symptom management, maintenance or enhancement of comfort and function, and amelioration of suffering.

ETHICAL PRINCIPLES

Patients alone—those without capacity, advance directives, family, or friends—present special challenges because their wishes are inaccessible and the usual sources of information about them are unavailable. In the clinical setting, the responsibility for making treatment decisions for this vulnerable population necessarily falls to the clinical and administrative staff of the health care institution. This decision-making authority is grounded in the following principles:

- The health care institution has an obligation to provide high-quality care that responds to the patient's medical needs. The institution assumes additional fiduciary responsibilities to protect vulnerable patients who cannot act in their own interest, have provided no expression of their wishes, and have no one to advocate for them.
- The goals and plan of care are informed by the patient's condition and prognosis, the benefits, burdens, and risks of the therapeutic options, and an assessment of what is in the patient's best interest. These considerations receive heightened scrutiny when the patient is without capacity or personal supports.
- The best interest of a patient, especially one at the end of life, does not always require aggressive therapeutic or diagnostic intervention. The threshold determination should be whether the overall goal of care is cure, improvement, remission, maintenance, or comfort, and the plan of care should reflect the indicated focus.
- It is the responsibility of the attending physician, in consultation with the health care team, to make a medical assessment, including a determination of whether the patient is dying, develop a plan of care, and make medical recommendations.
- Respect for persons requires that their wishes about their own care be accorded as much deference as possible. Patients with decisional capacity who understand their treatment options and their implications should have their refusals of treatment honored so long as they understand the consequences of their decisions. Patients alone, although lacking the capacity to make care decisions for themselves, should not be subjected to treatment over their active objections. When the best interests of vulnerable patients are in tension with their "spoken choice," the institution has a heightened responsibility to exercise protective clinical and administrative judgment.
- In its dual role as health care provider and surrogate decision maker, the institution has a responsibility to use all appropriate clinical and administrative resources in making and reviewing decisions that affect the treatment of patients alone.

PROTOCOL

There is no such thing as administrative consent. Consent that is provided by a surrogate or a health care agent when a patient is not able to make decisions for himself or herself is a form of consent that is widely accepted as legitimate in a variety of situations. Administrative consent, however, is not a form of surrogate consent; indeed, it is not really any type of consent. What is misleadingly labeled *administrative consent* is actually a process of *review* by the medical director, or by a physician who is designated by the medical director, to determine if the medical case meets certain criteria. These criteria are discussed below.

The office of the medical director will perform the following functions:

- Consult with any attending physician who recommends that a patient without capacity, advance directive, or identifiable surrogate (a patient alone) undergo a specific procedure that requires signed informed consent. Review with the attending the proposed procedure, including its indications, the potential risks and benefits, and the alternatives, including no treatment.
- Request clinical consultations that may inform the decision by clarifying the goals and plan of care.
- Review efforts to identify a surrogate for the patient and, if indicated, make additional efforts, including contacting the patient's nursing home or prior treating physician(s).
- Ascertain whether
  —the patient alone is refusing recommended treatment or is merely unresponsive, especially the patient whose refusal appears focused and consistent
  —ethical, clinical, or legal concerns, uncertainties, or disagreements have been raised by the patient's care team
  —the decision generates conflict with administrative and clinical goals related to length of stay
  —disagreement exists within the health care team regarding the necessity of the intervention

In any of these circumstances, the office of the medical director will arrange for multidisciplinary case review by the medical director or designee, the patient's attending physician, another physician in the attending's department, Risk Management, the Legal Department, and Bioethics. This review may reveal the need for a dispute resolution process.

- Refer the decision to the medical director, or his or her designee when no surrogate has been identified, no objections have been raised by the clinical team, and the attending physician wishes to proceed. The medical director/designee reviews the patient's medical record and examines the patient.

- If the medical director/designee *concurs* with the attending physician that the proposed procedure is medically indicated and in the patient's best interest, based on the options available to the patient at the time, the medical director/designee so indicates in the remarks section of the informed consent form. Administrative authorization to proceed with treatment is provided in lieu of the consent of the patient or surrogate.

- If the medical director/designee *does not agree* that the procedure is indicated and/or in the patient's best interests, he or she may discuss with the attending physician consideration of an alternative approach to treating/caring for the patient or request a multidisciplinary review, if needed, to clarify the issues further.

PART IV

Sample Policies and Procedures

Access to bioethics consultation

Advance directives

Determination of brain death

Do-not-intubate (DNI) orders

Do-not-resuscitate (DNR) orders

Forgoing life-extending treatment

The review of institutional policies and procedures is one of the ethics committee's most important functions. Because of its interdisciplinary membership and focus, the committee brings a critical perspective to the analysis of the templates for clinical and organizational action. Of particular ethics concern is whether the policies and procedures effectively implement the values and mission of the institution, while maintaining the accepted standards of health care and business endeavor.

Policy and procedure documents can function in different ways, depending on their objectives, the needs of the institution, and the laws and regulations of the state in which the institution is located. All are intended to provide guidance for the staff in responding consistently to specific situations. Some are sets of instructions about what steps should be taken. Others list the forms that should be used in implementing a process. Still others identify the health care professionals responsible for certain activities. The most useful provide both education and direction, explaining the purpose and underlying principles of the policy, as well as the institutionally agreed-upon plan of action. Some policies begin with an abstract or statement of purpose that summarizes the function, underlying reasoning, and, in some cases, the principles that ground their analytic structure.

The following policies are presented as samples with the permission of several health care institutions around the country. No attempt has been made to survey care-providing organizations about their policies or to collect data on how they are drafted or implemented. Rather, these policies were selected because they address clinical issues that have ethical implications and because most health care organizations have adopted some version of them, allowing for comparison of how different institutions address the same situations. In each instance, a policy from a particular institution ("Medical Center") has been annotated in boxed text to indicate its noteworthy features, as well as those of similar policies from other institutions. As noted elsewhere in this book, health care delivery is regulated by each state's law, and these differences are reflected in the policies that govern institutional procedures. Where the differences are notable, they are highlighted in the annotations.

ACCESS TO BIOETHICS CONSULTATION

> Several institutions have separate policies that address clinical ethics consultation. Others include ethics consultation in their policies on the function of an ethics committee.

PURPOSE

1. To ensure that patients, their families and designated representatives, and the caregiving staff are provided the opportunity to participate in the deliberation of the Bioethics Consultation Service and Bioethics Committee on issues that affect patient care.

2. To establish a process for timely access to the Bioethics Consultation Service for the analysis and resolution of ethical problems and conflicts in patient care.

3. To establish a process for access to the full Bioethics Committee when, in the judgment of the Bioethics Consultation Service, patient care issues would benefit from wider deliberation.

4. To establish a process whereby the Bioethics Committee is available to the Medical Center caregiving and administrative staff for education and review of policies related to bioethical issues.

> One policy explains the purpose of the consultation service: "The Ethics Consultation Service is primarily intended as a resource when patients, family members or health professionals may feel that they have reached the limits of their own personal or professional ability to address ethical questions."

SCOPE

This policy extends to all Medical Center caregiving and administrative staff, patients, families, and designated representatives throughout the integrated delivery system.

FUNCTION

1. All ethical issues in the clinical setting are appropriately addressed by the Bioethics Consultation Service, comprised of members of the Division of Bioethics at the Medical Center. Members of the Consultation Service are available whenever a consult is requested to provide timely and continued assistance in clarifying and resolving ethical dilemmas. A summary of the consult is documented in the patient's chart.

Two institutions whose policies were reviewed have clinical ethics consultation services staffed by trained ethicists. Most policies describe clinical consultation as a responsibility of a consultation service, team, or subcommittee of the ethics committee and staffed by committee members. As an example, "In order to fulfill its mandate to facilitate ethical decision-making in specific cases, the Ethics Committee provides an Ethics Consultation Service. The Ethics Consultation Service is staffed with Ethics Committee members in accordance with guidelines put forth by the American Society for Bioethics and Humanities in its most recent *Core Competencies for Health Care Ethics Consultation* (2000)."

One policy distinguishes between two types of consultation:

"Informal Consultation: one that can be handled by one or two committee members and the individual seeking information by informal discussion and referral (as needed) to other appropriate resources or actions."

"Formal Consultation: one that necessitates a formal meeting of the individuals and health care providers who are most directly involved in the patient's situation in order to help resolve the ethical issue at hand. A minimum of two members from the [ethics committee] shall be present during the consult. The consult is formally documented in the patient's medical record using the standard [institution] consultation form."

Most policies provide for ethics consultations to be documented in the medical record.

One policy states that members of the ethics committee will conduct the initial evaluation and consultation, and provide verbal and written recommendations to the party or parties requesting consultation. This policy provides that medical ethicists are available on call twenty-four hours a day.

One institution has six ethics committees—a hospital-wide committee of the Medical Board and five multidisciplinary Departmental Ethics Committees. The Medical Board Committee reviews any clinical, policy, or administrative matter with interdepartmental or larger institutional implications. Other ethical issues are referred to the respective Departmental Ethics Committees.

Ethical issues for which consultation might be sought include, but are not limited to:

- developing, signing, and honoring of advance directives
- participation in the health care decision-making process
- withholding and withdrawing life-sustaining treatment
- do-not-resuscitate orders
- informed consent to and refusal of treatment
- patient dignity, confidentiality, and privacy
- patient rights and responsibilities

2. The Bioethics Committee, including members of the Division of Bioethics, as well as representatives of the caregiving and administrative staff, is available when a wider ethical analysis would be helpful. The interdisciplinary committee meets on a regular and ad hoc basis to:

- provide advisory and nonbinding recommendations for resolution of conflicts in care decisions
- participate in developing and reviewing Medical Center policy when matters of ethics are involved
- provide educational programs in bioethical issues, both within the Medical Center and for the wider community.

One policy defines ethical problems: "In general, an ethical problem exists when it is not clear what is the ethically sound action or course of action or when people disagree about what is best for a patient."

One policy identifies the scope of ethics committee consultation: "The Ethics Committee will provide consultative services when requested for assistance with a patient-related problem identified as an ethical issue. The medical ethics consult offers recommendations about patient care decisions that have an ethical dimension. Often, this may also include aggressiveness of treatment, questions of consent, alternative treatment options. In addition to consultative services, the Ethics Committee establishes guidelines, policies, and procedures regarding the withholding or withdrawal of life-sustaining treatments."

ACCESS

Anyone involved in patient care associated with the Medical Center—patient, family member or designated representative, or staff member, regardless of site—with an ethical concern or problem can access the Bioethics Consultation Service by contacting the Division of Bioethics. This service is normally available Monday through Friday from 9:00 a.m. to 5:00 p.m. Requests for consultation may also be referred to the Bioethics Consultation Service by the Office of the Medical Director. At other times, request for ethics consultations requiring immediate attention will be handled by the appropriate administrative nursing coordinator. If the patient care issue does not require immediate attention, a message can be left at the offices of the Division of Bioethics and will be responded to during the next working day.

> One policy provides for the availability of an ethics committee member "24 hours a day, 365 days a year to initiate a consultation." Other policies provide the telephone numbers of the Bioethics office or service, the ethics committee chair, the patient representative, or a bioethics pager number.

> One institution assigns to other departments key functions that are usually included within the responsibility of a bioethics consultation service. The patient advocate is the party initially notified of an ethical issue. The patient advocate interviews the patient and/or surrogate, speaks with the health care team, and informs Risk Management that a bioethics meeting needs to be scheduled, including a recommendation about the appropriate time. The risk manager reviews the medical record and documentation, speaks with the health care team, patient, and family as necessary, arranges the meeting, and notifies the bioethics committee members about the time and location.

Requests for consultation will be responded to within twenty-four hours. Depending on the nature of the patient care issue, the bioethics consultant(s) may convene a conference of the patient's caregiving team and selected members of the Bioethics Committee to evaluate relevant issues. On occasion, a case may also be presented to a full meeting of the committee for review.

> Other policies require a response within seventy-two hours of a consultation request. One policy provides for "STAT" consultations when immediate attention is required.

Caregiving and administrative staff members who wish to present bioethical issues, policies, and educational matters to the Bioethics Committee should directly contact the committee chair or co-chair through the Division of Bioethics.

> One policy addresses the issue of attending physician permission: "If the Committee believes a consult is necessary and the attending physician declines to permit Committee consultation with the patient or the patient's family, the Committee shall review this matter with the appropriate Director or Section Chief."

NOTIFICATION OF PATIENT, FAMILY, OR DESIGNATED REPRESENTATIVE

When the request for bioethics consultation comes from a patient, family member, or designated representative and the case will be presented to the full Bioethics Committee as part of the clinical consultation, those requesting will be notified and invited to participate in deliberations.

> One policy states, "The patient's attending physician and, when appropriate, the patient, or the patient's family, health care proxy or surrogate, the nursing staff, and other clinical staff caring for the patient will be advised that an ethics consultation has been requested and will be given every reasonable opportunity to participate in the consultation."

Permission of the patient, family, or designated representative is not required for either a consultation or full committee review.

CONFIDENTIALITY

All deliberations of the Bioethics Consultation Service and the Bioethics Committee are confidential, and all records and documentation are protected.

ADVANCE DIRECTIVES

PURPOSE

This policy informs associates and medical staff about federal and state laws that govern patients' rights to make advance health care decisions, including consent to or refusal of medical, surgical, or diagnostic interventions. Staff members are required to provide patients with (1) information about advance directives, (2) the opportunity to formulate advance directives, and (3) the offer of assistance in doing so. Care providers are required to be aware of and respect patient care wishes expressed in advance directives. Patients will not be discriminated against based on whether they have advance directives.

> Most policies amplify the last sentence above with some variation of "The hospital shall not condition the provision of care or otherwise discriminate against a patient based on whether or not the patient has executed an advance directive."

SCOPE

Applies to all Medical Center associates in the network and affiliated physicians and their staffs in other clinical settings.

DEFINITIONS

> Most policies define the different types of advance directives and other relevant terms. These definitions, taken together, provide a useful summary and comparison of the purpose, features, standards, and authority of the directives.

Advance directive: A written or oral expression of a capacitated individual's health care instructions, including general preferences and consent to or refusal of specified treatments or interventions. These instructions, including living wills and health care proxy appointments, are recognized by state law as constituting evidence of a person's health care wishes, stated in advance of decisional incapacity. They take effect only when the individual is deemed to have lost the capacity to make health care decisions. (Do-not-resuscitate [DNR] orders are considered a specific type of advance directive and are covered in a separate Medical Center policy.)

Living will: A list of instructions, written by a capacitated individual, about therapeutic interventions that he or she does or does not want under specified conditions, usually at the end of life. A living will is used as guidance in making health care decisions for an incapacitated patient and is especially useful for those without other persons who can make decisions for them. It may constitute clear and convincing evidence of a patient's wishes.

Health care proxy: A document in which a capacitated individual delegates health care decision-making authority to another person (a health care agent), in accordance with the Health Care Proxy Law.

> One policy also defines "Documented Oral Instructions—An adult's spoken wishes concerning life-sustaining issues expressed in a clear and convincing manner."

Health care agent: An adult, 18 years of age or older, who has been authorized through a health care proxy appointment to make health care decisions on behalf of a temporarily or permanently incapacitated patient, with exceptions listed below (see section II—Provisions of the Health Care Proxy Law). An alternate agent is also appointed by the patient to assume decision-making responsibilities in the event the primary agent is unable or unwilling to do so.

Family members, even next of kin, do not automatically assume the responsibility or authority of a health care proxy agent. *Only the appointment by a capable individual authorizes a person to be an agent and only a valid proxy document provides evidence of that appointment.*

> Not all policies include this important clarification, which alerts staff to the critical distinction between family members, whose decision-making authority may be limited, and the health care agent, whose authority is the same as the patient's.

Decision-making capacity: The ability to understand and appreciate the nature and consequences of health care decisions, including the benefits, burdens, and risks of therapeutic and diagnostic interventions, the alternatives to proposed health care, and the ability to make and communicate an informed decision about treatment.

> A helpful addition to this definition, which is referred to later in the policy, would be that a lower level of capacity is required to appoint a health care agent than to make the health care decisions the agent will be responsible for making.

Reasonably available agent: A health care agent who can be contacted with diligent efforts by the attending physician or someone acting on behalf of the attending or the Medical Center.

I. Policy Implementation

Health care providers are responsible for the close scrutiny and interpretation of the provisions of their patients' advance directives. Patients who are currently incapable of making their own decisions and have left explicit written or verbal instructions, in a living will or in a health care proxy, depend on their care providers to be aware of and respect their treatment wishes. The provisions of advance directives are activated only when patients have lost decisional capacity and are in specified conditions. For this reason, it is essential to determine whether the incapacitated patient meets those criteria before treatment decisions by others are based on the patient's advance directive.

> Not all policies explicitly state the circumstances under which the authority of advance directives is activated. These criteria provide important guidance for care professionals in determining when to rely on and follow advance directives.

> Some policies are limited to describing the process by which the execution of advance directives is initiated and followed up. Others provide detailed explanation of the purpose, scope, and implementation of directives, including how care professionals evaluate and honor their provisions.

A. Medical Center associates are responsible for implementing this policy as follows:

1. Upon admission to the Medical Center or new patient registration in the Ambulatory Care Network, other ambulatory care facility/program, or the Home Health Agency, all capacitated adult patients will be given or otherwise made aware of the following materials:

   a summary of state law concerning advance directives
   an explanation of the role of advance directives
   a summary of patient rights in this state

2. For the Ambulatory Care Network, "Health Care Proxy—Appointing Your Health Care Agent" or similar information from a nationally recognized source is used for patient education.

   If the patient lacks capacity upon admission/new patient registration, these materials will be given to the person who makes health care decisions on behalf of the patient. If the patient regains capacity during the hospitalization, he or she will be given the opportunity to execute an advance directive at that time.

B. For hospitalized patients:

1. After the above, all patients or their decision makers will be contacted by the admissions office before planned admission and reminded to bring copies of any advance directive documentation they may have.

2. During the admission process on the units, the nurse (RN/LPN) will ask the patient if he or she has executed a health care proxy or a living will or has a nonhospital DNR. If the patient lacks decisional capacity, the family/ significant other will be asked about the existence of advance directive(s).

3. The conversation with the patient (and others, as appropriate) requires sensitivity to the patient's values, culture, ethnicity, and religion when discussing care issues, especially those related to end-of-life care.

4. If the patient has brought an advance directive to the hospital, the RN/ LPN will place a *copy* of it in the medical record and inform the attending physician or designee. This includes a copy of a nonhospital DNR. If the patient has an advance directive but the document is not immediately available, the RN/LPN will ask the patient/family to bring it to the hospital as soon as possible.

5. If the patient does not have a health care proxy and indicates a desire to execute one, the RN/LPN may answer questions and provide a blank proxy form for the patient to complete. The patient should be advised of the importance of discussing the appointment with the persons he or she has selected as proxy and alternate proxy. The patient/family should be advised to retain the *original* advance directive and give copies to the proxy, alternate proxy, and the patient's PMD. A copy of the form should be placed in the patient's medical record as soon as it is completed. If the patient needs *additional* assistance completing a health care proxy form, the RN/LPN will refer the patient to Social Services for assistance.

6. If there is any question about the patient's decisional capacity to execute an advance directive, a formal capacity determination should be made by the attending or, if necessary, a psychiatric consult.

7. If there are conflicts or uncertainty about the patient's wishes, contact Bioethics or the Office of the Medical Director.

8. A patient who has no one to appoint as a health care proxy but wants to articulate care wishes in advance of incapacity may want to complete a living will. Social Services may review with the patient general issues about living wills, but should also notify the attending to discuss medical specifics and complete documentation with the patient.

9. If the patient or family member has questions about DNR, DNI, or the clinical substance of a living will, the social worker will clarify issues but should contact the attending or designee for further discussion and a consideration of medical appropriateness. Bioethics and the Office of the Medical Director are available for assistance.

10. If the patient does not have an advance directive and does not wish to have one, that preference must be respected. The RN/LPN will document in the medical record the patient's decision not to have an advance directive and will notify the patient that assistance will be available in the future if requested. At that point, no further follow-up is necessary.

11. If referrals are indicated to either the MD or Social Services, the RN/LPN will complete the admission database and make the appropriate referrals.

12. When Social Services has followed up with a patient who decides not to pursue a health care proxy appointment, Social Services will so document in the medical record and no further follow-up is needed. The case will be closed in CIS.

Institutions differ in terms of who assumes responsibility for initiating and following up discussions about advance directives. Some policies make inquiring about and explaining advance directives the responsibility of the registrar at the time of admission. Further information may be available from patient representatives, physicians, or nurses. Some policies make follow-up the responsibility of social workers or nurses.

---

13. For patients admitted to the in-patient psychiatric unit, a copy of "Planning for Your Mental and Physical Health Care and Treatment" is given. Questions are answered and assistance provided.

C. Medical Group (Outpatient)

After receiving information about advance directives, the patient is asked to sign a sticker stating that he or she has received information and that all questions should be referred to the patient's health care provider. Advance directives, when known, will be honored.

D. Home Health Agency

On each new admission, the nurse or therapist must explain advance directives to the patient and ask if the patient has a health care proxy or living will. If the patient has one, then the nurse asks for a copy of the proxy or living will to be kept in the patient's medical record. If the patient is not able to provide a copy, the clinician notes the names of the health care agents and their telephone numbers and/or any specific wishes for artificial feeding and similar interventions. Some patients may have a nonhospital DNR order that is signed by the MD at the time that the patient is coming onto the home care program. The nonhospital DNR order must be reviewed every ninety days, so the home care nurse adds the order "DNR in effect" on the MD orders that are sent every sixty days. The patients are also instructed that they may revoke these advance directives at any time.

E. Medical Center Physicians' Responsibilities

1. Attending physicians and other licensed independent practitioners should routinely discuss advance directives with capacitated patients and encourage them to appoint health care agents or, if they have no one to appoint, to complete living wills. (When clinically indicated, the risks, benefits, and burdens of a do-not-resuscitate [DNR] order, another form of advance directive, should also be discussed.)

2. The house staff should include discussion of advance directives in the history and physical completed for all in-patient admissions.

3. When clinically indicated, the attending physician makes a capacity determination and documents the determination in the patient's medical record.

4. Whenever a decision requiring informed consent is needed, the attending physician must reevaluate the patient's capacity to make that specific decision.

5. If the attending physician determines that the patient lacks the capacity to make health care decisions but has sufficient capacity to appoint a health care agent, he or she should encourage the patient to do so. The attending physician's documentation should reflect the judgment that the patient has the required level of capacity to appoint an agent. If the patient requires assistance completing a health care proxy, a referral to Social Services should be made through the computerized information system.

6. If the attending has determined that the patient lacks decisional capacity and the patient has a health care agent, the attending will discuss with the health care agent the benefits, burdens, risks, and the alternatives to any proposed procedure. The agent has the right to receive any and all medical information that the patient would have received if capacitated.

7. The physician is required to honor in good faith the health care agent's decisions as if made by the patient. If, however, the physician has concerns about the health care agent's understanding of the patient's wishes, the agent's capacity to make decisions on the patient's behalf, or other questions about the health care proxy decision process, Bioethics or the Medical Director's Office should be consulted.

8. When a physician becomes aware that the patient has revoked the proxy appointment, the physician must document the revocation in the patient's medical record and, if appropriate, discuss this action with the agent.

9. If a physician is unable to honor a health care agent's decision(s) based on the physician's sincerely held religious or moral beliefs, the physician must con-

tact the medical director or designee, to transfer the patient to a physician willing to abide by the agent's decision(s), and so advise the agent.

The foregoing section provides a useful explanation of the physician's responsibilities for discussing, facilitating, and honoring advance directives. One policy adds language stipulating that the agent's authority equals but does not exceed that of the capable patient, here referred to as the *principal*:

"The Hospital does not have to honor an agent's decision:

1. if it would not have honored the decision had it been made by the principal; and

2. if the Hospital would be permitted by law to refuse to honor the decision if made by the principal; and

3. if the decision is contrary to a formally adopted policy of the Board of Trustees . . .

4. if the Hospital informed the principal or the agent of the Hospital's policy at the time of admission, if reasonably possible; . . ."

One policy includes a little gentle encouragement for staff to complete advance directives: "The hospital provides in-service education to staff concerning advance directives and related hospital policies and procedures. All staff members are encouraged to consider completion of a health care proxy."

Care providers are encouraged to contact either or both of the following available resources with any questions or concerns about advance directives:

1. Bioethics
2. Office of the Medical Director

During evenings, weekends, and holidays, the associate director of nursing (A.D.N.) should be contacted via the page operator.

II. Legal Authority
    A. The Patient Self-Determination Act is a federal law that requires all Medical Center staff to determine whether patients have advance directives, inform them of their right to execute advance directives, and provide them with assistance in doing so.
    B. The Health Care Proxy Law is a state law that allows a capable patient to appoint a health care agent with legal authority to make health care decisions for the pa-

tient after capacity has lapsed. A health care agent's decision-making authority has priority over that of any other surrogate.

The Health Care Proxy Law permits a patient to delegate to another person (health care agent) all or part of the patient's authority to make health care decisions in the event he or she loses decisional capacity. Unless specifically limited in the appointment document, the agent is authorized to make all decisions the patient would make, including decisions about life-sustaining treatment. The agent is required to make determinations consistent with what the patient would have chosen if he or she had decision-making capacity or, when the patient's wishes are unknown, with what is in the patient's best interest.

One policy specifies what the proxy appointment document *must* and *may* include:

"A. A properly executed proxy appoints the health care decision-making agent without the need for further proceedings.

B. The proxy document must:
   1. identify the principal and the agent
   2. indicate that the principal intends to confer health care decision-making authority to the agent to act on the principal's behalf
   3. be signed and dated by the competent adult principal in the presence of two adult witnesses
   4. be signed and dated by two adult witnesses (the person appointed agent or alternate agent cannot be a witness)
   5. include a statement from the witness that the principal completed the proxy willingly and free from duress.

C. The proxy may:
   1. include special wishes or instructions of the principal and/or
   2. include limits on the agent's authority and/or
   3. contain an expiration date or specify that it expires upon the occurrence of a stated condition and/or
   4. provide for the appointment of an alternate agent and/or alternate(s)
   5. include the principal's wishes or instructions regarding organ and tissue donation. Failure to state wishes or instructions shall not be construed to imply a wish not to donate."

Decisions about artificial nutrition and hydration may be made by the agent, but *only* if he or she knows or can ascertain the patient's wishes about these interventions.

> This state-specific limitation on the powers of the agent to make decisions about artificial nutrition and hydration is not included in all policies.

An agent may not make decisions about autopsy or organ donation, unless he or she is otherwise authorized to do so.

A living will can be used in conjunction with a health care proxy to provide the agent with additional guidance about the patient's wishes. In the event that the agent's decisions are inconsistent with the terms of the living will, Bioethics or the Medical Director's Office should be consulted.

> One policy includes a section that addresses possible inconsistencies between a patient's previously stated wishes and the agent's current decisions. This language reflects the frequent need for agents to respond to circumstances not anticipated by patients, which may be significant later when care decisions must be made.
>
> "The agent has no authority to rescind or override the principal's prior expressed wishes as memorialized in the proxy or expressed in another form, unless the agent can substantiate this through
>
> 1. a conversation the agent had with the principal in which the principal told the agent that he or she wanted different treatment than what he or she previously indicated; or
> 2. a change in medical circumstances, such as improvement in the principal's medical condition or the unexpected availability of a significant new treatment option, that would suggest that the principal would reverse his or her decision under the same circumstance."

If a patient has specified health care instructions in an advance directive and neither the agent nor the alternate agent is available, Bioethics or the Medical Director's Office should be contacted for assistance in reviewing the patient's instructions.

A copy of the health care proxy should be placed in the patient's medical record upon admission/new patient registration or as soon thereafter as possible.

III. Health Care Proxies and Agents
  A. Who May Appoint a Health Care Agent?
     Any competent person 18 years old or older, any married person, or any parent may appoint a health care agent. Adults are presumed competent to appoint a health care agent, unless they have been deemed incompetent by a court.

B. Who May Be Appointed a Health Care Agent?

Any competent adult (18 years of age or older) may serve as a health care agent, with the following exceptions: a hospital employee may not serve as agent for any patient at the hospital, unless he or she is related to the patient, or the patient appointed the agent before admission to the hospital. Physicians are the only exception to this rule.

A patient may appoint his or her physician as agent, but the physician may not serve as both agent and attending physician once the agent's decision-making authority begins.

A physician who has been appointed as a patient's agent may not determine the patient's capacity to make health care decisions.

A person not related to the patient may not be appointed as agent if, at the time of the appointment, he or she is serving as health care agent for ten or more other people.

C. Lack-of-capacity Determinations

> Most policies include a detailed explanation of incapacity and the process for its clinical assessment.

A patient may have the capacity to appoint an agent to make decisions on his or her behalf, yet lack the capacity to make the more complex treatment decisions the agent will make.

> By stipulating that a relatively low level of capacity will suffice to appoint a health care agent, the policy encourages the care team to consider the potential for patients with diminished or fluctuating capacity to appoint agents while they are still able to do so.

The decision-making authority of the health care agent is activated *only* when it is determined that the patient is temporarily or permanently incapacitated and ends when capacity is regained.

> The policy emphasizes that, even if an advance directive has been executed and even if a health care proxy agent has been appointed, decision-making authority remains with the patient unless and until incapacity has been determined. Explicit mention of the permanent or temporary nature of the inca-

pacity is an important safeguard against the misconception that decisional authority, once assumed by the agent, remains with the agent. This reinforces the
important notion that the patient resumes decision making whenever sufficient
capacity is demonstrated.

A determination that the patient lacks the capacity to make specific health
care decisions must be made by the *attending* physician, with a reasonable degree
of medical certainty.

When the attending physician is also the patient's proxy, another attending
physician must make the determination of capacity.

a. For a health care decision that *does not require forgoing life-sustaining* treatment, the *determination of incapacity need only be made by one attending*
   physician.
b. If the agent is to make a decision about forgoing (withholding or withdrawing) life-sustaining treatment, the attending physician must *consult with an-*
   other physician to confirm the patient's lack of capacity. The consultation must be
   recorded in the patient's medical record.

Notice of a determination of incapacity must be given verbally to the agent. If
the patient is able to comprehend, verbal and written notice of an incapacity
determination must also be given to the patient. If the patient opposes the lack-
of-capacity determination or the health care decision(s) made by the agent, the
objection or decision of the patient prevails, unless a judge confirms that the
patient lacks capacity.

If family members or significant others object to the determination of incapacity, or the health care decision(s) made by the agent, but the patient does not
object, the person objecting must obtain a court order to overturn the incapacity
determination or health care decision. Unless or until a court order is obtained,
the health care agent's decisions prevail.

If and when the patient regains decision-making capacity, the agent's authority ceases. The physician should notify the agent and document the change in
the chart.

The attending physician's determination of incapacity must be documented
in the patient's medical record. The entry should describe the cause, nature,
extent, and probable duration of the incapacity, within a reasonable degree of
medical certainty.

Each time a major decision is to be made and consent is needed from the
agent, the patient's lack of capacity to make that specific decision must be recon-
firmed by the attending physician and documented in the chart.

Mentally Ill Patients

Mental illness does not by itself constitute or indicate decisional incapacity. However, if lack of capacity is due to mental illness, the attending physician making the incapacity determination must be (or consult with) a board-certified psychiatrist. The consultation must be documented in the patient's medical record.

Mental illness (under the Health Care Proxy Law) does not include dementia, such as Alzheimer's disease.

Mentally Disabled Patients

If lack of capacity is due to mental retardation and/or developmental disability, the attending physician making the incapacity determination must be (or consult with) a physician or clinical psychologist who is employed at a school for the developmentally disabled; or has been employed for at least two years and is qualified to render care in an Office of Mental Retardation and Developmental Disabilities (OMRDD) facility; or has had special training or at least three years' experience in treating developmental disabilities and meets other criteria to be established in ORMDD regulations.

The consultation must be documented in the patient's medical record.

Once lack of capacity has been determined, the physician must give notice to:

a. the agent, orally

b. the patient, orally and in writing, if there is any indication that the patient can comprehend the notice

c. the mental health facility director, if the patient is a resident in or has been transferred from such a facility

d. legal guardian, if applicable

Some policies require the attending physician to notify only the agent when the patient has been determined to lack capacity.

D. The Health Care Agent's Decision-making Authority

Some policies describe in detail the scope of the agent's decision-making authority, providing useful guidance to care professionals about the decisions the agent is empowered to make.

When the patient is not capable, the decisions of an appointed agent take precedence over the decisions of any other person (e.g., a surrogate appointed under the DNR law), unless the health care proxy document indicates that the patient limited the agent's authority at the time of appointment, or the court appoints a guardian to make decisions about the patient's health care. Unless otherwise limited, the agent is authorized to make any and all health care decisions that the patient would make if capacitated. If, however, forgoing of nutrition and/or hydration is contemplated, the agent must have specific knowledge of the patient's previously expressed wishes regarding nutrition and/or hydration.

Before making any decisions on behalf of an incapacitated patient, the agent must consult with a physician, registered nurse, licensed psychologist, or certified social worker, as indicated by the nature of the decision to be made.

The agent must carry out the patient's previously expressed specific wishes and act in accordance with the patient's religious or moral beliefs to the extent that they are known or can reasonably be determined. If the patient's previously expressed instructions are inconsistent with the plan of care considered by the treating team to be clinically appropriate for his or her current medical condition, the agent should confer with the attending physician and make decisions consistent with what the patient would likely decide under the unanticipated circumstances. If the patient's wishes, religious beliefs, or moral beliefs cannot be ascertained, the agent must act in the patient's best interest.

To make informed decisions on behalf of an incapacitated patient, the agent should be provided with all information about diagnosis, prognosis, and therapeutic alternatives that would normally be provided to the patient if capacitated. The attending physician may share with the agent any relevant communications he or she previously had with the patient.

E. Out-of-state Proxy

A health care proxy or similar document (e.g., a *durable power of attorney for health care*) executed in another state is valid in this state as long as it complies with the laws of the state in which it was executed. (*Note*: A power of attorney document is authorization for legal and financial decision making and is *not* the same as a health care proxy.) Any questions about the validity of out-of-state proxies or other legal documents should be referred to the clinical assistant to the medical director, who will review any questions with the Legal Department.

All policies reviewed state that their institutions will honor valid out-of-state proxies, although they do not all make the important distinction between powers of attorney and health care proxies.

F. Witnessing the Health Care Proxy Appointment

The proxy form is valid when signed *by the patient* before two witnesses, neither of whom can be the person appointed to be the agent or the alternate. The witnesses attest to the patient's signature and willingness to execute the proxy. If requested,

Medical Center employees are encouraged to witness health care proxies for capacitated patients.

Any concerns regarding witnessing or completeness of the health care proxy form should be referred to the Medical Director's Office as it sometimes possible to clarify matters sufficiently to honor the patient's health care proxy designation.

See section III-N for witnessing guidelines for a patient in a mental health facility regulated by the Office of Mental Hygiene (OMH).

G. Revocation of a Proxy Appointment

1. Every adult is presumed competent to revoke a proxy appointment, unless he or she is found incompetent by a court.

2. A patient may revoke the proxy designation at any time in writing, orally, or with any other action that indicates a specific intent to revoke.

3. The execution of a second proxy appointment automatically revokes one executed at an earlier time.

4. Divorce or legal separation renders the proxy invalid if the agent is the divorced spouse, unless the proxy states otherwise.

H. Dispute Management

Disputes, such as those regarding determinations of capacity, between or among the agent, family/surrogate, and doctor require consultation. Bioethics or the Office of the Medical Director or Risk Management should be contacted. They will contact the Legal Department if a legal opinion from a Medical Center counsel is required.

I. Alternate Agent

The alternate agent takes the primary agent's place under certain conditions specified in the appointment document or when the patient's attending physician concludes that the primary agent is not reasonably available, willing, or competent to serve, and is not expected to become reasonably available to make timely decisions.

If the alternate agent has begun to serve and the primary agent becomes available, willing, and competent, the primary agent automatically replaces the alternate.

J. Health Care Proxy and Do-not-resuscitate (DNR) Orders

When the patient lacks decisional capacity, the health care agent's decision(s) takes precedence over the decisions of any other person (e.g., a surrogate under the DNR law). The existence of a health care proxy document does not negate the need for a DNR order or for DNR attending physician documentation and consent forms.

Before consulting a health care agent about DNR decisions, two physicians must confirm and document the patient's lack of capacity, utilizing the attending physician's DNR documentation form. Thereafter, the agent may be asked to consent to a DNR order in accordance with the do-not-resuscitate (DNR) policy.

If the agent agrees to consent to a DNR order, the oral or written consent to DNR form should also be completed and the DNR order (either electronic or written) should be entered.

If conflict exists between a DNR form previously signed by the patient and the agent's current instructions, Bioethics or the Office of the Medical Director should be consulted.

K. In the Emergency Department

If a delay in determining whether an agent has been appointed or in contacting the agent will harm the patient, treatment should be provided in accordance with accepted emergency medical standards.

Nevertheless, when an incapacitated patient's diagnosis and prognosis can be determined in the Emergency Department, the information should be provided to the agent to allow an informed decision. Physicians should honor decisions by a health care agent in the Emergency Department in the same way they would honor the decisions of a capacitated patient.

L. Psychiatry

In a facility regulated by the Office of Mental Hygiene (OMH), when a patient signs a health care proxy, one witness must be a person who is not affiliated with the facility, and one witness must be a physician certified by the American Board of Psychiatry and Neurology.

DETERMINATION OF BRAIN DEATH

An individual is dead if he or she has sustained irreversible cessation of circulatory and respiratory function or irreversible cessation of all brain function, including the brainstem.

One policy's Background section describes the clinical and state-specific legal context of brain death and ends by distinguishing brain death from other forms of patient unresponsiveness: "Following the published guidelines assures that a patient who is still alive will not be misdiagnosed as dead. The patient in coma with some remaining brain-related bodily functions is not dead. Either behavioral or brain stem reflexes indicate that brain death has not occurred. A patient in a chronic vegetative state may remain in a prolonged coma indefinitely, yet not meet the criteria for brain death."

PRINCIPLES

- A patient determined to meet the clinical criteria for brain death as outlined in this policy is both physiologically and legally dead.

> This is the only policy reviewed to emphasize explicitly that brain death is both a physiological and a legal definition of death.

- All religious or moral objections to the brain death standard as a basis for declaring the individual dead will be treated with equal respect and, whenever possible, reasonable accommodation.
- Families will be allowed a reasonable amount of time and support to reach understanding and acceptance of the fact that the patient has died.
- Families may require supportive services provided by a multidisciplinary team to help them understand the brain death determination.

PROCEDURE

The procedure for determining whether brain death has occurred should be initiated when a patient has suffered such a severe and extensive brain injury as to cause irreversible brain damage. If brain death is suspected, the attending physician shall discuss with the family:

- the procedures for determining brain death
- the meaning of brain death as death
- the futility of further treatment measures
- the consequent termination of all treatment measures if brain death is determined and confirmed (see section VII on reasonable accommodation)

Families may need time to understand and accept the prognosis. The determination of brain death is a multistep process. At each step, families are given adequate time to understand and process information. As brain death is a medical determination, the clinical evaluation does not require specific consent from the patient's next-of-kin or health care agent. However, reasonable efforts must be made to notify them.

- Whenever possible, the patient's nurse, social worker, or other member of the team is part of discussions with the family to promote continuity of support. The attending physician shall maintain communication with the other members of the team regarding discussions with the family.

The team should contact the state Organ Procurement Organization (OPO) for possible organ and tissue procurement. The law mandates that all death and imminent death be referred to the OPO in a timely manner. Communication with the OPO should be ongoing throughout the brain death determination process.

> One policy begins by stating, "The Brain Death Protocol is applicable to all patients, whether they *are* or *are not* organ donors." Such a statement provides clarification and reassurance that no separate set of criteria or procedures are in place to expedite the brain death determination of specific patients because they are likely organ donors.

I. Determination of Brain Death in Adults (Age 18 Years Old)

    The clinical evaluation of brain death is to be made by two attending physicians credentialed to do brain death determination. At least one of the evaluations should be done by a neurologist or neurosurgeon.

    • Neither of the above physicians can participate in the procedure for the removal or transplantation of organ or tissues.

    Each attending evaluates the patient's brain function and writes one of the two required notes. The order of the evaluation is of no consequence provided both evaluations conclude the patient meets the criteria and the documentation states the patient is brain dead. The period of observation required to confirm the diagnosis will vary depending on clinical circumstances. For adults, a six-hour interval between clinical evaluations is recommended but not required if there is a known cause and ancillary testing is performed.

> Most reviewed policies require that brain death be determined by two physicians, one of whom must be a neurologist or neurosurgeon. One policy states that brain death can be certified by a single physician but that two physicians are necessary when the patient is a potential organ and/or tissue donor. This provides another safeguard against the possibility or even the perception that brain death might be determined more readily in potential organ donors.

    A. Clinical Evaluation

> This policy sets out the process for clinically determining brain death in adults and children in considerably greater detail than the other policies reviewed.

When there is a known cause for the patient's condition, the determination of brain death may be made if:

1. There is no clinical evidence of toxic or chemical depression of the nervous system.
2. The patient is not in cardiovascular collapse. Shock, as defined as a mean arterial blood pressure (MAP) less than 55 mm Hg, prohibits the declaration of brain death. Pressors to support arterial blood pressure may be used (mean BP = (2 * BP diastolic + BP systolic) / 3).
3. The patient is not hypothermic (T < 90 degrees F/32.2 degrees C).

The neurologic examination consistent with brain death includes:

1. Coma or unresponsiveness—no cerebral motor response to pain in all extremities (no response to nail bed pressure and supraorbital pressure)
2. Absence of brainstem reflexes:
   a. absence of pupillary light reflex
   b. absence of oculocephalic reflexes
   c. absence of oculovestibular reflexes
   d. absence of corneal reflexes
   e. absence of pharyngeal and tracheal reflexes

If, in the clinical judgment of the attending physician, an exogenous source of intoxication is suspected, toxicological studies are mandatory. If the patient has been on hypnotic/sedative type or other CNS depressant medication, it must be determined that these drugs are not involved in producing the coma. When neuromuscular blockers have been used, normal neuromuscular transmission must be present.

- If the attending physicians do not agree that the criteria for brain death have been met, the criteria are not considered met and appropriate ancillary studies should be done to resolve the discrepancy.

B. Apnea Test

The apnea test can be performed after the first clinical evaluation. During the apnea test, the patient must be on continuous oxygen saturation monitoring and blood pressure monitoring. To perform the apnea test:

1. Perform a baseline arterial blood gas (ABG) and hypersaturation of blood, giving 100 percent oxygen via the respirator for ten minutes.
2. Disconnect patient from the respirator, but supply 100 percent oxygen (6 liters/minute) via nasal cannula secured in the endotracheal tube.
3. Repeat ABG after approximately eight minutes and reconnect the respirator.

The apnea test is positive (supports diagnosis of brain death) if respiratory movements are absent and the repeat arterial PCO_2 is greater than 60mm or shows a 20mm increase from baseline.

- If the patient becomes hemodynamically unstable or develops bradycardia, the patient is reconnected to the respirator. A repeat ABG should be drawn immediately and, if it meets the above criteria and a minimum of five minutes has elapsed, the test is considered positive. If not, the apnea test should be repeated or ancillary testing done.

  In situations where apnea testing cannot be initiated, such as in hemodynamic/respiratory instability (i.e., ARDS or hypoxemia), see use of ancillary studies (below).

C. Ancillary Studies

  When, in the judgment of one of the physicians performing the evaluation, the clinical examination is not sufficient to make a declaration of brain death, there is no known cause, and/or when apnea testing cannot be done, one of the following tests should be considered:

  - *Nuclear medicine brain scan*—No uptake of isotope in brain parenchyma. Written consent is not required for a nuclear medicine brain scan.
  - *Cerebral angiography*—No intracerebral filling at the level of the carotid bifurcation or circle of Willis. Four-vessel intracranial angiography is definitive in diagnosing cessation of circulation to the entire brain (both cerebrum and brainstem). Written consent is required.
  - *Electroencephalogram (EEG)*—The EEG can demonstrate electrocerebral silence. Written consent is not required.
  - *Transcranial doppler*—No diastolic or reverberating flow and documentation of small systolic peaks in early systole. Written consent is not required.

  The ancillary testing and determination of brain death can be performed even if the family expresses religious, moral, or emotional objections to brain death. Confirmatory determination provides medical certainty about the clinical condition of the patient. If the family refuses consent for ancillary testing, notify administration, which may seek guidance from Bioethics and the Legal Department.

This section emphasizes that confirmatory testing must be conducted—even over families' religious or moral objections. This is in contrast to the section below, which discusses termination of treatment measures after brain death has been confirmed, and which may require reasonably accommodating families' sensibilities.

Note: Complete cessation of circulation to the normothermic adult brain for more than ten minutes is incompatible with survival of brain tissue. Documentation of this circulatory failure is evidence of death of the entire brain.

II. Determination of Brain Death in Children and Infants

The attending physicians must demonstrate that all of the following criteria have been met to determine brain death:

1. Absence of confounding drug levels
2. Absence of clinical signs of cerebral responsiveness and brainstem activity
3. Apnea
4. Electrocerebral silence ($<$ one year old)

To fulfill the above criteria, the following procedures are required:

1. Demonstrated absence of confounding drug levels
2. Clinical examination to demonstrate absence of cerebral responsiveness and brainstem activity

During all testing, the patient must be maintained normothermic and as normotensive as possible. The examining physician must demonstrate:

1. Total unresponsiveness to verbal, auditory, and painful stimuli
2. No spontaneous vocalization and no voluntary activity
3. Fixed, dilated pupils, unresponsive to light
4. Absence of eye movements induced by oculocephalic and ice cold caloric irritation of the ear canals
5. Absence of facial and oropharyngeal responses to stimulation
6. Absence of corneal, gag, cough, sucking, and rooting reflexes
7. Tone is flaccid, with no spontaneous or induced movement (excluding spinal cord movements such as reflex, withdrawal, or spinal myoclonus)

All examinations and tests must be documented in the medical record by each attending. The age-related procedures are outlined below (see observation requirements).

A. Determination of Apnea in Children:

These procedures must be administered jointly by a neurology or neurosurgery attending physician and a pediatric critical care attending physician.

a. Determine that the patient is normocapnic by blood gas measurement.
b. Give 100 percent oxygen for ten minutes while the patient is on a respirator.
c. Remove the patient from the respirator while continuing 100 percent oxygen by catheter to the endotracheal tube.
d. Obtain blood gases every five minutes.
e. Demonstrate that the patient does not breathe spontaneously during an eight-minute test period, or that the PCO_2 reaches a level greater than 59 torr.

If the patient becomes hemodynamically unstable or develops bradycardia, the patient is reconnected to the respirator. A repeat ABG should be drawn immediately and, if it meets the above criteria and a minimum of five minutes has elapsed, the test is considered positive. If not, the apnea test should be repeated or ancillary testing done.

B. Electroencephalographic Testing for Electrocerebral Silence

The EEG testing is to be interpreted by an attending neurologist in accordance with American Clinical Neurophysiology Society Guidelines.

C. Observation Requirements:

a. Below age 7 days: No determination of brain death may be made.

b. Age 7 days to 2 months: Two complete examinations (includes apnea testing) and two EEGs separated by at least forty-eight hours are required.

c. Age 2 months to one year:

Either (1) or (2):

1. Two complete examinations and two EEGs separated by at least twenty-four hours.

2. One complete examination and one EEG, and either one concomitant cerebral-radionuclide angiographic study (CRAG), conducted by an attending nuclear medicine physician, or one contrast angiography study conducted by an attending neuroradiologist, which study demonstrates arrest of carotid circulation at the base of the skull and absence of intracranial arterial circulation.

d. Over one year:

Either (1) or (2):

1. Two complete examinations separated by at least twenty-four hours.

2. When an irreversible cause exists, one complete examination and one EEG and either a confirmatory CRAG study conducted by an attending nuclear medicine physician or a contrast angiographic study conducted by an attending pediatric radiologist, which study demonstrates arrest of carotid circulation at the base of the skull and absence of intracranial arterial circulation.

III. Pronouncement of Death

After the attendings have determined and documented that the patient is brain dead, the pronouncement of death is made and the family is notified.

IV. Informing the Family/Significant Other(s) of Final Determination of Death

The family/significant other(s) shall be notified as soon as the criteria for brain death have been met. The unit clinical team and attending physician(s) should be available to provide support for the family.

Families will require multidisciplinary support:

• The nursing, social services, palliative care, and/or chaplaincy may provide bereavement support for the family.

• Families, including those who object to a brain death determination, will be offered additional emotional support.

• An ethics consultation may assist family in accepting brain death.

> Some policies require notifying the patient's family, but do not explicitly address the need for coordinated and ongoing communication with the family. For example, "Whenever possible the family should be fully informed about the patient's condition. Family members should be afforded a brief time to adjust to the impending determination of death, the resultant removal of the respirator, and have their questions answered."

V. Organ and Tissue Donation

The responsibility for discussing organ donation with the legal next of kin and obtaining consent for donation rests with the procurement coordinator of the state OPO. The coordinator collaborates with the clinical team throughout the brain death determination and consent process. The explanation of brain death should be understood and accepted by the family before any mention of organ donation.

VI. Management

1. Therapeutic modalities should be continued after the pronouncement of death for *organ* support if organ/tissue donation is being considered. Unless there is a need for reasonable accommodation (see section VII), if there is no possibility of organ/tissue donation, upon pronouncement of death, all organ support interventions shall be discontinued on the unit upon the *written order* of the attending physician.

2. If the patient is a potential organ donor and not already in an ICU setting, arrangements may be made to transfer the patient to an ICU setting for appropriate management.

3. The deceased patient's family and significant other(s) should be treated with sensitivity and respect and should be offered the opportunity to be present when the ventilator is disconnected. If they wish to be present, they should be advised of the possible occurrence of isolated spinal movements.

   a. If the family requests a reasonable time delay before disconnecting the ventilator, efforts should be made to accommodate the request.

   b. The family should be informed that the ventilator will not be disconnected immediately in the face of religious, moral, or other objection to brain death determination unless continued utilization deprives other patients who require these resources (see section VII).

> This is the only policy reviewed to detail the nature of and responsibility for informing the family that brain death has been confirmed and that, therefore, interventions will be discontinued. An important feature is the explanation that

even temporary continuation of the ventilator will not be possible if it deprives a patient who can benefit from the resource.

VII. Reasonable Accommodation of Moral or Religious or Other Objection to Brain Death

State-specific requirements that "reasonable accommodation" be made for families' religious or moral objections to brain death standards do not appear in other policies. State policies address the accommodation in varying degrees of detail.

Efforts shall be made to provide a sensitive compromise that balances respect for the religious or moral beliefs, feelings of families and care providers, the legal and medical standard of care, and the interests of other patients.

If a family expresses objection to a brain death determination or there is knowledge of the patient's objection to a brain death determination prior to the loss of decision-making capabilities, the attending physician shall immediately notify the administration and Risk Management. An ethics and/or palliative care consultation or a member of the chaplaincy may provide support and counseling for the family and assist members in accepting the death of their loved one. The attending physician informs the family that the following interventions may be withheld or withdrawn:

  a. treatment in an intensive care unit
  b. medications or other treatment
  c. blood or blood products
  d. care by a private duty nurse paid for by the hospital
  e. nasogastric or intravenous nutrition or hydration

If, in spite of bereavement support and ethics involvement, the family continues to express religious, moral, or other objections to the brain death determination and discontinuation of interventions, the attending physician shall fully inform the family of the following:

  a. The family may arrange for a second opinion by appropriate outside medical specialists and staff will make reasonable efforts to facilitate such consultations.
  b. The family may arrange for transfer to another facility willing to accept the deceased patient. Reasonable efforts will be made to facilitate such a transfer. A brief extension will be allowed if arrangements for transfer are being completed.
  c. The family may seek judicial review.

If continuation of any treatment measures, including the use of the ventilator, causes that treatment to be withheld from another patient, administration must be notified. In such cases, all such measures, including the ventilator, may be withdrawn without waiting for court authorization. The attending will so document in the medical record. The deceased patient may be removed from the intensive care unit if the medical staff determines that the bed is necessary to provide appropriate medical care for other patients and the deceased patient is not a potential organ donor.

Three days after the final determination of brain death, if the family persists in objecting to the brain death determination, the Legal Department may consider whether to seek court authorization to withdraw the ventilatory support.

VIII. Medical Record Documentation

The results of the brain death evaluation shall be documented in the medical record by both attendings. Discussion with family concerning the evaluation, the criteria used, and the specific results of the tests done and the time of final brain death declaration should be documented.

- The time of death is the time of the second note that states that the patient is brain dead.

IX. Conscientious Exemption for Physicians/Associates

All reasonable efforts shall be made to reassign a nurse, physician, or other associate who has a strongly held cultural, ethical, or religious objection to carrying out the provisions of this policy.

This is the only policy reviewed that contains provisions to exempt physicians and other staff who hold cultural, religious, or moral objections to participating in the brain death protocol.

One policy reviewed addresses the matter of legal liability: "A physician who makes a determination of death in accordance with this section and accepted medical standards is not liable for damages in any civil action or subject to prosecution in any criminal proceedings for his acts or the acts of others based on that determination." The policy further states that any person who in good faith relies on a medical determination of brain death is not civilly or criminally liable.

DO-NOT-INTUBATE (DNI) ORDERS

PURPOSE

To clarify the policy and procedure for forgoing (withholding) intubation for patients at the Medical Center.

> This is the only policy reviewed that deals separately with forgoing intubation for adults in situations other than cardiopulmonary arrest. One institution has a separate set of DNI Guidelines for Infants, Children and Adolescents. One institution addresses forgoing intubation in nonarrest situations in a separate section in its policy on forgoing life-extending treatments.

SCOPE

All Medical Center associates involved in providing patient care services.

I. Application: A do-not-intubate (DNI) order should be used to forgo intubation in circumstances *other* than cardiopulmonary arrest.

> One institution's policy, DNI Guidelines for Infants, Children and Adolescents, specifies what will and will not be done for a minor patient with a DNI order. Some excerpts:
> "DNI - In the event of respiratory insufficiency or arrest, no endotracheal intubation for the purpose of sustained mechanical ventilation or for the purpose of establishing a patent airway will be initiated and/or continued.
> Considerations:
> 1. The presence of a DNI order does not prohibit the use of an endotracheal tube for:
>   a. Controlling the airway for surgical procedures
>   b. Use in suctioning
>   c. Use in acute reversible upper airway obstruction, i.e., choking
>   d. Use in temporary hypoventilation, i.e., narcotic overdose
>   e. As an adjunct for pain relief or relief of dyspnea
> 2. DNI does not prohibit the use of cardiopulmonary resuscitation (CPR)....
> 3. The concept of DNI is compatible with maximal therapeutic care. The patient

may be receiving vigorous support in all therapeutic modalities and yet justi-
fiably be considered DNI." The last point, also emphasized in several DNR
policies, reinforces the notion that forgoing any intervention, even one that
is life-sustaining, does not determine the overall care plan or alter the team's
attention to the patient.

II. Procedure for Entering a DNI Order

DNI orders are *separate* from DNR orders.

In a cardiac and/or pulmonary *ARREST* a DNR order *includes not intubating*
the patient.

• However, in *NONARREST* conditions requiring intubation, including moderate
to severe respiratory distress, a *separate DNI order* is required to forgo intubation.
Nonarrest situations are *not* covered by the DNR law.

The policy on forgoing life-extending treatments that addresses DNI orders
covers only "an adult patient without capacity and without a health care agent."

A. DNI Order for a Capacitated Patient

A patient *WITH* decisional capacity may choose not to be intubated at any time
in the future *or* only under certain specified conditions after full discussion with
the attending physician.

1. If the patient *wants to be intubated* in *all circumstances except a cardiopulmonary
arrest, no separate* DNI order is needed, and a DNR order will suffice.

2. If the patient has consented to a do-not-resuscitate (DNR) order and also
requests not to be intubated or reintubated for respiratory distress, a *do-
not-intubate order should also be entered.* The Attending Physician's Do-Not-
Intubate (DNI) Documentation Form should be completed and a written or
electronic do-not-intubate (DNI) order entered. *Note: When the patient already
has a DNR order, a separate DNI consent form is NOT needed.*

3. In the rarer circumstance that a patient does not wish to have a do-not-
resuscitate (DNR) order but requests not to be intubated under any circumstance, *both* the Attending Physician's Do-Not-Intubate (DNI) Documentation
Form *and an additional form,* Patient Surrogate Consent to Do-Not-Intubate
(DNI) Order, must be completed and a written or electronic do-not-intubate
order entered. The patient should be advised that having a DNI order without
an accompanying DNR order would severely limit the physicians' ability to
provide effective resuscitation if CPR were required.

B. DNI Order for an Incapacitated Patient with a Health Care Agent

If the patient has an appointed health care agent, the agent may request that the patient not be intubated for significant respiratory distress or other noncardiac and/or pulmonary arrest condition, just as the patient would if the patient had decisional capacity. The attending physician must document the patient's lack of capacity, obtain a concurring attending's opinion as to lack of capacity, and fully document the discussion with the agent about the patient's condition and prognosis. The attending physician should then follow the instructions in A-1, 2, or 3 above as relevant to the patient.

C. DNI Order for Patient without Capacity, with Surrogate

When an incapacitated patient has a surrogate who is not an appointed health care agent, the attending may *ONLY* enter a do-not-intubate (DNI) order to forgo intubation for significant respiratory distress or in another *NONARREST* situation under the following conditions:

1. A *DNR order has been entered,* based on one of the *four medical conditions* stipulated in the DNR policy *(i.e., terminal condition, permanent unconsciousness, medical futility, or extraordinary burden) and*

2. The patient's family or other surrogate are in agreement about the patient's wishes and are able to clearly *describe to the attending physician* the patient's prior wishes. (This constitutes clear and convincing evidence of the patient's prior wishes not to be intubated in the present circumstances.) *and*

3. The attending physician completes his or her portions of the Attending Physician's DNI Documentation Form.

4. A second attending physician, the concurring attending, completes the two "Concurring Attending" sections of the Attending Physician's DNI Documentation Form, entering a concurring opinion about the patient's lack of decisional capacity and the patient's medical condition.

5. The attending physician should complete the required documentation and enter either a written or an electronic DNI order.

(*Note: If the above conditions for a DNI order have been met, there is NO need to obtain written evidence from family/surrogate and/or review by the Legal Department and the medical director.*)

The policy on forgoing life-extending treatment that includes DNI orders stipulates, "The attending shall ask family members and friends to document their evidence in writing, when feasible, and enter such depositions in the chart."

III. Review, Modification, or Revocation of a Do-not-intubate (DNI) Order

A. The attending physician should review the DNI order every seven days for inpatients and every sixty days for ALOC patients and whenever the patient's condition materially changes, to determine if the order is still appropriate in light of the patient's condition. The review, however, does not require the physician to obtain consent each time the order is renewed.

   B. If a patient *regains decisional capacity,* the DNI order authorized by the agent or other surrogate *must be revoked* and the attending must discuss treatment options with the *patient.*

   C. If the *patient's condition improves,* the attending physician must *reassess* the patient's prior declared choices in light of the patient's changed condition to determine whether forgoing intubation is still indicated. The attending should discuss this assessment with the patient/agent or other surrogate, as medically indicated.

   D. If the *patient, agent, or other surrogate revokes or otherwise modifies his or her consent* to a do-not-intubate order, any health professional who becomes aware of this change must contact the attending physician immediately. The attending *must cancel the order* and document in the medical record and on the Attending Physician's DNI Documentation Form any modifications or revocation of the order and the reasons given for the change. Thereafter, if indicated, dispute mediation may be initiated by contacting Bioethics or the Medical Director's Office.

IV. Contact for Assistance Regarding This Policy

   Any *questions concerning this policy* should be directed to the Office of the Medical Director or to the Division of Bioethics during the daytime from Monday through Friday and to the on-call associate director of nursing (A.D.N.) at all other times. The A.D.N. will involve the appropriate resource department.

DO-NOT-RESUSCITATE (DNR) ORDERS

PURPOSE

To set forth policies and procedures for deciding to forgo cardiopulmonary resuscitation (CPR) in the event of a cardiac and/or respiratory arrest and entering a DNR order. A DNR order does not limit any other care and can be consistent with aggressive treatment. If there is no DNR order, the law assumes the patient wants and consents to CPR, and a code must be called. (The extent and duration of the code are based on the medical judgment of the physician(s) present.)

> A policy, beginning with a statement of purpose, can be used to meet educational as well as compliance objectives. This policy articulates an institutional philosophy about the purpose and procedures of do-not-resuscitate (DNR) orders; establishes and explains standards for decision making about resuscitation; and provides guidance in obtaining informed consent for, writing, and documenting DNR orders.

One policy, Do Not Attempt to Resuscitate, emphasizes in its title and its content that it is the *attempt* to resuscitate, not the successful resuscitation, that will be forgone. The policy begins with an abstract that says, in part, "Resuscitation may not benefit patients who are permanently unconscious, suffering with terminal illness (if death is anticipated within a relatively short time), or who have debilitating irreversible conditions. The primary principles that should govern decisions to issue DNAR orders are self-determination, patient welfare, and the futility of medical treatment."

This DNR policy meets medical, legal, ethical, and accreditation standards to help Medical Center physicians and other associates provide optimal patient care and protect patients' rights. Any questions concerning this policy should be directed to the Office of the Medical Director or Bioethics. Attached to this policy are forms that must be completed before a DNR order is issued.

Most DNR policies include the various forms that must be completed in different circumstances when DNR orders are authorized. Some policies also include a statement about the purpose of the paperwork, for example: "To simplify compliance with the requirements of state law, eight documentation sheets have been developed. These documentation sheets set forth the steps the responsible physician must take before he or she can issue a DNR order, and the appropriate sheet for the patient must be completed before the responsible physician can issue a DNR order. Attached to each documentation sheet are any consent forms that may be necessary before a DNR order is issued."

Note: DO-NOT-INTUBATE (DNI) orders are closely associated with but distinct from DO-NOT-RESUSCITATE (DNR) orders. (See the Do-not-intubate (DNI) Policy.) In summary:

In a cardiopulmonary *arrest,* a DNR order permits withholding both intubation and other components of CPR. A separate DNI order is not needed.

In situations *other than an arrest,* a separate DNI order is needed to forgo intubation since a DNR order *only* applies to cardiopulmonary arrest. A DNI order is appropriate when a patient/surrogate chooses to forgo intubation or reintubation for present or future moderate to severe respiratory distress or when a patient has requested not to be intubated under *any* future circumstance.

Clear and convincing evidence of the patient's wishes regarding resuscitation is required if the patient lacks decisional capacity. DNI orders in nonarrest situations are fully covered in the Do-not-intubate (DNI) Policy.

> No other DNR policy reviewed distinguishes and explains the relationship between do-not-resuscitate (DNR) and do-not-intubate (DNI) orders. One policy on forgoing life-extending treatment, however, contains a separate section devoted to forgoing intubation by means of DNI orders. (See Forgoing Life-extending Treatment Policy.)

TABLE OF CONTENTS: DO-NOT-RESUSCITATE (DNR) POLICY

> Because the process of considering, executing, and implementing DNR orders involves matters addressed in other policies (decisional capacity, advance directives, informed consent), those matters are discussed in several DNR policies as well.

E. Physician Documentation and Surrogate Consent to DNR

F. Concerns about Surrogate Decision Making

G. Procedure for Obtaining a DNR Order for Incapacitated Patients *without* Health Care Proxies or DNR Surrogates When There is *NO Objection*

H. Procedure for Obtaining a DNR Order for Incapacitated Patients When Patient, Agent, or Possible Surrogate *Objects*

I. Patients Who Are Minors

J. Special Situations: Patients with Mental Illness, Mental Retardation, and/or Developmental Disability

> Because of the complexity of the DNR process, including determination of decisional capacity and decision-making authority, one policy includes two flow charts, one for the adult and one for the minor patient.

IV. Notification of the Patient, Health Care Proxy, or DNR Surrogate and the Health Care Team

V. Renewing DNR Orders

VI. Revoking Consent to a DNR Order

VII. Canceling DNR Orders

VIII. Nonhospital DNR Orders

IX. Transfers

A. To the Medical Center

B. From the Medical Center

C. To Another Attending Physician

X. Dispute Mediation and Judicial Review

A. Dispute Mediation Process and Judicial Review

B. Dispute Mediation Committee Membership

C. Mandatory Mediation

XI. Other Issues/Concerns about DNR Orders or DNR Policies and Procedures (P&P)

XII. Appendices: DNR Documentation and Consent Forms

A. DNR Documentation Form

B. Oral Consent to DNR Form

C. Written Consent to DNR Form

D. Affidavit of Close Friend Consenting to a Do-Not-Resuscitate Order

E. Nonhospital DNR Order Form

(The five DNR order forms listed above are available on every unit.)

DNR POLICY AND PROCEDURES

I. Definitions

Adult: Any person who is 18 years of age or older, has custody of a child, or has married.

Attending physician: The physician with primary responsibility for the patient's treatment and care. More than one physician, sharing responsibility, may be the attending physician.

Capacity: Capacity to make a DNR decision means the ability to understand and appreciate the nature and consequences of a DNR order, including the benefits, burdens, and risks of CPR, and to reach an informed decision regarding a DNR order. Every adult is presumed to have decisional capacity unless there has been a *clinical determination of incapacity* or a *legal determination of incompetence.*

Cardiopulmonary resuscitation (CPR): Measures to restore cardiac function and/or to support ventilation in the event of a cardiac or respiratory arrest. These measures include manual chest compression, intubation, artificial respirations, direct cardiac injection, intravenous medications, electrical defibrillation, and open-chest cardiac massage. CPR excludes measures taken in the absence of an arrest, such as intubation to improve ventilation and cardiac function.

Close friend acting as surrogate: Any adult who knows the patient and presents a completed affidavit (as set forth in Appendix D) to the attending physician.

Concurring physician: An attending physician, selected by the patient's attending physician, to provide a concurring opinion about the patient's diagnosis, prognosis, and/or decisional capacity.

Dispute mediation process: A mechanism for resolving conflicts arising between or among health care professional(s), the patient, and/or patient's family or surrogates. Any disagreement about entering a DNR order must be referred to mediation, during which time the order may not be written and an existing DNR order must be suspended. If the patient (or someone purporting to speak on the patient's behalf) objects to the DNR order, the staff member hearing the objection should document the objection in the patient's medical record. The order should not be written without consulting with the medical director/designee.

DNR surrogate: An adult, other than a health care agent, selected in accordance with the State Public Health Law and section III-D-2 of this policy, to make decisions about a DNR order on behalf of an incapacitated patient. The list of potential surrogates and order of priority is found on both the oral DNR consent form, Appendix B, and the written DNR consent form, Appendix C.

Do-not-resuscitate (DNR) order: An order not to attempt CPR in the event of a cardiac or respiratory arrest. Such an order may include all CPR measures or may be limited to specific procedures. A DNR order for an outpatient requires a separate order. (See Nonhospital DNR Order, Appendix E.)

Emergency medical services personnel: The personnel of an agency providing initial emergency medical assistance, including but not limited to first responders, emergency medical technicians, and advanced emergency technicians. These personnel are legally required to honor nonhospital DNR orders when called to attend a patient who has experienced a cardiopulmonary arrest in the field.

Extraordinary burden: In determining whether CPR would be an extraordinary burden under section II-D-2 of this policy, factors to be considered include but are not limited to whether CPR would cause more harm than benefit because of a patient's frailty, debility, or illness.

Health care agent: An adult to whom health care decision-making authority has been delegated through a health care proxy, in accordance with the Medical Center's Administrative P&P, entitled Advance Directives: Health Care Proxies and Living Wills. The agent's powers are only activated by a determination that the patient lacks decisional capacity. The decisions of the agent supersede those of any other person. If, however, the agent's decision seems contrary to the patient's previously expressed wishes, the agent must indicate what changed wishes of the patient support the agent's decision. A copy of the Health Care Proxy Form should be placed in the patient's medical record.

Hospital emergency service personnel: The personnel of the Emergency Department of the Medical Center, including but not limited to, attending physicians, registered professional nurses, other nursing staff, and registered physicians assistants assigned to the Medical Center's Emergency Department.

DNR based on medical futility: The DNR law defines CPR medical futility as follows: (1) CPR will be unsuccessful in restoring cardiac and/or respiratory function, or (2) the patient will experience repeated arrests in a short period of time before death occurs.

> These futility criteria, stipulated in the state law with its narrow physiologic definition of DNR futility, are not found in the reviewed policies from other states. The policies of other states provide for physicians to assess resuscitation according to the same futility criteria as other treatments. For example, one policy defines futile treatment as one that has "no realistic chance of providing a benefit that the patient has the capacity to perceive and appreciate, such as merely preserving the physiological functions of a permanently unconscious patient or has no realistic chance of achieving the medical goal of returning the patient to a level of health that permits survival outside the acute care setting. . . ."

Mental illness: An affliction manifested by a disorder or disturbance in behavior, feeling, thinking, or judgment to such an extent that the patient requires care, treatment, and rehabilitation. Mental illness does not include delirium or dementia, such as Alzheimer's disease, or other disorders related to delirium or dementia.

Minor: Any person under 18 years of age except one who has custody of a child or who has married or is serving in the Armed Services.

Nonhospital DNR order: An order that directs emergency medical services personnel and Medical Center Emergency Department staff not to attempt CPR if the patient suffers a cardiac or respiratory arrest in the field or in the Emergency Department or other ambulatory area.

Permanently unconscious: Irreversibly unconscious, without thought, sensation, or awareness of self or environment, including an irreversible coma, persistent vegetative state, or the end stage of certain degenerative neurological conditions.

Terminal condition: An illness or injury from which there is no recovery and which reasonably can be expected to cause death within three months to two years, depending on the underlying diagnosis.

Witness: Any capacitated adult who attests to the validity of a verbal consent or written signature.

II. General Guidelines

    A. Overview

        The DNR law established rules under which capacitated patients and, in appropriate circumstances, others speaking on behalf of the incapacitated patient, may consent to issuing a DNR order. This policy describes the circumstances under which DNR orders should be entered and reviewed.

Every patient is presumed to consent to the administration of CPR in the event of cardiac or respiratory arrest, unless a DNR order is written.

To forgo *other* life-sustaining treatments, see the Forgoing Life-sustaining Treatment Policy. When patients/surrogates choose *in advance to forgo intubation* in non-cardiopulmonary arrest situations, see the Do-not-intubate (DNI) Policy.

All patients, even those with DNR orders, should receive care that is appropriate to their medical conditions. A DNR order refers only to cardiopulmonary resuscitation (CPR) and does not limit any other care or treatment for the patient or authorize denial or withdrawal of treatments other than CPR.

This type of overview, which establishes the clinical and legal context, the presumption of capacity, and the notion that DNR refers only to CPR and does not limit other care, appears in some but not all DNR policies. One policy emphasizes the specificity of the order by stating, "Maximal therapeutic efforts in all other areas of care, especially with regard to improving patient comfort, which includes relief of pain and fear and supplying fluids and nutrition, will be provided as appropriate."

Under its state law, one policy permits DNR orders to be tailored to the individual needs of patients: "The diversity of patients, illnesses, and therapies requires that DNR orders be adaptable to specific circumstances. To ensure flexibility, three types of DNR orders may be given . . .

- 'DNR Comfort Care' orders activate the DNR Protocol at the time the order is given. DNR Comfort Care orders permit comfort care only both *before and during* a cardiac or respiratory arrest. . . .
- 'DNR Comfort Care-Arrest' orders activate the DNR Protocol at the time of a cardiac or respiratory arrest. . . . Resuscitative therapies will be administered before an arrest but not during an arrest. . . .
- All other DNR orders are 'DNR Specified' orders. DNR Specified orders modify the DNR Protocol in some respect, either in treatment modalities or in the timing of the protocol activation."

This policy also requires that all patients with DNR orders wear DNR identification bracelets to "facilitate communication and direct care to comply with DNR orders previously given, especially in emergencies."

Summary of Steps for Attending Physicians for Obtaining a DNR Consent and Entering a DNR Order

1. Determine that the patient meets the criteria for a DNR order. (See Criteria for Surrogate Consent to DNR, section III-D-3b, 1–4, below.)

2. Assess the patient's decisional capacity to consent to or refuse consent to a DNR order. (See Capacity.) The capacity assessment must be thoroughly documented in a progress note.

3. *Procedure for Patients with Capacity*:

   a. Discuss the DNR order with the patient.

   b. Obtain the patient's oral consent (see Appendix B) or written consent (see Appendix C) to a DNR order, and place the consent form in the medical record.

   c. Complete the Attending Physician's Do-Not-Resuscitate (DNR) Documentation Form and place it in the medical record. (See Appendix A.)

   d. Enter a DNR order. This may be done by entering a written doctor's order or an electronic order on CIS.

4. *Procedure for Patients without Capacity, with a Surrogate:*

   a. Discuss DNR with the health care agent or other DNR surrogate.

   b. Obtain the health care agent's or other surrogate's oral consent (see Appendix B) or written consent to a DNR order to a DNR order, and place the consent form in the medical record. (See Appendix C.)

   c. Complete the Attending Physician's Do-Not-Resuscitate (DNR) Documentation Form, which includes obtaining the required signatures of a concurring attending physician as to the patient's lack of capacity and medical condition. Place the form in the medical record. (See Appendix A.)

   d. Notify the patient of the lack of capacity determination and the consent of the health care agent or other surrogate to the DNR order. (See section IV-A.)

   e. Enter a DNR order. This may be done by entering a written DNR order or an electronic DNR order on CIS.

5. *Procedure for Patient without Capacity Who Has NO Surrogate to Consent to a DNR Order*

   Consider whether the patient meets the criteria for a medical futility DNR (for a patient who has no health care agent or DNR surrogate or when the agent or potential DNR surrogate is unwilling or unable to consent but does not object to a DNR order). If there is objection to entering a DNR order, see f-2 below.

   a. *No Available or Willing Health Care Agent or DNR Surrogate*

   If the patient has no health care agent or other DNR surrogate to consent to a DNR order, or if the patient has a potential surrogate/relative who is unwilling or unable to consent but *does not object*, a DNR order may be written, based on medical futility. In order to enter a DNR based on medical futility, the patient must meet one of the following criteria, as determined by the attending physician: either the patient would not survive an arrest or would have multiple arrests in a short period of time, that is, that CPR would fail/ be medically futile. *For a medical futility DNR order to be entered when there is no one to consent to DNR, two additional concurring physician signatures are required.* Both a concurring attending physician *and* the medical director/ designee must sign the appropriate sections of the Attending Physician's DNR Documentation Form and document the rationale for their opinions about capacity and futility in the progress notes. (See section III-D-3.)

b. *Objection by Patient, Agent, or Other DNR Surrogate to a DNR Order Based on Medical Futility*

If the patient, the patient's health care agent, or other potential DNR surrogate objects to the attending physician's entering a DNR order based on medical futility, the matter must be submitted to dispute mediation, and the order may not be entered until the mediation is completed. (See Dispute Mediation, section X.) If the Dispute Mediation Committee agrees that a DNR order based on medical futility may be written, the steps in section II-B-3-f-1, directly above, should be followed.

f. Other Considerations in Consent to DNR

- A DNR surrogate (who is not the health care agent) may consent to a DNR order only if the patient is in one of the four medical conditions listed in section III-D-b-1–4.

- A health care agent may consent to a DNR order under the same circumstances as the patient would, if the patient were capacitated.

- Consent to a DNR order may be authorized by a DNR surrogate, based on instructions in the patient's living will. If there is no health care agent or DNR surrogate available, the attending should contact Bioethics or the Office of the Medical Director for assistance in reviewing the living will, to determine if the patient's medical condition corresponds with the information in the living will.

B. Role of House Staff in Obtaining Consent to and Entering DNR Orders

> Other policies do not distinguish in such detail the DNR responsibilities of attending physicians and house officers.

As described in section II-B above, obtaining consent to and entering a DNR order is primarily an attending physician responsibility. However, the house staff, in conjunction with the attending physician, may perform the following steps in the policy and procedure: (*House staff*: See specific instructions to attending physicians in section II-B above for detailed instructions about each step in the DNR procedure.)

1. Discuss the patient's suitability for a DNR order with the attending physician.

2. Request psychiatric consultation or involvement of a concurring attending physician as requested by the patient's attending physician.

3. Discuss risks, benefits, and burdens of CPR with the capacitated patient, health care agent, or DNR surrogate, as appropriate.

In addition to the above delegated responsibilities, fellows and senior house staff who are licensed in this state may serve as concurring physicians for DNR orders on evenings, nights, weekends, or holidays when waiting for a concurring attending physician to come to the hospital would be unrealistic in light of the patient's condition. Otherwise, house staff may not act in place of attending physicians.

C. Limited DNR Orders

1. DNR orders *may* be limited to certain types of procedures or to specific conditions if, after full explanation of the benefits and burdens, the patient or surrogate will *only* consent to orders forgoing specific resuscitation measures or under specific conditions.

2. DNR in the OR/PACU or other specific locations (e.g., the Dialysis Unit, Radiology Department):

A DNR order is valid and must be respected by all health care providers even if an arrest occurs away from the patient care unit, in a diagnostic and treatment area such as the operating room, dialysis unit, or radiology department. The involved physician(s) must discuss with the patient (or surrogate for an incapacitated patient) whether the existing DNR order should be suspended for surgery or another procedure and, if so, specify the duration of the suspension. The attending surgeon, the attending anesthesiologist, and the patient or surrogate must be in agreement. The joint decision either to continue or to suspend the DNR order should then be documented in the progress notes, as well as in the anesthesia documentation, and fully communicated to the health care team.

> The importance of clarifying the DNR status during the perioperative period is emphasized in most, but not all, policies.

D. Health Care Providers Objecting to a DNR Order

1. *Attending Physicians*: An attending physician who becomes aware of a patient or family request for a DNR order and who objects to a DNR should promptly make known to the person requesting the DNR order his or her objection to the issuance of such an order and the reason(s) for this objection. The physician should either submit the matter to dispute mediation or make all reasonable efforts to arrange to transfer the patient to another attending physician.

2. *Other Medical Center Physicians and Associates*: If a Medical Center physician or associate, other than the attending physician responsible for the care of a patient with a DNR order, objects to providing care in accordance with the DNR order, he or she should inform the attending physician and his or her immediate supervisor, who will take reasonable steps, including adjusting staff assignments, consistent with patient needs, to accommodate the staff member's objection.

III. Consent for DNR Orders

A. Elements of Informed Consent to a DNR Order

Before a DNR order may be entered, the attending physician or other responsible physician must obtain either oral or written consent to a DNR order from the patient or a legally authorized agent or other surrogate. The person consenting should be provided with information about the patient's diagnosis and prognosis, the reasonably foreseeable risks and benefits of CPR for the patient, and the consequences of a DNR order. Oral consent should be documented on the Oral Consent to DNR Form, Appendix B. Written consent must be documented using the Written Consent to DNR Form, Appendix C.

Note: An adult patient with capacity or a health care agent may consent to a DNR order regardless of the patient's medical condition. A DNR surrogate may only consent if one of four medical conditions is present. (See section III-D-2-b-1–4.)

B. DNR Consent for Adults with Capacity

Consent to a DNR order must be obtained from the capacitated patient. Oral consent requires the signatures of two witnesses, one of whom must be a physician affiliated with the Medical Center. The Oral Consent to DNR Form (Appendix B) must be completed and placed in the medical record. If written consent is obtained, the Written Consent to DNR Form (Appendix C) must be signed in the presence of one witness, and the form completed and placed in the medical record.

If the attending physician determines that the patient would suffer significant and imminent harm from a discussion of CPR ("therapeutic exception" to the disclosure requirement), he or she should contact Bioethics or the Medical Director's Office for further direction before entering the DNR order. *The signature of the medical director/designee is required for a "therapeutic exception" to discussing a DNR order with a capacitated patient.*

Some policies provide a full and detailed discussion of the therapeutic exception, including the criteria, strictness of the standards, and the procedure. For example:

"If the attending physician determines that an adult patient with capacity would suffer *immediate and severe injury* from a discussion of CPR, the attending physician may write a DNR order without first obtaining the patient's consent, but only after:

1. obtaining written concurrence of another physician who has personally examined the patient; AND

2. ascertaining the wishes of the patient to the extent possible without subjecting the patient to the risk of immediate and severe injury; AND

3. obtaining the consent of an available health care agent, or, if none, then the consent of a surrogate, unless the order is entered based on the patient's previous consent; AND

4. documenting the reasons for invoking the therapeutic privilege.

5. When the therapeutic exception provision is invoked, the attending physician shall reassess the patient's risk of injury from a discussion of cardiopulmonary resuscitation on a regular basis and shall consult the patient regarding resuscitation as soon as the medical basis for not consulting the patient no longer exists.

6. 'Immediate and severe injury' is a strict standard and should only be invoked when serious medical consequences may reasonably be expected to result from informing the patient, such as a heart attack or suicide attempt."

C. Determination of Incapacity

An attending physician and a concurring physician must determine that a patient lacks capacity and must document this opinion on the Attending Physician's DNR Documentation Form (Appendix A). While house staff may not act in place of the attending physician, fellows and senior house staff licensed in this state may act as concurring physicians on evenings, weekends, or holidays when delaying the DNR order to wait for a concurring attending physician would be harmful in light of the patient's condition.

"Capacity" to make a DNR decision means the ability to understand and appreciate the nature and consequences of a DNR order, including the risks and benefits of CPR, and to reach an informed decision. Every adult patient is presumed to have decisional capacity unless there has been a clinical determination of incapacity in accordance with this section, section III-C, or a court determination of incompetence. A finding that a patient lacks capacity to make a decision about DNR does *not* necessarily mean that the patient lacks capacity for other decisions since capacity is decision-specific.

Some policies limit the discussion of decisional capacity to the definition section and provide steps for determining capacity on the appropriate documentation sheet.

D. Specific Consent Requirements for Patients without Decisional Capacity

    1. *Exception for Adults without Decisional Capacity Who (When Capacitated) Previously Consented to DNR*

    A DNR order may be written if a copy of the previously signed DNR consent form is in the medical record and lack of capacity is documented on the Attending Physician's DNR Documentation Form (Appendix A).

Some policies also require that, before a DNR order may be written for a patient who previously consented to such an order, the responsible physician must determine "the existence of any medical condition specified in the patient's PREVIOUS CONSENT."

---

    2. *Patients without Capacity, with Health Care Agents*

    Once a health care agent has been identified and the health care proxy is in the patient's medical record, the agent has the same authority to make decisions about CPR as would a patient with capacity. The Office of the Medical Director or Bioethics should be contacted with any additional questions about the authority of a health care agent to make CPR decisions.

    3. *Patients without Capacity, with a DNR Surrogate (Who is Not an Appointed Health Care Agent)*

      a. *Surrogate Priority*

      In order of priority, the following individuals, who must be reasonably available, willing, and competent to make a decision about a DNR order, may serve as a patient's DNR surrogate:

        (1) a court-appointed individual

        (2) a spouse

        (3) a son or daughter, 18 years or older

        (4) a parent

        (5) a brother or sister, 18 years or older

        (6) a close friend (Close Friend Affidavit, Appendix D, must be completed)

This DNR surrogate hierarchy, specified in state law, is not found in other policies, which refer to surrogates in terms of their formal appointment (health care agent, court appointment), oral appointment, or relationship to the patient (next of kin, close friend).

---

      b. *Criteria for Surrogate Consent to DNR*

      A DNR order based on a surrogate's consent may not be issued unless an attending physician and concurring physician determine and document in the DNR order that the patient has *at least one* of the following medical conditions (terms defined in section I):

(1) the patient has a terminal condition; *or*

(2) the patient is permanently unconscious; *or*

(3) CPR would be medically futile; *or*

(4) CPR would impose an extraordinary burden on the patient in light of the patient's medical condition and the expected outcome of the CPR (e.g., the patient is so frail, debilitated, or ill that CPR would cause more harm than benefit; however, advanced age and infirmity alone do not constitute sufficient basis for this determination).

These state-specific criteria do not appear in other policies, which do not list the conditions under which resuscitation would be considered nonbeneficial or futile. For example, one policy states, "The medical conditions under which the DNI/DNR order may be applicable shall be left to the judgment of the responsible resident physician in conjunction with the assigned attending physician."

E. Physician Documentation of Surrogate Consent to DNR

A DNR order may be written for patients with surrogate consent if either the Oral or the Written Consent to DNR Form is completed, and the Attending Physician's DNR Documentation Form (which includes determination of lack of capacity and the patient's medical condition by the attending and concurring attending) is also completed and both forms are placed in the medical record.

An Affidavit of a Close Friend must be completed, *only if* the surrogate is a common law spouse, a nonrelated significant other, a niece, nephew, cousin, clergy person, neighbor, or other friend.

F. Concerns about Surrogate Decision Making

The Office of the Medical Director or Bioethics should be contacted immediately if:

1. There is a question about whether a surrogate is available, willing, and competent to act.

2. There is any reason to question whether the surrogate's decision is based on the patient's wishes, including a consideration of the patient's religious or moral beliefs.

3. There is any reason to question whether the surrogate is making the decision based on the patient's best interests if the patient's wishes are not known and cannot be ascertained.

4. There is any reason to believe that there is anyone higher on the surrogate list who is available, willing, and competent to act on behalf of the patient.

5. The surrogate consents to a DNR order and the patient objects, in which case a

DNR order should not be written and the Office of the Medical Director or Bioethics should be contacted.

6. There is conflict about the DNR consent between or among the following individuals: the patient, anyone on the surrogate list, and/or the care providers. (See Dispute Mediation, section VIII.)

G. Procedure for Entering a DNR Order Based on Medical Futility for Incapacitated Patients Who Do Not Have an Available or Willing Health Care Agent or DNR Surrogate and There is No Objection to a DNR Order

A DNR order may be entered for these patients in the following circumstances:

1. when lack of capacity is documented on the Attending Physician's DNR Documentation Form; *and*

2. the attending physician has documented in the progress notes that he or she has determined that no competent health care agent or DNR surrogate is reasonably *available and/or willing to make a DNR decision for the patient* and the reasons for this conclusion; *and*

3. the attending physician *and* the concurring attending physician have documented that, after personally examining the patient, they have determined that CPR would be medically futile and their reasons for that conclusion and signed the Attending Physician's DNR Documentation Form; *and*

4. the medical director or his or her physician designee has also documented in the progress notes that, after personally examining the patient, he or she has determined that CPR would be medically futile and the reasons for that conclusion and has signed the Attending Physician's DNR Documentation Form.

H. Medical Futility DNR Order for an Incapacitated Patient When Patient, Health Care Agent, or Other Surrogate OBJECTS to a DNR Order

If a patient, health care agent, or DNR surrogate objects to a DNR order, the order may not be written and the Office of the Medical Director or Bioethics or Risk Management should be contacted. (See Dispute Mediation, section VIII.)

Some policies do not discuss the medical futility that can justify a DNR order, other than to define it in the definitions section.

Other policies address DNR orders based on futility in greater detail, for example:

"1. If the physician determines that CPR would be medically futile, as NARROWLY defined in the definitions section of this policy, the physician may, BUT IS NOT OBLIGED TO, enter a DNR order on that basis, provided that he or she takes the following steps:

a. the physician must discuss the DNR order with the patient, agent, or surrogate, if possible;

b. the judgment of futility must be confirmed by a second physician, and;

c. the physician enters the order in the patient's chart and informs the patient, agent, or surrogate. The consent of the patient, agent, or surrogate is not required; however, if there is an objection, follow the provision outlined in section VII2 below.

2. If the patient, health care agent, or surrogate refuses to consent to a DNR order and the physician believes that CPR would be futile for the patient, the physician must seek a second opinion before issuing a DNR order. If the second physician concurs that CPR will be futile, as futility is defined in the definitions section of the policy, and the concurrence is written in the chart, the attending physician shall inform the patient, agent, or surrogate of this medical judgment. If the patient, agent, or surrogate continues to request CPR and the patient's treatment team has exhausted all efforts to achieve concurrence and understanding, the dispute mediation should be convened."

I. Patients Who Are Minors

One institution provides a separate policy, DNR Guidelines for Infants, Children and Adolescents.

In order to write a DNR order for a patient who is a minor, the following steps are required:

1. The attending physician must determine that, to a reasonable degree of medical certainty, the patient is in at least *one* of the following categories (see definitions in section I) and document this determination in the patient's medical record:

   a. the patient has a terminal condition; *or*

   b. the patient is permanently unconscious; *or*

   c. resuscitation would be medically futile; *or*

   d. resuscitation would impose an extraordinary burden on the patient in light of the patient's medical condition and the expected outcome of resuscitation for the patient.

This repeats the criteria that justify a DNR order for an adult lacking capacity.

2. After the attending physician has determined that a patient is in one of the requisite categories, the attending will ask another attending physician to

examine the patient personally and make an entry in the progress notes documenting his or her judgment and the basis for that judgment. The attending physician and the concurring attending will each complete the designated sections of the Attending Physician's DNR Documentation Form (Appendix A), which also includes sections for capacity determination by both the attending and the concurring attending.

3. A parent or legal guardian of the patient must consent to a DNR order before the order may be issued. Consent may be *either* oral *or* written.

   a. Oral consent must be witnessed by two adults, one of whom is a Medical Center-affiliated physician, using the Oral Consent to DNR Form, which must then be placed in the medical record.

   b. Written consent must be witnessed by two adults, using the Written Consent to DNR Form, which must then be placed in the medical record.

4. The parent or legal guardian of a minor shall consider the minor's wishes and religious and moral beliefs in making a decision about consenting to a DNR order.

5. If the minor patient is able to understand the consequences of a DNR order and expresses a preference, the assent of the patient should be obtained before a DNR order is written. If it appears that the minor patient has capacity sufficient to provide consent, the determination of capacity must be made by the attending physician in consultation with the parent or guardian and must be documented in the patient's medical record. The parent(s) of a minor patient must also consent if the minor is under 18 years of age. Written consent must be witnessed by two adults, using the Written Consent to DNR Form, Appendix B, which must be placed in the medical record.

> Some policies do not address the characteristics or determination of decisional capacity in minors, and consider only the informed consent of the parent(s) or guardian(s).

6. Prior to entering the DNR order, the attending physician or a designee must make diligent efforts to inform a noncustodial parent of the proposed DNR order if that parent has maintained substantial and continuous contact with the child. These efforts must be documented in the medical record.

7. If either parent or the minor OBJECTS to entering a DNR order, or the attending physician has questions about a parent or guardian's authority to consent to a DNR order, the order must not be written, and the Office of the Medical Director, Bioethics, or Risk Management should be called. (See Dispute Mediation, section VIII.)

J. Special Situations: Patients with Mental Illness, Mental Retardation, and/or Developmental Disability

Bioethics or the Office of the Medical Director should be contacted for additional special requirements for any patient who resides in a facility regulated by the Office of Mental Hygiene (OMH) or who has mental illness, mental retardation, and/or developmental disability.

IV. Notification of the Patient, Health Care Agent or DNR Surrogate, and the Health Care Team

After the DNR consent has been obtained and documented, the attending physician must complete the notification section of the Attending Physician's DNR Documentation Form, enter a written or electronic DNR order, and notify the patient, health care agent, or DNR surrogate, as appropriate.

The attending physician (or designee) should notify the team caring for the patient as soon as a DNR order is in effect.

V. Renewing DNR Orders

The attending physician should review the DNR order whenever the patient's medical condition materially changes to determine if the order is still appropriate in light of the patient's condition. Such review, however, does *not* require the physician to obtain consent each time the order is renewed.

If there is concern about a possible delay in renewing the DNR order, the physician in charge of the patient care unit/service should be consulted to expedite the matter.

Even without changes in the patient's condition, the following *renewal requirements* apply:

A. Inpatients

1. Acute level of care patients: at least every seven days
2. Alternate level of care (ALC) patients: every sixty days

B. Outpatients

Nonhospital DNR order: Each time the attending physician examines the outpatient. (See section VI below.)

Review of a nonhospital DNR order need not occur more than once every seven days, but at least every ninety days. The attending physician (or a registered nurse who provides direct care to the patient at the attending physician's direction) must enter the review in the patient's record on the DNR order. When the nurse enters the review, the attending physician must enter a confirmation of the review in the patient's record within fourteen days of the nurse's review. The attending physician who issues the nonhospital DNR order need not be the same physician who reviews the order, but the physician who issues the order should give a copy of the order to the new physician (e.g., patient's private physician or physician affiliated with the home health agency).

The patient/surrogate should be given a copy of the nonhospital DNR order reflecting the current review each time the order is renewed and instructed to keep the order in an easily accessible place at all times.

VI. Revoking Consent to a DNR Order

A capacitated patient, a health care agent, or a DNR surrogate who has consented to a DNR order may revoke the consent at any time by notifying the attending physician or a member of the clinical staff orally or in writing or by *any* act evidencing a specific intent to revoke the consent.

Any health care professional who becomes aware of a revocation must notify the attending physician of the revocation.

However, if a health care agent or DNR surrogate for an incapacitated patient wishes to revoke a DNR order to which the patient (when capacitated) had consented, Bioethics or the Office of the Medical Director should be consulted.

> Some policies do not address the authority of the DNR surrogate to revoke a DNR to which the patient had previously consented.

Whenever a DNR consent has been revoked, the following steps should be taken by the attending physician:

1. Confirm the intent to revoke.
2. Cancel the written or electronic DNR order.
3. Draw an "X" across the Attending Physician's DNR Documentation Form and write "Revoked as of" and print the date and sign below. (*Do NOT remove the form from the medical record.*)
4. Document in the progress notes the reason for the revocation.
5. Notify the team caring for the patient.
6. If indicated, consult with Bioethics or the Office of the Medical Director.

VII. Canceling DNR Orders

A. General Rule

The attending physician is responsible for canceling any DNR order that should no longer be in effect, whether because consent was revoked or the patient's condition changed. The attending physician must do the following to cancel a DNR order:

1. Cancel the written or electronic physician's DNR order.
2. Draw an "X" across the Attending Physician's DNR Documentation Form and write "Canceled as of" or "Revoked as of" and print the date and sign below.
3. Document the reason for cancellation/revocation in the progress notes.
4. Notify the person who consented to the DNR order and the team caring for the patient.

B. Patient Who Regains Decisional Capacity after a Surrogate Consented for the Patient to a DNR Order

Medical Center associates who believe that a patient (who had previously been determined to be without capacity) has regained capacity should immediately contact that patient's attending physician. The attending physician should review the patient's condition and document any change in the patient's decisional capacity in the progress notes. If the patient has indeed regained capacity, the attending physician should cancel the DNR order. If the patient's medical condition is such that a DNR order is still indicated, the attending physician should seek consent to a DNR order from the now-capacitated patient, as set forth in section III-A.

VIII. Nonhospital DNR Orders

A. Honoring a Nonhospital DNR Order

A nonhospital DNR order is an order that directs emergency medical services personnel and Emergency Department staff *not to attempt CPR if the patient suffers a cardiac or respiratory arrest* in the community, in the hospital's ambulatory departments, including the Emergency Department, or in a nonhospital health care facility.

A nonhospital DNR order should be honored as if it were a hospital-initiated DNR or a DNR order for a patient transferred from another hospital or health care facility. (See section IX-A—Transfers.) The Emergency Department attending and/or the inpatient attending physician should evaluate the patient's suitability for a DNR order. The attending physician should honor the patient's DNR decision unless "other significant and exceptional medical circumstances warrant disregarding the order."

Other policies have additional exceptions to the imperative to honor a nonhospital DNR, for example:

"[emergency medical service personnel or hospital emergency service personnel] believe in good faith that the order has been revoked or canceled;

family members or others on the scene object to the order and physical confrontation appears likely."

To continue the DNR status, the attending physician should:

1. Attach a copy of the nonhospital DNR order to the Medical Center Attending Physician's DNR Documentation Form, with a notation reading "See attached nonhospital DNR form."

2. Review the DNR status with the patient/surrogate, as indicated and document any discussion.

3. Enter a written or electronic DNR order.

B. Writing a Nonhospital DNR Order

A nonhospital DNR order may be issued in the hospital upon discharge or in the community/ambulatory care setting. In either case, *the attending physician must enter the nonhospital DNR order on the State Department of Health Nonhospital Order Not to Resuscitate (DNR) Form,* which is available on all Medical Center inpatient units and at the ambulatory care sites.

When the nonhospital DNR order is written in the inpatient setting by a licensed physician, the order is effective upon discharge. *If the order is initiated in the hospital,* consent should be obtained from the capacitated patient (or the surrogate for an incapacitated patient), *using a hospital consent to DNR form.* The physician must sign and date the order form and the consent form. The original order should be sent home with the patient/surrogate and a copy of the order and the completed consent form placed in the medical record.

When the nonhospital DNR order is issued in a physician's office, ambulatory care center, or elsewhere in the community, consent is governed by the same sections of the DNR Law as apply to hospital-initiated consents as described in this policy, provided that the adult patient with capacity may also consent to a nonhospital DNR order orally to the attending physician.

C. Renewal Requirements for Nonhospital DNR Orders

The attending physician must review whether a nonhospital DNR order is still appropriate in light of the patient's condition each time he or she examines the patient, whether in the hospital or elsewhere. The review need not occur more than once every seven days but must be done at least every ninety days. A new form is not required after such review. The attending physician should record the review in the patient's medical record. If, however, a registered nurse provides direct care to the patient, the nurse may record the review in the medical record at the direction of the physician. In such case, the attending physician must confirm the review in the record within fourteen days.

Note: Once signed by a physician, a nonhospital DNR order is valid, even if not reviewed within ninety days. Thus, if a signed nonhospital DNR order is presented, it must be honored unless it is known that the order has been revoked or if the hospital Emergency Department attending physician determines that other significant and exceptional medical circumstances warrant disregarding the order. As with patients transferred from another hospital with a DNR order in place, the non-hospital DNR order remains effective until it is reviewed by a Medical Center attending who either renews it or cancels it.

IX. Transfers

    A. To the Medical Center

Unless revoked by the person who consented, *DNR orders for patients transferred to the Medical Center from another facility or nonhospital DNR orders from the community remain in effect until the attending physician examines the patient.* Thereafter, the attending must either: (1) issue a DNR order continuing the prior order (no further consent is needed), or (2) cancel the order under exceptional medical circumstances and immediately notify the person who consented to the order and the hospital staff directly responsible for the patient's care of the cancellation. Such cancellation does not prevent entry of a DNR order at a later time. A DNR order should accompany any patient who is reported to have a DNR order upon transfer from another hospital or health care facility. (If evidence of the DNR order does not accompany the patient, Medical Center physicians and staff should make all efforts to obtain the order from the transferring facility.)

    B. From the Medical Center

Whenever a patient with a DNR order is transferred from the Medical Center to another location, the attending physician should inform EMS personnel (or others transporting the patient) and the receiving hospital/facility of the patient's DNR status, and provide a copy of the DNR order to the transporter and the receiving hospital/facility.

    C. To Another Attending Physician

Any attending physician who transfers the care of a patient with a DNR order to another physician must inform the new attending of the DNR order and ensure that a copy of the order is part of the patient's medical record.

X. Dispute Mediation and Judicial Review

    A. Dispute Mediation Process

A dispute mediation process will be employed to resolve any conflict concerning a DNR order. Any interested person may submit a DNR issue to dispute mediation. To submit a case to an ad hoc dispute mediation committee the person requesting the dispute mediation should notify the Office of the Medical Director, who must then notify the attending physician and Bioethics. Once notified, the attending physician must ensure that no DNR is written or, if written, the DNR is suspended, until: (1) the issue is resolved, (2) the mediation process has concluded its efforts to resolve the dispute, or (3) seventy-two hours have elapsed from the time the dispute is submitted, whichever occurs first. When the dispute mediation process has been concluded, the decision should be implemented in accordance with this policy.

> Policies in states that do not require dispute mediation have a different approach to consensus about DNR orders. For example, "In the absence of medical futility, the principles of self-determination and informed consent shall apply to the DNI/DNR decision-making process. When the patient has decision-making capacity, the DNI/DNR decision shall be reached consensually by the patient and resident and attending physician. If the patient is without decision-making capacity, this decision shall be reached consensually by the family and the resident and attending physician. If the patient or family disagrees, the DNI/DNR order shall not be implemented."

A representative of the committee should enter in the progress notes: (1) when and by whom the request for dispute mediation was received; (2) when dispute mediation occurred; and (3) the outcome of the dispute mediation process.

Persons participating in dispute mediation must be informed of their right to judicial review at the conclusion of the process. If disagreements persist after the above time frame, the Legal Department must be contacted to bring the matter to resolution.

B. Dispute Mediation Committee Membership

1. The ad hoc dispute mediation committee should include representatives from Bioethics, the Medical Director's Office, Risk Management, and other resources, as indicated. If required, the Medical Center's Dispute Mediation Committee will be convened and will be comprised of members of the Medical Center's Bioethics Committee selected by the Medical Center president or his or her designee, and must include an administrative representative, a physician, and a registered nurse. Special membership requirements obtain when the case involves lack of capacity due to mental illness, mental retardation, or developmental disability.

2. In situations involving patients with mental illness, mental retardation, and/or developmental disability, the committee must also include a board-certified psychiatrist.

> Some policies describe the composition of the dispute mediation committee but not its responsibility or scope of authority.

C. Mandatory Dispute Mediation

The following are situations in which the attending physician must submit the matter to dispute mediation:

1. When the attending physician has actual notice that any persons on the sur-

rogate list (or, if the patient is from an Office of Mental Hygiene–regulated facility, the facility director) opposes a DNR decision by another surrogate, even if the person objecting is lower on the surrogate list.

2. A physician or the Medical Center administration opposes a patient's or surrogate's DNR consent, and the physician has chosen not to transfer care of the patient before dispute mediation.

3. One parent objects to a DNR order for a minor.

4. When the patient resides in a facility regulated by the Office of Mental Hygiene (OMH).

XI. Other Issues or Concerns about DNR Orders or the DNR Policy and Procedure
The Office of the Medical Director or Bioethics or should be contacted during the daytime Monday through Friday for any other issues or concerns about DNR orders. At all other times, the associate director of nursing (A.D.N.) should be contacted. The A.D.N. will contact the appropriate resource department in a timely manner.

Other policies address issues of immunity, for example:

"1. No physician, health care professional, nursing assistant, hospital, or person employed by or under contract with the Hospital, shall be civilly or criminally liable or be deemed to have engaged in unprofessional conduct for carrying out any decision regarding CPR, or for applying standards and procedures, if done in accordance with the requirements of this policy.

2. The same immunity applies to the above persons for performing CPR when a DNR has been issued as long as the person reasonably and in good faith:

   a. was unaware of the DNR order; OR

   b. believed that consent to the order had been revoked or canceled.

3. No person shall be subject to civil or criminal liability for consenting or refusing to consent in good faith to a DNR order on behalf of a patient.

4. No person acting in good faith as a participant in dispute mediation shall be subject to civil or criminal liability or be deemed to have engaged in unprofessional conduct."

FORGOING LIFE-EXTENDING TREATMENT

Some policies begin with an abstract or statement of general guidelines that summarizes their underlying philosophy and reasoning. For example, one policy explains the sometimes necessary departure from the presumption favoring the preservation of life: "Clearly, however, avoiding death should not always be the preeminent goal. Not all technologically possible means of prolonging life need be or should be used in every case." The point is underscored by the title: "Policy on Forgoing Life-Sustaining or Death-Prolonging Therapy."

Another policy's preamble includes the principles that ground its analytic structure. "The primary principles that should govern decisions to issue withhold or withdraw orders are self-determination, patient welfare, and the futility of medical treatment."

PURPOSE

To delineate the roles of the physician and the members of the health care team in guiding patients, their health care agents, or family or other surrogates in end-of-life decision making. This policy summarizes procedures to follow when decisions to forgo treatment are made by/for the following:

1. *Patients with decisional capacity* (section II-A)
2. *Incapacitated patients with health care agents (designated in health care proxies)* (section II-B)
3. *Incapacitated patients without health care agents but with family or other surrogate(s)* (section II-C)
4. *Incapacitated patients who have NO known family or other surrogate decision maker* (section II-D)
5. *Minor patients' parent(s) and/or legal guardian(s)* (section II-E)

Some policies begin with a section that defines relevant terms, including forgoing life-sustaining or life-extending treatment, decision-making capacity, surrogate, futile treatment, and clear and convincing evidence. For example, one policy defines life-sustaining treatment as "any medical intervention, technology, procedure or medication that forestalls the moment of death, whether or not the treatment affects the underlying life-threatening disease or biological process."

SCOPE

All Medical Center associates involved in providing patient care services.

I. Principles
  - *Physicians and other providers have no medical, legal, or ethical obligation to offer or provide treatment(s) that are not medically indicated.*

> One policy refers to the concept of medical futility to explain why certain treatment should not be provided: "A physician has no ethical duty to continue treatment once it has been judged to be futile and ineffective nor to initiate or recommend futile treatment."

  - *Capacitated* patients *may refuse any treatment,* including treatments that are life sustaining.

> One policy begins with a more expanded statement of its general underlying principles:
>
> "A. All decisions about life-extending treatment shall be based on a careful determination of what is in accordance with the patient's declared choices and best interests.
>
> B. There is a presumption in favor of providing life-extending treatment.
>
> C. Adults with mental capacity have a right to reject any life-extending treatment.
>
> D. Surrogates have the authority to reject life-extending treatment on behalf of patients without mental capacity if acting in accordance with the declared choices and the best interests of the patients.
>
> E. Physicians and other health care providers should initiate discussions with patients and family members regarding treatment preferences and executing health care proxies or other written expressions of health care preferences before decisional incapacity occurs. Patients should be encouraged to have open discussions with family members about treatment preferences.
>
> F. A surrogate who has been authorized pursuant to this policy to make health care decisions for the patient has the same right as the patient to receive medical information and to access medical records necessary to make informed decisions regarding the patient's health.
>
> G. Rejecting life-extending treatment is not suicide and complying with the patient's wishes is not assisting or aiding in suicide.

H. The right to reject applies to all life-extending treatment, including artificial nutrition and hydration for adult patients.

I. There is no legal or ethical distinction among withholding and withdrawing and limiting life-extending treatment.

J. An individual health care provider may be relieved from carrying out a health care decision made pursuant to this policy if he or she has a 'conscience objection,' that is, the decision is contrary to the individual's religious beliefs or moral convictions."

- Most treatment decisions for patients who do not have decisional capacity are made by the attending physician in conjunction with the patient's family, taking into consideration the patient's wishes and best interests.

II. Procedures for Responding to Requests to Forgo Life-sustaining Treatment(s)
    Questions about forgoing life-sustaining treatment may be raised by a capacitated patient, a health care agent, family member or other surrogate, the attending physician, or any other care provider. Any decision to forgo life-sustaining treatment, either by a capacitated patient or on behalf of an incapacitated patient, should trigger a process of discussion about the reasons for the decision, the consequences of forgoing treatment, and the full range of therapeutic options, including palliative care. A palliative care consult may be helpful to ensure that all measures to promote comfort, including adequate pain and symptom management, have been addressed.

Several policies discuss the critical role of palliation, including management of pain and other symptoms, in the care of patients who are dying or whose life-sustaining treatment will be forgone.

One policy includes a detailed section on communication, including the physician's obligation to elicit the patient's values and avoid imposing his or her own values, initiating a discussion of forgoing life-sustaining treatment soon after a poor prognosis has been confirmed, communicating a terminal diagnosis while the patient still has decisional capacity, and sharing with the patient or surrogate the responsibility for decision making.

One policy establishes the criteria that must be met before life-sustaining treatment may be forgone:

"a. A patient *may* be considered an appropriate candidate for withholding or withdrawing treatment if any one or more of the below-listed conditions are present. The patient must be evaluated and documented evidence of at least one of the following conditions must be present before consideration of withholding or withdrawing life-sustaining treatment can be made:

i. In the attending physician's opinion, the patient is irreversibly terminally ill or,

ii. In the attending physician's opinion, the patient is in a vegetative state with no reasonable hope that the patient will return to a cognitive state, or

iii. A patient with the capacity to make such decisions has expressed the desire to have treatment withheld or withdrawn.

iv. The healthcare agent or guardian of an incompetent patient requests withdrawal or withholding of treatment.

v. The patient has completed an advance directive providing clear and convincing evidence of his or her wishes concerning treatment.

b. In cases where the prognosis is uncertain, consultation with a second physician is recommended. . . ."

One policy individually addresses specific life-sustaining interventions, including CPR, mechanical ventilation, dialysis, transfusion of blood and blood products, antibiotics and other medications, nutrition, and hydration. The interventions are discussed in terms of their purposes, and how and why they can be forgone.

One policy on forgoing life-extending treatment includes a section that deals specifically with orders that authorize the forgoing of intubation in situations other than cardiopulmonary arrest. (See policy on Do-not-intubate [DNI] orders.)

One institution has a separate policy, Terminal Withdrawal of Ventilator Support and Extubation, which begins with the following definition: "Terminal Withdrawal of Ventilator Support ('TWVS') refers to the process of withdrawing ventilator support when the patient or surrogate has determined that continued or prolonged ventilation is not an acceptable outcome. The patient or surrogate has chosen comfort over extending life. With regular ventilator weaning, death is neither expected nor accepted. TWVS differs from traditional weaning in that the withdrawal process proceeds regardless of the patient's vital signs, and comfort measures such as anxiolytics or narcotics may be given regardless of adverse impact on vital signs. The outcome of TWVS is often the patient's natural death; however, this is not always the case. This policy does not permit euthanasia, but does permit allowing a patient to die when appropriate."

Several policies organize the discussion in terms of who assumes the responsibility for the decision to forgo life-sustaining treatment. For example, some policies distinguish the decision-making process according to the following categories: the adult patient has clear capacity, the adult patient's capacity is unclear, or the adult patient has a clear lack of capacity. Decisions about forgoing life-sustaining treatment in the care of children are usually addressed in separate sections.

A. Patients with Capacity

1. *Forgoing Treatment*

    A patient with capacity may refuse any life-sustaining intervention after full discussion with the attending physician of condition and prognosis as well as the benefits, burdens, and risks of the full range of medical interventions, including the option of no treatment. If the patient refuses specific life-sustaining treatment(s) and the *attending physician has determined that forgoing the treatment(s) is medically appropriate* based on the patient's condition and poor prognosis, the attending should fully document the discussion(s) with the patient and the medical assessment in the progress notes. The attending should proceed with the requested plan, including providing pain and other symptom management.

2. *Forgoing Medically Indicated Treatment*

    If a capacitated patient refuses life-sustaining treatment that the physician believes to be *medically indicated,* further efforts should be made to ascertain the patient's understanding of the proposed treatment(s) and to provide assistance when the patient indicates that there are family and other social concerns that may be resolved. The risks and benefits of refusing treatment should be clarified.

    If there is any question about the patient's capacity to make an informed refusal, a psychiatric consult should be requested.

When a capacitated patient who has been fully informed of the consequences of refusal continues to refuse medically indicated life-sustaining treatment, the patient's decision must be honored. The patient should be encouraged to sign the refusal of treatment section on the back of the Medical Center informed consent form.

Oral refusal may be accepted but must be given to the attending in person and before another adult witness. The attending should then thoroughly document the refusal on the consent form and in the progress notes.

B. Patients without Decisional Capacity, with a Health Care Agent (Designated in a Health Care Proxy) (*Note:* A copy of the health care proxy must be in the patient's record.)

 1. Forgoing Treatment

A health care agent, designated by the patient to make *all* health care decisions if the patient becomes incapacitated, may request that specific life-sustaining treatment(s) be forgone. The agent's decision to forgo treatment, if medically indicated, must be honored after full discussion with the attending of the benefits, burdens, and risks to the patient of such a decision. Before acting on an agent's request to forgo life-sustaining treatment(s), the attending physician should:

   a. Obtain a concurring opinion as to lack of capacity from another attending, and

   b. Document the following information in the progress notes:
      (1) the patient's condition and prognosis
      (2) the patient's incapacity
      (3) the fact that a copy of the health care proxy is in the chart
      (4) the agent's decision (based on knowledge of the patient's wishes or the patient's best interest)
      (5) the plan for implementing the agent's decision, including provision for pain and other symptom management

 2. Forgoing Medically Indicated Treatment

Any decision to forgo life-sustaining or other medically indicated treatment(s) should trigger a process of discussion about the reasons for the decision, the consequences of forgoing treatment, and the range of therapeutic options, including palliative care.

If a health care agent for an incapacitated patient refuses *medically indicated* treatment and there is any question as to whether the agent's decision is in accord with the patient's wishes or best interest, the refusal of treatment should be referred to Risk Management for multidisciplinary review, in accordance with Medical Center's Consent Policy.

All discussions about and decisions to forgo or continue treatment should be appropriately documented.

This is the only policy reviewed to discuss both forgoing treatment considered medically indicated and forgoing treatment not considered medically indicated.

One institution has a separate Policy on Patient Refusal of Life-Sustaining Treatment, which addresses the patient's refusal of *recommended* treatment. The policy begins by setting out the ethical issue: "When a patient, or surrogate(s) acting on behalf of a patient, refuses recommended treatment, a dilemma can be created for health care professionals: respect for a patient's wishes can conflict with the obligation to help and not to harm the patient." The policy also states that the decision to refuse specific treatment(s), by itself, does not indicate lack of capacity, a wish to die, or a refusal of any other treatment.

In contrast, another institution has a separate policy that deals with patient requests for treatment that is *not recommended*. Managing Requests for Treatment Judged Medically Futile or Harmful addresses the process for responding to requests for interventions that are not clinically indicated. The policy distinguishes treatments that are medically futile ("offer no reasonable possibility of a meaningful extension of life or improvement of the patient's quality of life or other significant benefit for the patient") and medically harmful ("reasonably expected to produce significant suffering or other burdens for the patient, and which offer no reasonable possibility of producing any benefit sufficient to justify the suffering or other burdens"). It also emphasizes the balance between honoring patient and family requests and promoting the best interests of the patient, and provides a ten-step process for interdisciplinary management.

C. Patients without Capacity, and without an Appointed Health Care Agent But with Family or Other Surrogate
   1. Physicians caring for an incapacitated patient who is terminally ill should discuss a palliative care plan or limited trials of certain treatment modalities (e.g., dialysis) with the family or other surrogate. This discussion should include review of the patient's prior declared health choices as well as the patient's condition and prognosis. A palliative care or a bioethics consult and/or a family meeting may be helpful in clarifying the plan.
   2. If family/surrogate for an incapacitated patient chooses to forgo life-sustaining treatment that the attending physician believes is clearly medically indi-

cated, the refusal should be referred to Risk Management for multidisciplinary review.

3. If the family of an incapacitated patient (when there is *no* appointed health care agent) asks to withdraw or withhold life-sustaining treatment, the family must provide clear and convincing evidence of the patient's prior wishes to forgo such treatment(s). The Medical Director's Office must be contacted and will coordinate the steps in the process.

4. The following steps should be taken for family/surrogate's requests to forgo life-sustaining treatment(s) for an incapacitated patient:

    a. *Attending Physician's Review of Patient's Medical Condition and Prognosis*

       The attending physician must review and document the family's request and concur that forgoing the specific treatment is medically appropriate, based on the patient's medical condition and prognosis. If indicated, additional clinical consults (e.g., neurological or pulmonary consults) should be obtained to clarify the prognosis. The attending should also document the patient's lack of capacity and obtain a concurring attending opinion as to incapacity.

    b. *Identifying Surrogate(s) for Incapacitated Patients*

       The health care team should ascertain who is available, knowledgeable, and willing to speak for the patient. While the DNR law *does* specify a hierarchy for consenting to a DNR order, state law does *not* specify a hierarchy of surrogates to make decisions about forgoing life-sustaining treatment for the incapacitated patient. Therefore, the team may obtain information from anyone who knows the patient's preferences, including the patient's primary care physician or friends of the patient. There should be agreement among family/surrogates as to the substance of the patient's wishes.

In states that provide for a hierarchy of surrogates who can make health care decisions for patients without capacity, policies on forgoing life-sustaining treatment may include a priority list such as the following:

"Patient Without Decisional Capacity: In those instances in which the patient lacks decisional capacity, the patient's representative shall make the decision regarding forgoing life-sustaining treatment. In the usual order of priority, the following individuals may act as the patient's representative:

1. In the case of a minor, the child's parents or legal guardian.

2. In the case of an adult,

    a. the individual designated by the patient in a health care directive as his or her agent or a legal guardian appointed by a court;

b. the spouse;

c. an adult son or daughter;

d. either parent;

e. an adult brother or sister;

f. other close family members; and

g. in some circumstances a close personal friend of the patient."

c. *Supporting Family/Surrogate(s) in Making Treatment Decisions for the Patient*
The attending physician must fully discuss with the patient's family/surrogate(s) the patient's condition, prognosis, and treatment options. It should be emphasized that decisions to forgo life-sustaining treatment must be based on the patient's wishes. Family/surrogates should be reassured that measures will be taken to *ensure appropriate sedation and analgesia and all necessary comfort measures for the patient and to provide emotional support for the family/surrogate(s).*

d. The *medical director's staff (or a member of the Bioethics Division) must be contacted to coordinate the necessary steps in assisting the family and the health care team* if the family/surrogate wishes to forgo life-sustaining treatment.

All reviewed policies require the involvement of the Bioethics Committee or Consultation Service when requests are made to forgo life-extending treatment. For example, one policy includes a section that details the role of the Bioethics Committee in decisions about forgoing life-sustaining treatment. In other sections, the policy states that the Bioethics Committee is to be contacted in cases of disagreement between the capacitated patient and the physician, or when an individual other than a health care agent requests that life-sustaining treatment be withheld or withdrawn from a patient without capacity.

One policy details the role of the patient advocate, in addition to the ethics committee, in the process of considering and making decisions about forgoing life-sustaining treatment.

Another policy specifies the need to consider the patient's spiritual values at the end of life and recommends the involvement of the Pastoral Care Department when requests are made to forgo life-sustaining treatment. "The spiritual values of the patient at the end of life should be addressed and the consultative services of the Pastoral Care Department utilized as appropriate."

e. *Family/Surrogate(s) Documentation of Patient's Wishes*

The family/surrogate(s) will be asked to provide written information about the patient's prior declared treatment wishes. Bioethics or the medical director's staff may be asked to assist families and other surrogate(s) in documenting the patient's previous life choices and experiences.

If family/surrogate is unable to provide written documentation, an administrative progress note may be substituted. This note documents the family's/surrogate's verbal description of the patient's wishes. The note should include the names and relationship to the patient of all involved family, as well as quotes or paraphrases of their description of the patient's prior declared wishes.

In order for the Medical Center to proceed with the request, all family/surrogate(s) must be in *agreement* as to the *substance* of the patient's prior declared choices. The health care team should help family/surrogate(s) to clarify their understanding of the patient's wishes in the context of the patient's condition and prognosis. A bioethics consult may be helpful in this regard.

f. *Legal Department Review*

The Legal Department, in conjunction with the Office of the Medical Director, reviews the documentation for clear and convincing evidence of the patient's wishes.

g. *Administrative Note*

An administrative note is entered in the medical record, documenting that clear and convincing evidence of the patient's wishes has been provided. The surrogate letter(s) and/or any other written evidence is placed in the medical record.

h. *Medical Director/Physician Designee Review*

The medical director or the medical director's physician designee reviews the attending physician's (and consultants') documentation of the patient's condition and prognosis. If the medical director/designee agrees that the decision is medically appropriate, he or she documents concurrence in the progress notes.

i. *Implementing the Plan to Forgo Life-Sustaining Treatment*

The attending physician is responsible for coordinating the timing of and the activities related to withholding or withdrawing specific treatment(s) with the family/surrogate(s) and the health care team. Provision should be made for *relieving any pain and managing other symptoms,* including dyspnea, by administering sedatives and/or analgesia. Consultation with Palliative Care, Critical Care Medicine, and/or Respiratory Therapy may be helpful for symptom management and certain technical aspects of withdrawal.

j. *Dispute Mediation Process*

If there is disagreement between or among the patient's family members, surrogates, and/or care providers, the matter shall be referred to dispute mediation by notifying the Office of the Medical Director or Bioethics. Until the dispute has been mediated, no order to forgo life-sustaining treatment may be written.

> Some policies detail the dispute mediation function of the ethics committee when disputes arise about forgoing life-sustaining treatment.

D. Incapacitated Patients with No Available or Willing Health Care Agent, Family, or Other Surrogate Decision Maker

Incapacitated patients without family or other surrogate decision maker should be identified early in their hospital stays. *In the absence of surrogates, the Medical Director's Office coordinates the support required to make appropriate treatment decisions.* Multidisciplinary review, including a second opinion, when indicated, is utilized to provide medically appropriate interventions.

For these "patients alone," efforts are made to contact long-term care facilities and previous and current health care providers to try to ascertain the patient's prior life and treatment choices. When necessary, particularly when an incapacitated patient refuses medically indicated, life-sustaining treatment, a decision may be made to apply for guardianship or to submit specific treatment decisions for court-ordered decision making.

III. Conscientious Objection to Implementing a Request to Forgo
Life-Sustaining Treatment

Any attending physician or other health care provider who has strong moral or religious objection to honoring the decision of a patient or surrogate to forgo life-sustaining treatment must make his or her objections known immediately, to the department chairperson for attending physicians and the immediate supervisor for other associates. The attending physician may be excused from participating if a medically adequate transfer of care can be arranged. All reasonable efforts will be made to reassign other health care providers who have strongly held cultural, ethical, or religious objections to carrying out the provisions of this policy.

> All policies reviewed contain provisions for physicians who have moral or religious objections to forgoing life-sustaining measures to transfer their patients to other physicians who are more comfortable with the process. Continuity of care and nonabandonment are emphasized. One policy notes, "There is a dis-

tinction between treatment a doctor believes to be detrimental to a patient's best interest, and treatment to which a physician has a conscientious objection."

IV. Contact for Assistance Regarding this Policy

For assistance in responding to requests to withdraw life-sustaining treatment(s) from an adult patient without decisional capacity and without a health care agent, or from a minor patient at any Medical Center site, contact the Medical Director's Office. When indicated, Palliative Care, Bioethics, the Pediatric Ethics Program, and/or the Legal Department will also be involved.

Any *questions concerning this policy* should be directed to the Office of the Medical Director or to the Division of Bioethics during the daytime from Monday through Friday and to the on-call associate director of nursing (A.D.N.) at all other times. The A.D.N. will involve the appropriate resource department.

PART V

Institutional Code of Ethics

Many health care institutions now have adopted codes or statements of organizational ethics articulating the standards that govern behavior in the clinical, administrative, and research settings. Some provide an institutional road map, integrating and referencing the institution's other relevant policies.

As part of its focus on organizational ethics, the Division of Bioethics at Montefiore Medical Center developed a detailed code of ethics for the institution. The code represents the value framework for ethical decision making on the clinical and organizational levels, discussed in chapter 8. It is distinguished from the institution's JCAHO-mandated compliance code by its normative reach beyond the minimum demands for adherence to legal and regulatory requirements. The code sets the bar at a higher level—the ethical obligations of the institution as health care provider—and establishes the *desired* rather than the *required* standard of behavior. It is presented here as a suggested model for other ethics committees to modify in response to the needs of their institutions.

MONTEFIORE MEDICAL CENTER CODE OF ETHICS*

Montefiore Medical Center strives to abide by the ethical principles embodied in this Code of Ethics in all aspects of patient care, medical education, clinical research, and community service, and in all aspects of administrative functions related to those services. These ethical principles describe guidelines for honorable behavior for health care providers, managers, and all other associates and volunteers. Montefiore strives to realize these standards in all its clinical and organizational activities.

ORGANIZATIONAL PRINCIPLES

Montefiore Medical Center recognizes that managers and associates have ethical obligations to patients, staff, and the community. Therefore:

1. Montefiore creates an ethical organizational environment by:

*Copyright 2001, Montefiore Medical Center. Reprinted with permission.

- promoting ethical decision making through mechanisms that integrate ethical analysis into clinical and administrative deliberation and policy development
- protecting the rights of human subjects and promoting the welfare of animals in research protocols
- developing mechanisms for implementing the ethical principles in the code and establishing a process for resolving ethical disputes
- involving staff in ethical decision making on the organizational and clinical levels by promoting discussion of ethical issues, expression of ethical concerns without fear of reprisal, and consideration of whether behavior is ethical
- listening and attending to the concerns of patients and families
- reducing institutional barriers to patients and families receiving information and guidance from providers and making informed health care decisions
- creating effective, efficient, and confidential dispute resolution mechanisms to address ethical conflicts and concerns on the organizational, administrative, and clinical decision-making levels

2. Montefiore pursues a socially responsible agenda by:

- addressing the health of the community by working with individuals and groups to identify public health care needs, establish priorities, and provide adequate notice of available services
- promoting accessible, affordable, and convenient primary care
- building community alliances that work with community organizations and individuals to promote public health and safety, and coordinate health care delivery
- supporting teaching and research as important parts of its responsibility to the community and the larger society

3. Montefiore engages in responsible stewardship by:

- conserving limited health care resources by using them efficiently and responsibly, and distributing them beneficially and cost-effectively
- promoting cost-effective care through cooperative clinical decision making that uses resources wisely, by avoiding both under- and overtreatment, and encouraging patients to assume responsibility for monitoring and improving their health
- maintaining continuous quality review to assess the effectiveness of resource utilization and clinical outcomes
- incorporating ethical principles and reasoning into resource planning and utilization review in order to promote financial accountability at all organizational levels
- promoting measures, including incentive plans, to increase provider

productivity, motivate effective resource utilization, provide high-quality patient care, and enhance the work ethic
- providing the same standard of care, regardless of payment source, by enforcing policies that define equity and prohibit discriminatory provision of care
- identifying and cultivating potential sources of public and private funding for patient care, medical education and research
- devoting a portion of its institutional budget to funding uncompensated care for the uninsured and underserved

4. Montefiore supports fair marketing and communication practices by:

- promoting realistic consumer expectations by accurately reflecting the institution's health care delivery record and capabilities, and limiting promises to what the institution can actually provide
- promoting informed consumer choice by providing the public with accurate and balanced information about existing and planned institutional resources, treatment capabilities, and areas of specialization
- disclosing information to patients about institutional relationships that create actual, potential, or apparent conflicts of interest

CLINICAL PRINCIPLES

Montefiore Medical Center recognizes that its primary mission is to ensure the provision of high-quality, ethically based patient care. Therefore:

1. Montefiore monitors quality of care by:

- promoting best clinical practice by using measures of quality that reflect the current research on clinical outcomes and practice guidelines
- including all departments and disciplines in system-wide continuous quality improvement to improve the quality of care and promote clinical skills
- monitoring and reducing adverse clinical events by focusing on patient safety, and identifying and eliminating practice patterns and systems that deviate from accepted standards of care
- promoting continuity of care by sharing appropriate medical information, coordinating services among providers, and developing discharge plans that monitor the transition from hospital to the community or other care facilities
- abiding by the principle of truth telling and requiring appropriate personnel to disclose health-impairing mistakes to patients and, where indicated, their families, in order to respect autonomy and prevent or mitigate harm

2. Montefiore supports ethical clinical decision making by:

- stressing the importance of ethically based and informed health care decision making by requiring that providers confirm the patient's decisional capacity and, if the patient lacks capacity, identify the appropriate surrogate
- supporting informed choice by clearly informing patients, proxies or other surrogates about treatment options and their benefits, burdens, and risks, with special attention to decision making for patients incapable of making health care choices
- respecting the rights of all concerned parties by protecting patient and family interests, providing clinical information for informed consent and refusal, enhancing patient and family voice in clinical decision making, and addressing patient and family concerns and complaints
- supporting a principled dispute resolution system that addresses treatment and interpersonal conflicts, strives for consensus, and is based on ethical, medical, and legal principles
- recognizing that mediator neutrality is essential in addressing and resolving clinical disputes between and among staff, patients, families, and other surrogates

3. Montefiore promotes multidisciplinary clinical consultation by:

- promoting collaborative clinical management and supporting the authority of specific multidisciplinary teams
- supporting attending physicians' professional judgment and authority, while requiring institutional oversight and joint clinical management and implementing a plan of care that reflects the patient's best interest, regardless of financial compensation
- continuing its long-standing commitment to readily accessible comprehensive primary care services through its network of ambulatory care clinics, supplemented by specialty care services

4. Montefiore protects patient privacy and confidentiality by:

- making the protection of patient information central to patient care and related services
- creating mechanisms that provide authorized persons easy and timely access to computerized patient information, while safeguarding patient privacy and confidentiality
- restricting access to medical records and other health information, including billing information, to those with a "need to know" in order to provide direct patient care, review the quality of care, and pursue other legitimate clinical or organizational goals

- educating staff about their obligations regarding access to and disclosure of patient information
- advising patients that medical information will not be disclosed to others, including family and friends, without patient permission, except as permitted by law
- establishing policies and practices that protect against breaches of confidentiality and punish illegitimate access, use and/or disclosure of patient information

PART VI

Key Legal Cases in Bioethics

By including this section in the handbook, we are not suggesting that, in addition to its other responsibilities, your ethics committee should assume the functions of your institution's Legal Department. As emphasized throughout this handbook, the unique contribution of ethics committees is the application of ethical analysis to clinical and organizational issues. Nevertheless, it is important to recognize that the provision and assessment of health care takes place in a context shaped partly by the constraints of statutory and case law. This legal landscape, in turn, reflects the evolution of societal norms, judicial philosophies, governmental pragmatics, and, sometimes, political agendas. As noted in part I, almost all law governing health care is state-specific, and your committee will benefit from familiarity with how the relevant laws and regulations in your state affect the care provided in your institution.

This section, then, is intended not to teach law, but to provide an overview of key legal developments that inform your work. The following cases have been selected because they represent important legal rulings that have affected and, in some cases, profoundly altered health care and bioethics. In some instances, they illustrate the ways different courts address similar issues. In others, it is possible to see the disconnect between law and ethics that creates tensions addressed in ethics committee deliberation. Because of their historical significance, several of these cases are also referred to in the relevant chapters of part I.

The cases have been summarized to highlight the ethical issues they raise, keeping the legalese to a minimum. For those wishing to consult the original text, each case is presented with its legal citation, as well as a brief parenthetical statement of the holding, the legal principle derived from the court's opinion or decision. Further information about these and other pertinent cases and statutes can be found in the references at the end of this section. For example, a brief but very informative and accessible explanation of the American constitutional structure, including the relationship between federal and state courts, appears in *Law and Bioethics: An Introduction* by Jerry Menikoff.

INFORMED CONSENT

The doctrine of informed consent and refusal has its roots in the law of battery, which holds that unconsented-to touching, even treatment intended to be beneficial, is unlawful. The earliest, most well-known and widely quoted expression of this philosophy was by Justice Benjamin N. Cardozo, who said, "Every human being of adult years and sound mind has a right to determine what shall be done with his own body; and a surgeon who performs an operation without his patient's consent commits an assault for which he is liable in damages" (*Schloendorff v. Society of New York Hospital*, 105 N.E. 92, 93 (N.Y. 1914)).

The signal case establishing the principle of informed consent was *Canterbury v. Spence*, 464 F.2d 772 (D.C. 1969) (holding that the physician is obliged to provide sufficient information about a procedure's risks so that a reasonable patient can make an informed decision). The case concerned a patient who underwent surgery for back pain, fell out of bed during recovery, and suffered paralysis. Among the plaintiff's claims was that he had not been informed before surgery of the risk of paralysis. The court held that, not only consent, but *informed* consent is necessary before medical treatment is undertaken.

The issue before the court was the kind of risks that must be disclosed and here two opposing philosophies were articulated. One camp believed that the doctor should disclose risks considered standard by the medical community, a view that would require expert medical testimony during trial. The other camp held that the standard should be what the reasonable patient would consider a significant risk, requiring disclosure of a far greater range of risks. The *Canterbury* court held that the reasonable patient standard was more appropriate because it shaped the disclosure duty according to what the patient needed to know. Controversy remains about whether the nature and content of disclosure should be determined by the doctor's duty to inform or the patient's understanding of the disclosure. Although states are still about evenly split on which approach to follow, the medical community standard is the majority view.

More recently, two California cases further developed the doctrine of informed consent. *Moore v. Regents of the University of California*, 793 P.2d 479 (Cal. 1990) (holding that informed consent requires physician disclosure of "personal interests unrelated to the patient's health" but potentially affecting medical judgment) examined the doctor's conflict of interest. The case concerned the deliberate withholding from the patient of his doctors' plans to use tissue removed from his body for likely profitable research. Having made the diagnosis of hairy-cell leukemia and realizing the unique properties of Mr. Moore's tissue, the doctors applied for a patent on the cell line from the tissue before removing his spleen. On appeal, the court found that, even if the treatment had a therapeutic purpose, the patient's ignorance of the doctors' research and financial interest in his tissue, which may have affected their medical judgment, impaired his ability to give truly informed consent.

Arato v. Avedon, 858 P.2d 598 (Cal. 1993) (holding that the duty to obtain informed consent does not require a physician to disclose a patient's statistical life expectancy) concerned the nature of the patient's health-related information that is necessary for informed decision making. After being diagnosed with a virulent form of cancer, the patient consented to chemotherapy and radiation treatment. The doctors explained to the patient and his family the poor prognosis for this type of cancer and the experimental but promising nature of the chemotherapy; they did not, however, provide statistical information on his life expectancy. The suit brought following the patient's death claimed that, had he known the short life expectancy and the small chance of successful cure, he would not have undergone the treatment, and thus he had not given fully informed consent. The suit further claimed that his ignorance of his situation prevented him from adequately ordering his affairs, resulting in his family suffering financial hardship.

The *Arato* court found that the physicians had provided the patient with what was required to give an informed consent—sufficient information material to the treatment decision to enable the patient to make a knowledgeable choice. The unreliability of statistical morbidity data, plus the patient's apparent reluctance to learn his life expectancy, removed the physicians' burden to disclose the information. Because of its emphasis on not imposing unwanted, potentially distressing information, it has been suggested that *Arato* represents an expansion of the therapeutic exception to the disclosure obligation.

HEALTH CARE DECISION MAKING

Withholding or Withdrawing Life-sustaining Treatment

Among the most difficult bioethical dilemmas are decisions to refuse or terminate life-sustaining treatment, made either by capable patients or on behalf of patients without capacity. In 1975, what became known as the "right to die" was brought to national attention when 21-year-old Karen Ann Quinlan lapsed into a persistent vegetative state (PVS). Although doctors determined that her condition was irreversible, they were reluctant to accede to her family's wishes and discontinue life support measures. In a unanimous landmark decision, *In re Quinlan*, 355 A.2d 647 (N.J. 1976) (recognizing a constitutionally protected right to refuse life-sustaining treatment and upholding the exercise of that right by the family of a patient in PVS), the New Jersey Supreme Court held that removal of the respirator necessary to keep Ms. Quinlan alive would not constitute criminal homicide because death would result from existing natural causes.

In an analysis that weighed the interests of the state against the benefits and burdens to the patient, the *Quinlan* court noted that "the State's interest [in maintaining] life weakens and the individual's right to privacy grows as the degree of bodily invasion increases and the prognosis dims." Note that the court based its protection of the right to refuse treatment on the constitutionally protected right to privacy, what some commentators have called "privacy as autonomy."

Courts that have found persuasive evidence of terminal illness or unbearable suffering plus decision-making capacity have held that patients' decisions to terminate life-sustaining treatment are reasonable and supportable. *Satz v. Perlmutter*, 362 S.2d 160 (Fla.App. 1978) *aff'd* 379 S.2d 359 (Fla. 1980) (upholding a competent individual's right to refuse unwanted life-sustaining treatment) concerned a 73-year-old patient with amyotrophic lateral sclerosis, also known as Lou Gehrig's disease, a progressively debilitating and incurable disease. Although generally paralyzed and dependent on mechanical breathing assistance, he was alert, fully competent, and able to speak. He understood that his condition was terminal and he wanted to have the breathing tube removed from his trachea, knowing that this would cause almost immediate death. Indeed, he had attempted, unsuccessfully, to remove the tube himself. He was supported in this decision by his family.

The hospital, fearing both civil and criminal liability, refused to honor his request. The patient petitioned for a court order preventing the hospital from interfering with his decision. The state intervened, citing four state interests in keeping a patient alive, which had been articulated in an earlier case, *Superintendent of Belchertown State School v. Saikewicz*. These four justifications were the state's (1) interest in the preservation of life; (2) duty to prevent suicide; (3) need to protect innocent third parties; and (4) need to maintain the ethical integrity of the medical profession. The court found that "the condition is terminal, the patient's situation wretched, and the continuation of his life temporary and artificial." Accordingly, despite the state's four interests in maintaining life, the court held that the plaintiff's decision to terminate his life-supporting treatment was reasonable.

Refusal of life-sustaining treatment by a capable patient on religious grounds is illustrated by *Fosmire v. Nicoleau*, 551 N.Y.S.2d 876 (1990), in which a Jehovah's Witness refused the blood transfusions necessary to save her life during childbirth. The court held that, at the time of treatment, this patient was competent to express her wishes and make a health care decision. The court considered the four state interests in keeping a patient alive, especially the claim that preserving her life was for the benefit of her children, and found that the state had failed to show paramount interest in preventing the patient from exercising her right to refuse treatment.

A patient's right to refuse nutrition and hydration was addressed in *Bouvia v. Superior Court of Los Angeles County*, 225 Cal. Rptr. 297 (Cal.Ct.App. 1986) (holding that a decisionally capable person may refuse artificial feeding enforced to sustain life, even if the person is not terminally ill). Cerebral palsy and arthritis had slowly robbed the 28-year-old patient of the use of her limbs and she was completely dependent financially as well as physically. Nevertheless, she was intelligent and competent, and had graduated from college. When she tried to starve herself to death by refusing food, a nasogastric tube was inserted through which she was force fed. Her request to have the tube removed was denied by the lower court, which found that, because she was incurably but not terminally ill, she could potentially live for years.

The appellate court, however, held that a competent person's right to refuse unwanted life-sustaining treatment encompasses forced tube feedings, and that the absence of a terminal prognosis does not affect that right. The court emphasized that the right to refuse treatment belongs to the competent patient and is not to be limited or denied by physicians or courts. It is interesting that the concurring opinion foreshadowed the assisted suicide debate by saying that, rather than having to starve herself, Ms. Bouvia should have been able to call upon her doctors to help her achieve a painless death.

Surrogate Decisions to Forgo Life-sustaining Treatment

The substituted judgment standard of decision making for an incapacitated patient was first articulated in *Superintendent of Belchertown State School v. Saikewicz*, 370 N.E.2d 417 (1977) (holding that an individual incompetent from birth has the same right as competent individuals to refuse medical treatment and is not required to undergo unwanted life-sustaining treatment). The case concerned Joseph Saikewicz, a profoundly retarded 67-year-old man with the mental age of less than 3 years. The issue before the court was whether to treat his leukemia with chemotherapy, which would cause him considerable discomfort and had a 30 to 50 percent chance of extending his life for two to thirteen months, or forgo therapy, in which case he would die within weeks.

In reaching its ruling, the *Saikewicz* court began by recognizing the patient's lifelong incapacity to make decisions and using an objective standard to consider what would be in his best interest. But then the court proposed an alternative method of decision making for this patient—substituted judgment—suggesting that the incompetent individual's choices could be inferred by a surrogate decision maker based on what is known about his wishes and values. The court's somewhat strained reasoning was that those who are and have always been legally incompetent still have the same right as others to refuse life-sustaining treatment, and to deny them that right just because they are incompetent devalues their worth.

Despite the utility of the substituted judgment standard in surrogate decision making, the way it was used by the *Saikewicz* court has been largely discredited by subsequent courts and commentators. Substituted judgment is typically reserved for those situations in which previously capable patients have a known history of preferences that can guide decision making on their behalf. Precisely because the profoundly retarded have no such history, decisions for them must rely on the best interest standard, drawing on what *others* believe will promote their well-being. The *Saikewicz* court blurred this distinction and relied on the fiction that the always-incompetent patient has values and wishes that can be divined by surrogate decision makers, explaining that "the decision . . . should be that which would be made by the incompetent person, if that person were competent, but taking into account the present and future incompetency of the individual. . . ." The risks of applying this contrived reasoning in the clinical setting are discussed in chapter 3 and were pointed out later by the *Storar* court considering a similar case.

The standards for making decisions on behalf of the never-competent and the formerly competent were more clearly distinguished in a pair of 1981 cases. *In re Storar*, 52 N.Y.2d 363 (N.Y. 1981) (holding that the guardian of a lifelong incompetent may not withhold medical treatment in a belief that such withholding is in the incompetent's best interest) concerned a profoundly retarded 52-year-old man with terminal bladder cancer whose mother petitioned for an order discontinuing the blood transfusions necessary to keep him alive. The patient had been from birth incapable of making a reasoned determination about his health care and his mother rejected the recommended transfusions because they caused him discomfort and would extend his life by only three to six months. Here, the question was whether the patient's best interests were served by allowing his mother or the hospital to have decision-making authority.

In its ruling, the court analogized the patient to a child incapable of exercising his autonomy, even though he was chronologically an adult. Note that, in contrast to the earlier *Saikewicz* court, the *Storar* court relied on the notion of best interest, rather than engaging in the fiction that the wishes of a never-competent person could be used to guide decision making. In explaining why it declined to use substituted judgment, the court said of the *Saikewicz* reasoning that asking what an incompetent person would decide if competent "would be similar to asking whether if it snowed all summer would it then be winter?" Relying on what it considered to be the patient's best interest, the *Storar* court held that, while a parent may consent to or refuse treatment on behalf of a child, the parent may not deprive a child of life-sustaining treatment.

The companion case to *Storar* was *Matter of Eichner*, 52 N.Y.2d 363 (N.Y. 1981) (holding that the agent of an incompetent may authorize the termination of life-sustaining measures if such termination is consistent with the prior wishes of the patient when competent). Also known as the Brother Fox case, the matter concerned an elderly priest who suffered brain damage and lapsed into a coma as a result of postoperative cardiac arrest. Brother Fox's guardian, Father Eichner, petitioned for an order discontinuing life support in accordance with Brother Fox's previously expressed wishes not to be kept alive artificially if he were in a vegetative state. Finding that Brother Fox's numerous statements at the time of the *Quinlan* case constituted clear and convincing evidence of his care preferences, the court held that the patient's wishes to have life-sustaining measures removed, as expressed through his representative, should be honored.

A pivotal case addressing both surrogate decision making and the right to refuse life-sustaining treatment was *In re Conroy*, 486 A.2d 1209 (N.J. 1985) (holding that an incompetent's life support may be removed if doing so is demonstrably in the incompetent's best interest). The case concerned an 83-year-old nursing home resident with multiple, serious, and irreversible physical and cognitive impairments that left her unable to do anything for herself and minimally responsive to her surroundings. Regardless of treatment, she was expected to live less than a year.

The court permitted removal of her feeding tube, articulating a range of surrogate decision-making standards for terminally ill patients. The court established three tests for determining when life-sustaining treatment may legitimately be withheld or withdrawn from an incapacitated patient: (1) *subjective test*—what is known about what the patient wanted, based on her prior explicit verbal or written statements; (2) *limited objective test*—"trustworthy evidence" about what the patient would have wanted plus clear indications that the treatment would only prolong suffering; and (3) *pure objective test*—without knowledge of what the patient would have wanted, but with clear indications that the burdens of the treatment "markedly outweigh" the benefits *and* that continuing treatment would be "inhumane."

Perhaps the most famous and precedentially important case of this kind was *Cruzan v. Director, Missouri Department of Health*, 497 U.S. 261(1990) (holding that the Constitution is not violated by a state statute requiring "clear and convincing evidence" of the prior consent of a comatose patient before terminating life-sustaining measures). The case concerned Nancy Beth Cruzan, a 25-year-old woman in PVS for seven years, whose parents petitioned for an order to discontinue artificial nutrition and hydration. The U.S. Supreme Court, in its only such decision, upheld Missouri's right to insist on the demanding "clear and convincing evidence" standard for determining the wishes of an incompetent patient regarding the termination of life support. Because it is the only Supreme Court decision regarding refusal of life-sustaining treatment, the *Cruzan* holding remains binding on all lower courts addressing these matters.

In a ruling with far-reaching implications, the *Cruzan* Court recognized the liberty interest of a competent individual to refuse unwanted treatment, but found insufficient evidence of the prior wishes of *this* patient. The Court noted that the grave and irreversible consequences of a decision to withdraw life-sustaining treatment justified refusing such a request without certainty about the patient's wishes when competent. The Court held that imposing the stringent clear and convincing evidence standard did not violate due process protections, partly because of the state's interest in preventing abuse when the family is unavailable, unable, or unwilling to act as surrogate decision maker. The Court noted that, because due process did not require the state to give decision-making authority for termination of life support to anyone but the patient, the state was not required to give family members the right of substituted judgment. The ruling *permits but does not require* states to insist that evidence of prior competent wishes to end life support meet the demanding clear and convincing standard of proof. Presently, Missouri and New York require application of this standard in the clinical setting, significantly limiting the ability of nonappointed surrogates in those states to make end-of-life decisions for incapacitated patients.

Finally, it is worth noting Justice O'Connor's dissent, in which she said that the clear and convincing standard denies many people the opportunity to refuse treatment because so few leave explicit instructions or indicate their wishes in the event of incapacity. Therefore, she predicted, the *Cruzan* decision did not foreclose the possibility that the constitutionality of surrogate decision making might be considered in the future. Indeed, it has been suggested that some state statutes authorizing health care proxy appointments represented, in part, a response to the uncertainty created by the clear and convincing evidence standard articulated in *Cruzan*.

Physician-assisted Suicide

Note that, while the *Cruzan* Court found that the Constitution protects an individual's liberty interest in refusing unwanted medical treatment, it did not find a constitutionally protected "right to die." In 1997, the U.S. Supreme Court ruled in two cases that sought to turn the right to refuse treatment into a right to assisted death. The plaintiffs in *Washington v. Glucksberg*, 521 U.S. 702 (1997) claimed that the Fourteenth Amendment Due Process Clause could encompass a protected right to determine the time and manner of one's death and to obtain physician assistance in doing so. The plaintiffs in *Vacco v. Quill*, 521 U.S. 793 (1997) claimed that, under the Fourteenth Amendment Equal Protection Clause, terminally ill patients not maintained on life support are treated unequally compared to terminally ill patients who *can discontinue* life support.

The Supreme Court rejected both arguments in two rulings that have more to do with palliative care than assisted suicide. The Court held that, while there is no constitutionally protected right to assisted suicide, there is a protected interest in pain relief. The Court reaffirmed the doctrine of double effect, saying that it is both legally and ethically appropriate to give terminally ill patients as much medication as necessary to relieve pain, even if the unintended effect is to hasten death. The Court also strongly reaffirmed the distinction between forgoing life-sustaining treatment and assisted suicide. Finally, the decisions indicated that, if states did not statutorily make it easier and less threatening for physicians to provide adequate analgesia to patients who need it, the Court would not rule out the possibility of revisiting the issue of assisted suicide in a future case. These rulings have far-reaching implications for palliation throughout the therapeutic continuum, especially at the end of life.

STATE ACTION TO PROTECT PUBLIC HEALTH

The authority of the state to safeguard the public health has traditionally been considered so vital that, in exchange for state protection, citizens have been required to relinquish specific individual liberties. For example, *Jacobson v. Massachusetts*, 197 U.S. 11 (1905) (holding that a statute mandating vaccination was justified even though it infringed on individual rights) established that, by its authority to safeguard public welfare, the state may use its police power to compel vaccination. In its ruling, the U.S.

Supreme Court also emphasized the state's reciprocal obligation to use its power discriminately, targeting its regulations to achieve only the identified state goal without unnecessary abridgment of individual liberties.

CONFIDENTIALITY

The need to protect the public health has also been invoked to justify breaching the professional duty of confidentiality, as in state laws requiring health care providers to report suspected cases of child abuse and neglect; wounds that are the result of gun shots, knives, or other pointed instruments; burn injuries of specified severity; and cases of reportable communicable diseases.

More recently, courts have recognized a professional obligation to disclose information that will protect identified third persons put at specific risk by patients' ability and intention to do harm. The legal duty to protect identified persons endangered by a foreseeable harm was first recognized in a negligence suit brought by the parents of a young woman murdered by her boyfriend. The case was *Tararsoff v. Regents of University of California*, 551 P.2d 334 (Cal. 1976) (holding that a therapist who concludes that a patient poses a foreseeable danger to a third person is under a duty to notify the potential victim). Even though Prosenjit Poddar had confided during his psychotherapy session his intention to kill Tatiana Tarasoff and the psychologist subsequently alerted the police, the therapist did nothing to warn the potential victim directly. The court reasoned that "the public policy favoring protection of the confidential character of patient-psychotherapist communications must yield to the extent to which disclosure is essential to avert danger to others. The protective privilege ends where the public peril begins."

The *Tarasoff* reasoning has been incorporated into the partner notification laws of most states, which now require that sexual and needle-sharing contacts of HIV-positive patients be informed that they have been exposed to the virus and should be tested. *Tarasoff* is also noteworthy because it significantly broadened the scope of professional duty to include not only the immediate patient, but an identified third party at risk who had no direct clinical connection to the care provider.

MEDICAL DECISION MAKING FOR MINORS

In general, the legal trend has traditionally favored the decisions of parents or guardians concerning a child's welfare. One landmark case illustrating this deference was *Parham v. J.R.*, 442 U.S. 584 (1979) (holding that a state may permit parents to have their child institutionalized without a formal hearing). A borderline retarded child manifesting aggressive and antisocial behavior petitioned the court through an appointed guardian, requesting that he be moved from Georgia's Central State Hospital to a less harshly restricted environment that would meet his needs. The court denied J.R.'s petition, holding that a minor's substantial liberty interest in avoiding unnecessary confinement is outweighed by the superior decision-making capacity of his parents who are presumed to act in their child's best interests.

In contrast was *Custody of a Minor*, 379 N.E.2d 1053 (Mass. 1979) (holding that, when even well-intentioned parental conduct threatens the welfare of a child, the interests of the child and the state may compel intervention). The case concerned 3-year-old Chad Green, a child suffering from acute lymphocytic leukemia. His parents believed that his best chance of cure lay in discontinuing standard chemotherapy and substituting metabolic therapy, including massive doses of vitamins and the drug laetrile. A lower court found that the child's condition required conventional therapy and warranted removing him from the legal custody of his parents. The appellate court affirmed, finding that, despite the traditional legal presumption that parents are the best judges of what is in their child's best interest, the compelling evidence here showed that Chad's well-being was seriously threatened by his parents' refusal to comply with medically proven therapy. The court held that the health and safety of a child must be the primary interest of the state, even when that interest overrides the authority of parents to care for their child.

The continuum of ethical decisions related to endangered or severely handicapped newborns is illustrated by two cases that captured national attention. At one end was the 1982 case of Baby Doe, who was born in Bloomington, Indiana, with tracheoesophageal fistula, a defect preventing the oral ingestion of food. While the condition is fatal, it is also easily remedied with surgery. However, the defect is more common in infants with Down's syndrome, as was true in this instance. Although Down's syndrome children run the gamut from profoundly retarded to educable and self-sufficient, the referring obstetrician testified that the infant would have a "minimally acceptable quality of life." The Indiana Supreme Court upheld the parents' refusal to permit surgical repair of the esophageal opening and the infant died. In this instance, the court did not elect to override parental decision even though the infant's life was at stake. Moreover, the only acknowledged reason for withholding treatment was the Down's syndrome. The resulting public outcry was based at least partly on the perception that, by withholding life-sustaining treatment, the parents were meeting their own needs to be relieved of the burden of a handicapped child.

The resulting Baby Doe regulations, issued in 1984, were intended to prevent seriously ill infants from being deprived of necessary medical attention. Drawing on existing law that made it illegal for agencies receiving federal funds to discriminate on the basis of handicap, these rules required hospitals to post notices stating that "nourishment and medically beneficial treatment (as determined with respect to reasonable medical judgments) should not be withheld from handicapped infants solely on the basis of their present or anticipated mental or physical impairments" (Furrow et al., 1991, p. 1184). The notices included a toll-free hotline number to facilitate reporting violations of the regulations, which would trigger intervention by "Baby Doe squads" of physicians, attorneys, and administrators. After several court challenges, the Baby Doe regulations were struck down by the U.S. Supreme Court, which ruled that parents had the right to refuse treatment for their children, regardless of handicap. Revised and less stringent regulations appeared in 1987 as amendments to the Child Abuse Prevention and Treatment Act.

At the other end of the spectrum was *In re Baby K*, 16 F.3rd 590 (4th Cir. 1994) (holding that life-sustaining treatment is required in an emergency setting, even if the treatment is medically futile). Baby K was an infant born with anencephaly, a condition that left her with a functioning brainstem that kept her body alive, but no upper brain function that would enable her to develop awareness or cognitive ability. In the opinion of treating physicians, providing ventilatory assistance was inappropriate, given the infant's limited life expectancy and dismal quality of existence. Nevertheless, the court upheld the mother's wishes for the infant to receive breathing assistance in the emergency room whenever she experienced respiratory distress. The court's reasoning was that, under the Emergency Medical Treatment and Active Labor Act (EMTALA), the Rehabilitation Act of 1973, and the Americans with Disabilities Act (ADA) of 1990, life-sustaining treatment is required in an emergency setting, even if that treatment is deemed medically futile. In this case, Baby K's breathing difficulty qualified as an emergency medical condition, the diagnosis of which triggered the hospital's duty to provide the infant with stabilizing treatment or transfer her to another facility in accordance with the provisions of EMTALA.

REPRODUCTIVE RIGHTS

Privacy

Historical and religious prohibitions against interfering with procreation were at the root of some states' statutory criminalization of contraception. These statutes were struck down in 1965 when the U.S. Supreme Court, in *Griswold v. Connecticut*, 381 U.S. 479 (1965), held that the constitutionally protected right to privacy of married persons was violated by laws restricting the use of or dissemination of information about contraception. The executive director and a physician at a Connecticut planned parenthood clinic were convicted under a state law that made it a criminal offense to provide counseling on contraception to married couples.

Griswold was a landmark case because it: (1) legalized the use of contraception by married couples and the freedom of their doctors to counsel them regarding its use; and (2) found in the Constitution a "penumbra" (or implication) of rights not specifically articulated in the text, but emanating from fundamental constitutional guarantees. These guarantees, according to the Court, included the very important zone of privacy in marital relations. This reasoning gave rise to the concept of privacy as autonomy, the protectable right to personal decision making. The far-reaching importance of this approach is that it allowed the *Griswold* Court, and subsequent Courts, to find a generalized right to privacy capable of accommodating a broadened scope of protected personal interests. The interests found to be protectable under the expanding right to privacy included those intimate areas of life related to personal decisions, such as marriage, procreation, child rearing, family definition, and abortion.

Griswold thus created a zone of privacy, which it accorded a high degree of protection. According to constitutional interpretation, fundamental rights are those that are so central to individual liberty that they can be abridged only when the state can demonstrate a compelling interest in doing so. The difficulty of overcoming this very high standard is the constitutional safeguard against arbitrary state intrusion in the lives of individuals. The *Griswold* line of reasoning, however, lost much of its vitality in *Bowers v. Hardwick*, 478 U.S.186 (1986) (holding that the right to privacy does not include a fundamental right to engage in consensual sodomy, even within the privacy of one's home), a decision considered to restrict privacy as autonomy. Based on homosexual activities, Hardwick was charged with violating the provisions of a Georgia state sodomy law. When the district attorney chose not to pursue the matter, Hardwick sued, challenging the constitutionality of a law that criminalized private, consensual sexual behavior. The Court distinguished consensual sodomy from any constitutionally protected right and clearly signaled its reluctance to expand further the definition of fundamental rights.

Nineteen years later, however, the Court overturned *Bowers* in *Lawrence and Garner v. Texas*, 539 U.S. 558 (2003) (holding that the Texas statute that criminalized sexual intimacy by same-sex couples, while not criminalizing the same behavior by different-sex couples, violates the Due Process Clause of the Fourteenth Amendment). The Court upheld the privacy and liberty rights of adults, ruling, "The Texas statute furthers no legitimate state interest which can justify its intrusion into the personal and private life of the individual." Nevertheless, in recent years, the Supreme Court has declined to expand the scope of individual privacy rights.

Abortion

The case that legalized abortion in the United States was *Roe v. Wade*, 410 U.S.113 (1973) (holding that a state antiabortion statute that prohibits abortion except to save the life of the mother, regardless of the stage of pregnancy or other factors, violates the Due Process Clause of the Fourteenth Amendment and denies a woman's right to privacy). The case was heard by the U.S. Supreme Court as the review of a challenge to a Texas law banning all abortions except those necessary to save the life of the mother. The Court held that the right of privacy "founded in" the Fourteenth Amendment's protection of "personal liberty and restriction of state action" was broad enough to encompass a woman's right to terminate her pregnancy under conditions limited only by the state's interest in her welfare and in the life of the unborn after viability. Moreover, the Court held these rights to be "fundamental" and "implicit in the concept of ordered liberty."

Roe represented a watershed in American legal, medical, and ethical thinking, and has had consequences far beyond the abortion issue. Considered by many to be the Court's most controversial ruling, the case was perceived as both a landmark for women's rights and an excessive level of judicial activism. To read the text of the remarkable Supreme Court opinion and concurrences is to read an encapsulation of the divisiveness and soul searching that marked—and still marks—this emotional issue.

Ultimately, the Court chose not to address the difficult issue of when life begins and declined to find that a fetus is a "person" within the meaning of the Fourteenth Amendment. To do so would have accorded the fetus due process protections that would have effectively invalidated the right to abortion. Instead, the Court referred throughout the opinion to "potential life," consistent with the trimester framework using viability as its standard.

The Court based its reasoning on the right to privacy in personal decisions it found in the Fourteenth Amendment and cited the inherent medical factors. Thus, the *Roe* Court held that a statute criminalizing abortion except as a life-saving measure regardless of other considerations violates the Due Process Clause of the Fourteenth Amendment. More specifically, the Court devised a regulatory scheme based on fetal development and viability, holding that during the first trimester, the decision to abort was within the zone of private decision making between the pregnant woman and her doctor; during the second trimester, the state may regulate abortion only to protect the health of the mother; and, during the third trimester, the state's interest in promoting life enables it to regulate and even prohibit abortion except to save the life of the mother. The policy was that the state's interest in promoting life and its associated right to intervene increases as the development and viability of the fetus advances.

The sweeping scope of *Roe* was modified in two subsequent Supreme Court decisions, although both reaffirmed a woman's right to an abortion. *Webster v. Reproductive Health Services*, 492 U.S. 490 (1989) (upholding a state's right not to fund abortion and to require viability testing) relaxed the rigid trimester framework, allowing states to focus on fetal viability in regulating abortion. The case was heard as a review of an order invalidating a Missouri state scheme to prohibit state-funded abortion. Finding that states were under no obligation to subsidize health care of any kind, the U.S. Supreme Court held that a state could refuse to fund any particular type of health care, such as abortion. The Court also did not find unconstitutional a state requirement that life can be protected after viability, the determination of which may be required as a condition of permitting an abortion. Accordingly, the ruling upheld the right of a state to withhold funding for abortion as it might for any other health care and to require viability testing prior to terminating any pregnancy of more than twenty weeks duration.

The second case was *Planned Parenthood of Southeastern Pennsylvania v. Casey*, 505 U.S. 833 (1992) (striking down state law provisions that unduly burden a woman's right to an abortion, discarding the trimester scheme entirely, and substituting the undue burden test to regulate abortion). Responding to the challenge of a Pennsylvania statute, the U.S. Supreme Court held that (1) it was necessary to reaffirm the essential holding of *Roe v. Wade* recognizing the right of a woman to have an abortion prior to the point of fetal viability; (2) the rigid trimester scheme adopted in *Roe* to regulate abortion should be replaced by a test to determine whether the restrictions on abortion placed an "undue burden" on a woman; (3) the medical emergency definition and the requirements for informed consent, twenty-four-hour waiting period, parental notification, and reporting and record keeping did not impose an undue burden, and were thus not invalid; and (4) the spousal notification provision did impose an undue burden and was, therefore, invalid.

The issue of abortion remains not only highly controversial, but central to much of the legal and political activity in this country. Opponents of abortion rights have as their stated goal the overturning of *Roe v. Wade* and, toward that end, they lobby for or against candidates for political and judicial positions. Seemingly unrelated matters, such as child health regulations, drug enforcement policies, stem cell research restrictions, and protections against domestic violence are perceived by many as efforts to chip away at the right to abortion without actually overturning *Roe*. Indeed, where one stands on the issue of abortion has become a litmus test of where one's social and political sympathies lie.

Surrogate Parenting

The most famous surrogacy case, and one that embodies all the potential risks and heartaches, was *In re Baby M*, 537 A.2d 1227 (N.J. 1988) (holding surrogate motherhood contracts void as against public policy because they extract payment of money for the termination of parental rights). Mr. and Mrs. Stern contracted with Mary Beth Whitehead, a married woman already a mother, to be impregnated by artificial donor insemination using Mr. Stern's sperm. After delivery, Ms. Whitehead reluctantly surrendered the baby, but then changed her mind, regaining the child and leaving the state. Although the trial court upheld the agreement, the appellate court found the contract void as a matter of public policy because it required payment of money for the termination of parental rights, and because it severed the relationship between a child and her natural parents, which is not in the best interests of the child. Ultimately, the court looked to the best interest of the child, as it would in any adoption, and awarded custody to the Sterns, with visitation rights to Ms. Whitehead.

Maternal-fetal Conflict

On occasion, a pregnant woman's assertion of autonomy brings her right to refuse unwanted treatment into conflict with the state's interest in protecting the life of the unborn. Courts have generally opted to save the fetus where possible, as illustrated by the case *In re A.C.*, 573 A.2d 1235 (D.C. 1990) (holding that a terminally ill woman must undergo a caesarean section to save her fetus). Although A.C. had agreed to a section at twenty-eight weeks gestation, the court approved the hospital's petition for surgery at twenty-six-and-a-half weeks. The baby died three hours after birth. The decision was subsequently vacated when it was shown that neither A.C.'s rights nor her decisional competence had been correctly evaluated because she had been so heavily medicated. Rather than offering the patient's dubious "informed consent" to authorize surgery, the treatment decision should have been based on substituted judgment, drawing on what was known of her prior wishes when she had unquestioned capacity.

Maternal-fetal conflict is also reflected in attempts to prosecute pregnant women for behavior that puts the fetus at risk. Some cases have argued that child abuse and neglect statutes include "fetus" within the meaning of the term *child* for purposes of finding liability for failure to protect the health and safety of the unborn. For example, *Jefferson v. Griffin Spalding County Hospital Authority*, 274 S.E.2d 457 (1981) held that rejection of necessary medical care, including a caesarean section, rendered a fetus a neglected unborn child. Likewise, *Whitner v. State*, 492 S.E.2d 777 (S.C.1997) found that the South Carolina state abuse statute included fetuses within the meaning of the term *child*. Although the ruling was subsequently reversed, this case represented the first time that a state's highest court upheld a woman's conviction for criminal neglect of her unborn child because she used cocaine while pregnant.

Sterilization

Perhaps the most egregious misuse of state power in the name of public protection was *Buck v. Bell*, 274 U.S. 200 (1927) (upholding the state's right to authorize forced sterilization of institutionalized persons afflicted with hereditary forms of mental retardation, provided that safeguards exist to prevent abuse). Carrie Buck, an 18-year-old involuntary inmate of a state mental institution, was the first person to be sterilized under the 1924 Virginia compulsory sterilization law. She was selected because of a perceived familial pattern of mental deficiency: she, her mother, and her daughter were all determined to be "feeble-minded." The U.S. Supreme Court upheld the state's involuntary sterilization of institutionalized mental defectives to prevent a future drain on society's resources. Justice Holmes' chilling assessment that "three generations of imbeciles are enough" is especially tragic in view of the later-suggested possibility that both Carrie Buck and her daughter were, in fact, mentally normal.

HEALTH CARE REIMBURSEMENT

The shifting of responsibility for treatment decisions was the focus in the first cost containment-related malpractice ruling in *Wickline v. State of California*, 228 Cal. Rptr. 661 (Cal.App. 1986) (holding that discharge decisions are the responsibility of the physician rather than the insurer). A patient sued the California state Medicaid program for injuries allegedly resulting from a premature hospital discharge following the program's refusal to authorize additional hospital days. The court held against the treating doctor for not challenging Medicaid's refusal to fund the necessary further hospitalization. Because the court did not specifically address the issue of how cost containment does or should affect medical judgment, this decision presented little guidance for physicians struggling with the balance of patient care and economics.

REFERENCES

Annas GJ, Law SA, Rosenblatt RE, Wing KR. 1990. *American Health Law.* Boston: Little, Brown and Company.

Becker S. 2004. *Health Care Law: A Practical Guide.* 2nd ed. Chicago: LexisNexis.

Furrow BR, Greaney TL, Johnson SH, Jost TS, Schwartz RL. 2001. *Bioethics: Health Care Law and Ethics.* 4th ed. St. Paul, MN: West Group.

Furrow BR, Johnson SH, Jost TS, Schwartz RL. 1991. *Health Care Law: Cases, Materials and Problems.* 2nd ed. St. Paul, MN: West Publishing Co.

Menikoff J. 2001. *Law and Bioethics: An Introduction.* Washington, DC: Georgetown University Press.

Pence GE. 2004. *Classic Cases in Medical Ethics: Accounts of Cases That Have Shaped Medical Ethics with Philosophical, Legal and Historical Backgrounds.* 4th ed. Boston: McGraw Hill.

PART VII

An Ethics Committee Meeting

The ethical principles, concepts, and strategies discussed in the preceding sections of this handbook can be seen in action during meetings of institutional ethics committees. Whatever the size and sophistication of your committee's membership, the frequency of its meetings, the scope of its responsibilities, and the complexity of the issues on its agenda, the utility of its work depends on the quality of committee deliberation. The effectiveness with which clinical and organizational matters are addressed is determined by the content and process of the committee meeting, including the engagement of its members and the expertise of its leadership.

This final section of the book illustrates how a committee might apply ethical theory and skills, awareness of organizational and legal imperatives, and sensitivity to group dynamics. What follows is an account of what a committee might sound like as it reviews a hypothetical clinical case and an institutional policy. As you listen in on this meeting, pay particular attention to how

- the issues are introduced and given context
- the members are provided with information and encouraged to consider different perspectives
- the group interacts
- the committee chair and vice chair clarify and reframe the issues, refocus the discussion, summarize the key points, and identify how the deliberations will inform future committee work

■

LEVIN: Because we have some guests at today's meeting, let's go around quickly and introduce ourselves. I'm Josh Levin, bioethicist in the Division of Bioethics.

KELLER: Dr. Sam Keller, physician liaison for Medical Center management. We're putting together a new initiative on end-of-life care for hospitalized patients, and we're looking at some of the ethical issues.

NORMAN: Dr. Peggy Norman, medical director of the Home Health Agency.

ROWAN: Gail Rowan, attorney.

SILVER: Ellen Silver, director of education.

POWELL: Dr. Eric Powell, Pediatrics.

MARTINEZ: Reva Martinez, social worker in Palliative Care.

CARRELTON: Rev. Ben Carrelton, chaplain.

BARNETT: Dr. Greg Barnett, Nuclear Medicine.

DOYLE: Barbara Doyle, nurse manager, Oncology.

RICE: Dr. Harriet Rice, Medicine and Hematology.

PRINCE: Abby Prince, community member.

WALTERS: Carol Walters, director, Division of Bioethics.

SEEGER: Dr. Michael Seeger, Cardiology.

LEVIN: Okay, I thought we would start with a case that Jill Carver called to discuss with me a couple of weeks ago. She is clinical director of nursing for Oncology and I hope she will join us during the meeting.

Jill called about a patient and a clinical situation that I thought raised some interesting ethical questions. Even though I understand that the problems have been resolved, it would be useful to think through some of the ethical issues and some of their implications.

Let me ask Barbara Doyle to present the case. And Dr. Barnett, maybe you could add anything you feel is pertinent, and then we could open it up for discussion.

DOYLE: We called Bioethics because we had a 68-year-old patient with metastatic thyroid cancer who was receiving radioactive therapy. He had undergone spinal fusion and radiation, and then presented with spinal cord compression and paraplegia. The only treatment Endocrinology felt would have any impact on his disease was radioactive iodine.

Prior to the patient's admission to our unit, we had a meeting with the head of nuclear medicine, Dr. Sandler, Dr. Rogers from Endocrinology, the nurse manager, the nurse taking care of the patient, Jill, and myself.

We met for one reason. We were concerned about giving radioactive iodine to a patient who wasn't able to take care of himself. He was dependent for all ADLs [activities of daily living]. Because of his disease, he was on a bowel regimen, had a Foley [catheter to collect urine], was immobile, and had a stage II pressure ulcer. In short, he needed full care for all his medical and personal needs. We were going to give him radioactive iodine and this would expose nursing staff to radioactive material in the course of their caring for the patient. We were concerned about the safety of the staff because there is an exposure limit, which, at that time was between six and ten minutes per person per shift.

WALTERS: Could you say more about why you were concerned?

DOYLE: Because spending any amount of time with a patient who has ingested radioactive iodine exposes you to the radioactive material.

LEVIN: Tell us a little bit more about the nature of the risk.

DOYLE: Our concern was about both the risk to staff and the possible effect on patient care. Jill called Bioethics because we thought, if staff are worried enough about the risk that they refuse to take care of the patient, then what happens? We weren't at that point yet, but we had to think ahead about possible problems.

LEVIN: This is how I saw the issue: the right of staff to decline to participate in the care of a patient out of concern for their own well-being or threats to their own health, when declining could jeopardize the patient's care. So there were two parts to the issue—the rights of staff and the well-being of the patient—that could be in conflict.

CARRELTON: Can I ask why he needed the treatment? Was it so that he wouldn't be paralyzed anymore?

DOYLE: No. His paralysis could not be changed. He will remain paralyzed.

NORMAN: So it wasn't curative?

DOYLE: It wasn't curative, but palliative, intended to slow down the progression of the disease. That was the only reason that he was getting the therapy.

LEVIN: In what way was it palliative?

DOYLE: Because the growth of the tumor eventually could lead to his death. So by slowing it down—this man wanted to live.

LEVIN: That's not really palliative, but aimed at arresting or slowing the disease. Palliative treatment is focused on managing pain and other symptoms, even while the disease progresses, which is very different.

BARNETT: We did refer to palliation, but probably incorrectly. We really questioned the efficacy of this plan. We gave him one of the highest doses we've ever given. We questioned whether what we were doing would really help him. But it was the only option left to him and he knew it. This is what he and his doctors wanted to do. This was his one shot. We knew we would not repeat it, and we wanted to make it count, so we gave the highest dose we felt we could give.

SEEGER: These are technical issues. We accept risk as caregivers in many different ways, some of which are better defined than others. There is a risk of blood contamination in any patient who has a transmissible disease in the blood. There is a risk of aerosol transmission from respiration. Even if you have gowns and masks, errors occur. People get stabbed with their own needles in the cath [cardiac catheterization] lab.

[TECHNICAL QUESTIONS ABOUT RADIATION DOSAGES]

BARNETT: First, Dr. Seeger, you're educated in dealing with radiation in the cath lab, so you're taking an educated risk. Your physicians and nurses are as well. The nurses on the medicine floors who don't deal with this every day are at an in-between level. They're knowledgeable, but they certainly don't have the risk-benefit understanding of radiation that you all have. That's why we spent time talking with them.

[TECHNICAL ANSWERS ABOUT RADIATION DOSAGES AND PROTECTIONS]

SILVER: Are we asking our nursing staff to expose themselves beyond the ten-minute recommendation?

DOYLE: We actually set the limit at six minutes. I got authorization to hire additional staff because of our concern that the patient is bed-bound and not able to do anything for himself. So we hired additional aides, who knew what was going on, to be on every shift and we clocked everyone to be sure no one exceeded six minutes.

[TECHNICAL DISCUSSION ABOUT THE RATE AT WHICH RADIOACTIVE MATERIAL IS ELIMINATED FROM THE BODY]

LEVIN: Barbara, let me say two things just to clarify the issue that was presented to me. First, if the patient were not turned and given other routine care by the nurses, his care would be compromised. I was told that a number of the nurses were very uneasy about doing this. The second point is that giving the radiation in the first place was something that was thought to have some benefit for the patient. I don't think we've yet clarified what that benefit was expected to be. Then we can look at the benefit-risk analysis.

DOYLE: We had one nurse who was breast feeding. A lot of nurses on my staff are in childbearing years, one who is actively seeking to get pregnant. I told them all that I didn't want them on that side of the hall. Anybody else who felt uncomfortable, I gave the option of not being assigned to care for the patient.

POWELL: Was there actually a risk to someone who is breast feeding or potentially pregnant? Is that risk real?

DOYLE: I wasn't willing to take it. One woman has been trying to get pregnant for a couple of years. I didn't want to put her in that position.

POWELL: But if you're telling them not to go to one side of the hall, what about all the other patients on that side of the hall? You're setting up parameters that may disadvantage other patients whose care may suffer if there is not enough staff.

DOYLE: I don't disagree with you.

[TECHNICAL DISCUSSION COMPARING RISKS AND PROTECTIONS WHEN PATIENTS RECEIVE OUTPATIENT TREATMENT FOR HYPERTHYROIDISM]

MARTINEZ: What about breast feeding?

[TECHNICAL DISCUSSION ABOUT RADIATION EXPOSURE AND THE LACK OF RISK TO BREAST-FEEDING WOMEN]

BARNETT: A breast-feeding nurse takes out a Foley bag full of urine with the hottest iodine there is, she's going to lactate pure breast milk. Being around the patient is not going to put radiation into her milk.

POWELL: So telling someone not to be in the room if she's lactating is more a comfort matter. It's not based on scientific evidence.

BARNETT: No, that's something that I didn't say.

KELLER: Just one more question. What's the medical evidence that this treatment was appropriate?

[TECHNICAL DISCUSSION OF THE MEDICAL JUSTIFICATION FOR THE TREATMENT, INCLUDING EVIDENCE THAT IT IS EFFECTIVE IN SLOWING THE DISEASE]

LEVIN: Was this symptom control? Was the patient in pain?

DOYLE: He was not in pain.

WALTERS: How old is this patient?

BARNETT: Sixty-eight.

WALTERS: Did he make the decision to have this treatment?

DOYLE: He did. He wanted the treatment.

WALTERS: You mean as debilitated as he was, he was still capable of making this choice?

DOYLE: Absolutely.

WALTERS: You've just defused all the arguments I was going to make. That's really interesting. What did the patient expect to get from this treatment?

DOYLE: He wanted to live and he thought this would enable him to live longer. He understood very clearly that he would remain paraplegic and that the treatment might have no effect on his cancer, but he wanted to take the chance. For that reason alone, I believe my staff was so supportive of the treatment.

KELLER: And you're saying that this kind of dose does prolong survival in studies.

BARNETT: Yes. But I don't know yet its effectiveness in this particular patient.

PRINCE: But for his stage of disease it was an appropriate option for him to consider and choose?

MARTINEZ: Perhaps the only option.

BARNETT: I think it *was* his only option.

POWELL: So it would possibly affect survival, but not quality of life. He's going to remain bed-bound, paralyzed, all those things.

DOYLE: Yes.

POWELL: Who determines the quality of the benefit and whether it justifies the risk? Is that what we're asking?

SEEGER: What I was going to raise was his capacity to participate in a decision about a Hail Mary therapy, a treatment of last resort. We take risks at our end, for example, radiation exposure in the cath lab, knowing that there is a concrete benefit for our patients.

SILVER: Sometimes. Sometimes we discover later that there might not be a benefit.

SEEGER: But we don't know that initially. We operate on our best information at the time. We're educated, but so is the staff. What often determines the difference is that some people are willing to take that risk. That's why they're in the cath lab and not up on the floors. I think what counts ethically about their participation is their perspective and their values as to the risk they take and why they choose to take it when they're in this profession.

LEVIN: Could you say more?

SEEGER: Because radiation injury or damage is a cumulative insult over a lifetime depending on tissue and type of radiation, any exposure is an increase in risk.
  Now if it's a particularly small risk, then some staff are able to say, "That is a risk I'm willing to take for the concrete benefit of this patient." But I view the professional

integrity and commitment of the caregiver as highly as I do the autonomy of the patient. I think we have to value the professional's commitment to a specific situation when it is outside normal practice, which, by all standards, this is.

WALTERS: I want to pick up on what Michael just said. I have argued that caregivers don't have autonomy, they have standards of professional conduct. Within those standards, they may disagree with or opt out of something. I would suggest that within professionalism there isn't a total lack of self-interest. But the professional cannot have the same degree of self-interest as the patient with full autonomy to consent or refuse or act in ways that are appropriate for him or her. I don't think professionals have that unlimited option to put their interests first because their professional obligations may conflict with what they personally would choose.

LEVIN: But you can make the point another way. If a patient is given a high dose of radioactive iodine and then has a cardiac arrest, that patient is going to be resuscitated. That's the training that nuclear medicine people and EMS and ER staff and other caregivers get. They are still required to take care of patients regardless of the risk. If that's what you're saying, then I understand.

WALTERS: I agree and I wondered if this therapy was so out of the line of general practice that it was exempt from caregiver obligations.

LEVIN: I think the question of whether, given this patient's particular medical condition, this was an appropriate treatment is a medical question. But the ethical question concerns the risk to the health professionals taking care of him. We might frame the question in terms of a benefit-risk analysis. Now, we usually talk about benefit, burden, and risk in terms of what the *patient* will experience. Here, we are asking whether the treatment is one whose benefit to the patient is sufficient to justify the risk it poses to the *professionals*.

I know a number of the nurses had questions and misgivings about the plan and were reluctant to participate in this patient's care. We should be clear, however, that these concerns were prospective. Despite their reluctance, none of the nurses actually refused and the patient's care was not compromised.

PRINCE: Outside the medical context, individuals are free to say, "No, I'm not going to endanger my health or safety by doing things that might harm me." But as a health professional, that right seems limited by obligations. One of the things that occurred to me in this case is what if most of the nurses had refused? What if they said, "Even though it's only a six-minute exposure, we're not going to do it"? What would you do then?

WALTERS: I'm just wondering if there are some other cases in the history of health care that are useful analogies. I'm thinking of two. For principled reasons, a nurse refuses to be involved in abortion cases.

ROWAN: Conscience clause cases.

WALTERS: Yes. And in the early 1980s, some health care providers didn't want to take care of AIDS patients because of what we didn't know about the disease and the risks. Is it useful to look back historically and find analogies?

KELLER: Actually, TB is a better example.

POWELL: SARS.

CARRELTON: Leprosy—the nuns used to put themselves at risk to care for people with leprosy.

MARTINEZ: Six or seven years ago, we had a family with two kids who had malaria. It was during the Ebola scare. There were some decisions made in our ER as far as who did and did not go to the floor because the care of patients in the ER would be compromised if the kids would have been quarantined there. So this isn't that far away.

PRINCE: Yes, and I would even expand the analogy to different professions, as Michael suggested. People who work with asbestos or wash those windows on the outside of skyscrapers are taking those risks, knowing that they come with the job they signed up for.

KELLER: The argument, I guess, is there are some people who said, "Yes, I want to be a nurse, but I didn't sign up for this one."

LEVIN: I'm not sure where this discussion is going. Perhaps someone can refocus us.

SILVER: Let me try. I think it's critical to educate the people involved in patient care about just what risks they face. I find that when nurses or doctors are exposed and they feel that people are giving them facts, they make informed decisions and they're more apt to cooperate. And when they feel they're not getting enough information and the issues are not being dealt with, then they feel that people are holding out on them and that's when rumors start and bad decisions are made.

LEVIN: For me, the central question here is, "What are the limits of professional obligation to take care of patients in light of what is thought to be risk to self?" Now this is a question we've visited before. It's not new, although it presents a bit differently here.

This was not actual caregiver refusal to give care. It wasn't based on religious values or ethics. It was reluctance based on concern about threat to self that seems, under the circumstances, to have been unfounded. I mean, there was no real threat to self, right? I guess that's a question, not a statement.

WALTERS: Can I just summarize? I think Josh clearly framed the issue. We've had certain analogous situations. Caregivers who have principled, philosophical, and religious objections to abortion do not participate in that procedure. When we started to withdraw and withhold life-sustaining treatment thirty years ago, people who had principled objections did not participate.

This case falls into a different category where the refusal or reluctance has to do with protecting one's health and safety rather than protecting one's values and principles. Here, there is an analogy to the AIDS epidemic, when we were very clear that the obligation was to care for patients and that the answer to caregiver risk was universal precautions, not opting out. It's worth noting that, as Reva pointed out, this is not confined to the past. When SARS patients in Toronto were intubated, 100 percent of the staff who were in the room during intubation got SARS. *100 percent.* We're going to face these situations and these issues in the future. We thought that this case presented an interesting variation on a familiar issue: the limits of professional choice in the face of risk and professional obligations.

LEVIN: So, Dr. Barnett, could you clarify whether there really was a risk to the nurses under these circumstances?

[TECHNICAL DISCUSSION EXPLAINING THAT STAFF HAD BEEN EXPOSED TO A VERY LOW LEVEL OF RADIATION]

[TECHNICAL DISCUSSION ABOUT HOW LEVELS OF EXPOSURE WERE MONITORED]

LEVIN: This is Jill Carver. Jill, I'm glad you're here. In light of the fact that the nurses were ultimately found not to have been at significant risk, do you feel that their reluctance to participate was reasonable?

CARVER: We had quite a few meetings with the nurses. Our approach was to give them all the information we had. If somebody was uncomfortable with the care plan, we had no problem saying, "We'll make sure you don't take care of the patient." Essentially, we asked for volunteers.

Many of the senior nurses were quite funny. They said, "Well, my ovaries don't work anymore anyway, so it's not a problem." We had staff on the floor volunteer to work overtime and then we got approval to hire extra staff.

PRINCE: What if your extra staff was not available?

DOYLE: They were available because we had them booked in advance. My fear was that everybody's six minutes would be up and there would be nobody to care for the patient.

WALTERS: Let me see if I can reframe the ethical question. First of all, I think you guys did a terrific job in taking a difficult circumstance and planning so that patient care would not be compromised.

But now I want to look at this in terms of bioterrorism, which we haven't talked about much in this committee but which is one of the big ethical debates. It seems inevitable that we will face a bioterror attack or an epidemic of avian flu. So, going forward, there are going to be situations in which staff will be asked to do things that may make them uncomfortable. It seems to me that this example of one patient in a difficult circumstance that was handled sensitively and effectively may not be a very good precedent for the uncertain times ahead.

POWELL: It sounds like the people part was handled beautifully. But if you're analyzing it in terms of a major disaster, I have questions about the decisions.

WALTERS: Because of their implications for other similar and not-so-similar circumstances?

POWELL: Yes. For example, in a mass attack, we would not have the luxury of planning ahead, asking for volunteers, or letting people who were uncomfortable opt out.

KELLER: Exactly. The concern with biochemical and nuclear terrorism is that it won't be one person coming into the hospital for elective treatment. The problem will be the masses of injured people who will need immediate and unanticipated attention. So it's easy to see how we'd deplete our staff very quickly, especially if they're only allowed ten minutes in a protective suit where the temperature gets up over 120 degrees. That type of training in those mock disasters is really very important.

WALTERS: I think that questioning the obligations of health care professionals to deal with very difficult circumstances that require personal sacrifice is high up on the list of things we need to do. I think we have to do this because hospitals will be the first responders.

KELLER: Just one last point about this case. Wouldn't it be useful to share this information with Janet Mandel in Occupational Health so that, if this ever comes up again in a similar or even different way, they don't have to rewrite the whole chapter? They'll already know.

WALTERS: That's a terrific suggestion.

KELLER: Janet probably wouldn't know more than you guys know about this, but at least she and her staff should learn from the body of information that you've developed.

WALTERS: This has been a very useful discussion. Thank you. I think the structural note that Sam just brought in of always involving Dr. Mandel in decisions about staff is an excellent one.

LEVIN: Let me bridge now to Sophia Lawrence, Office of the Medical Director. As you know, many of the requests for bioethics consults are triggered by end-of-life issues. We've had numerous discussions recently in this committee about our DNR order. But it's become clear that the larger context of the discussion really is our policy about forgoing life-sustaining treatment. Because Sophia is about to begin work on revising this policy, we thought we'd bring the matter to the ethics committee and ask her to open up the discussion.

LAWRENCE: The issue that I have been running up against—we've all been running up against—is the inconsistencies between the policy and the clinical situations it's intended to address. It's a very elegant policy but I think it does not always apply to the straightforward clinical situations.

As I've been thinking about the policy, it appears that we have two issues to address— one having to do with technology and the other, perhaps more challenging, having to do with decision-making authority. First, the cases that many of us get called on involve recent technologies, like ventricular assist devices and pacemakers, that are not addressed here because they were not in use when the original policy was drafted. A lot of things that we're able to do now were not included

in the category of "life-sustaining treatment." Moving forward, it seems important to be organizationally consistent in how we counsel a care team. It's not
helpful to say, "It's okay to do this with this equipment, but not okay to do that
with that equipment." At the very least, we should have some consensus on the
definition of life-sustaining treatment.

In terms of decision-making authority, I think we also need to step back and look at
whether the policy provides useful guidance. It seems that, during the past several years, we have responded to constraints in the law and increasingly complicated cases by adding layers to our decision-making process. We now have a fairly
elaborate and cumbersome protocol, involving the clinical team, the family, and
administration. The result is somewhat counterproductive from a bedside perspective. When you're looking at a patient who is actively dying and we're intervening with seemingly complicated administrative steps, it's just not useful. So
that's some of the context. I would appreciate feedback.

KELLER: I went through this policy last night. For the last three months, I have been
looking at patients who have been in the hospital for more than three weeks.
Many of the problems in those cases are end-of-life issues. Having had that experience, I find that it's very difficult to take what's in this policy, as Sophia said, and
try to apply it to real-life situations. I think it has to be totally revised to make it a
little more user-friendly.

I think that the average physician dealing with a difficult situation wouldn't know
where to go with this policy and what to do with it. One way of reading it is that
patients can't simply die anymore without having a medical director involved. I
mean, I read that and I thought to myself, "Well, can't people just die, or do I have
to call a medical director to discuss whether I have to intubate every single patient who is actively dying?"

LAWRENCE: That is the heart of the problem.

MARTINEZ: Is there something specific that you can point to in the policy that leads
you to think that?

KELLER: Let's see. I highlighted something on page 5D. "The medical director's staff (or
a member of the Bioethics service) must be contacted to coordinate the necessary
steps in assisting the family and the health care team if the family/surrogate
wishes to forgo ventilatory support, dialysis, artificial nutrition, and/or hydration." Why is that necessary?

WALTERS: From an ethics perspective, I don't think the law requires that strict a reading because you need to look at the context in which the law was developed and
how it is customarily applied in the clinical situation. A most narrow reading, I
would argue, is unnecessarily restrictive to physicians when patients are actively
dying. A good example would be a patient in the pulmonary care unit. Let's say
that he's in multiorgan system failure with end-stage AIDS. His kidneys are fail-

ing, and the decision is made not to start him on dialysis because he's dying. He has no advance directive and he's either alone in this world or he's never discussed his care wishes with his family. The fact that we don't know what he would want about dialysis is irrelevant because he's dying.

KELLER: I hear you saying we have no medical, legal, or ethical obligation to offer a treatment if it's not medically indicated.

RICE: How do you decide that something is not medically indicated?

KELLER: Because, in this hypothetical situation, it's not life-sustaining. That's one of the things that I find is difficult with this policy. Some of the terms that you guys use and are comfortable with, the average clinician finds confusing. "Capacity" I understand, but "life-sustaining" or "medically indicated," I don't know what those mean.

CARRELTON: Is there a difference between keeping alive and life-sustaining?

ROWAN: They are the same thing.

NORMAN: Are they? I don't know. I'm trying to think about a patient who is dying. It seems to me that there is a life that could be sustained versus a person who is dying. I guess I'm also thinking of ventricular assist devices. I'm thinking about what Sophia said. And it's going to get worse, not better. There are going to be more expensive, high-tech, invasive ways of postponing death.

SILVER: I think it's important to emphasize that we're trying to keep a balance between the requirements of the law and the clinical needs of dying patients. This is not a matter of seeing how we can get around the law. This is a matter of providing guidance to clinicians who want to practice well within the standard of medical care, the requirements of the law, and the ethical imperatives. Somehow, the policy has to convey that.

KELLER: I have to agree. The problem is that "life-sustaining" as a phrase applies to the case we discussed earlier. That radioactive iodine was a life-sustaining therapy. Yet at the other end we have the patient who, without dialysis, would be dead within two or three days. Well, you put him on dialysis and I bet I could stretch that time frame. We can keep tissue going for weeks in people with no viability. That's life-sustaining, but is it rational?

ROWAN: Well, for the legislature and the courts, the presumption is that people would want to be kept alive unless you have evidence of their wishes to the contrary. Because of that presumption, we always err in favor of providing life-sustaining treatment.

SEEGER: But the law also requires an understanding that patients know the burdens of what we're going to do them against the potential benefits. What we do is often abusive and painful and absolutely magnificent at prolonging dying and suffering.

POWELL: What's the difference between prolonging dying and prolonging life?

LAWRENCE: Where I have trouble as a frontline resource person is saying to professionals, who are inherently risk averse anyway, "You have no clinical, ethical, legal obligation to provide care that's not indicated."

RICE: I don't know how to define this, but I think that we are trying to decide whether patients are living or alive. I'm not quite sure about the semantics or whether we're getting too philosophical, but we are sustaining people who really aren't living. I don't know how we make that distinction. We have patients who are almost brain dead and we're forced by technology to sustain them. Is that really a life? Is that really what the patient would want? That's obviously a slippery slope and we're stuck.

WALTERS: What you have done is frame the discussion that usually takes place under a rubric of quality of life. That, I think, is a very different matter about which people of good will and intelligence can disagree.

I think what we're trying to grapple with is that people don't understand what this policy means. What about our pulmonary care unit [PCU] patient? What if he had told his family he would want everything done? At a certain point, the PCU people would say, "His kidneys are going. It would be crazy to dialyze a patient who is moribund, who has all of these other organ system failures and is crashing on 100 percent oxygen."

LAWRENCE: But the reason he isn't started on dialysis is not because he told us he didn't want it. It's because it doesn't make any clinical sense.

KELLER: But for patients who clearly fall into that actively dying category, isn't there a way to interpret the phrase "life-sustaining treatment" that permits us not to provide it?

POWELL: The problem is that, if you specify this in the policy and say that something doesn't make clinical sense, there is a danger that it will be interpreted in a quality-of-life sense, which is something we don't want.

KELLER: I think the real problem we have is not just the law or us or the wording of the policy, but that society hasn't come to grips with the reality of death. We have a nation that can't recognize that death is the inevitable consequence of birth. Sooner or later, it's going to happen. If society wants, we can allocate resources indefinitely. We can put LVADs in every one of the patients who has end-stage heart failure. We can then put them all on transplant lists and we can put them in ICUs and on ventilators.

What I'm saying is that we have to be able to define a group of patients who are actively dying. This is not somebody with COPD who you are going to intubate and prolong life or not, or somebody with end-stage dementia who you're going to feed or not. The patients we are talking about have multiorgan system failure. They are dying and they will be dead within a matter of days to a week.

RICE: Maybe it's like the judge said about pornography, "I can't define it, but I know it when I see it." I know a dying patient when I see one. But what do we or don't we have to do to a patient who is actively dying?

SEEGER: For those patients, I would say that nothing is life-sustaining.

POWELL: It's palliation.

PRINCE: But who decides that?

NORMAN: It's not like a definitive point. It's often a continuum and sometimes we're wrong. I have to tell you, just to humble myself, I made a home visit to a patient with a systolic pressure of 80. His mouth was open, he hadn't eaten in thirty-six hours. I called the family and said, "I just want to let you know it's going to happen soon." I don't usually say that and I don't say it lightly. Twenty-four hours later he woke up. He was diabetic and his sugars were all over the place. He woke up and two weeks later he is eating and his sugars are fine. I don't know what happened, but I was humbled.

RICE: But that's the slippery slope. That's the problem.

SEEGER: I know, but we've got to start somewhere. If somebody raised the issue in that kind of patient, "Should we intubate?" and we didn't have this policy, we would have a tube in that patient, which I think is not what we're trying to do here.

KELLER: The other thing about the policy is that most of it deals with patients or families wanting to abuse treatment, as opposed to the team's questions about how aggressive to be. The policy doesn't really deal with that issue, which is, I think, much more common.

WALTERS: Say a little bit more.

KELLER: The typical scenario concerns the desperately ill patient whose family wants to continue aggressive measures, usually antibiotics. Again and again recurrent sepsis, resistant organisms, more antibiotics, and it just goes on and on. At some point, the physicians say, "We just can't keep doing this forever," and the family says, "Oh yes you can." Is there some way to address that issue? Does that fall under the rubric of life-sustaining?

WALTERS: That falls under the rubric of futility and, if we ever solve this problem, we'll get to that problem.

KELLER: Well, we have a patient in the hospital for five months now. That's our current long stay. Recurrent infections, different antibiotics, round and round—it's just very difficult to watch.

MARTINEZ: The only reason that we're doing this is because the family wants it, not because it makes clinical sense.

KELLER: The son, who is having a very difficult time with his father's illness, keeps insisting that we need to go forward. The attending physician is finding the situation hard to negotiate, and the hospital is stuck.

CARRELTON: Would it be helpful for me to spend some time with the family? Sometimes a new face who just wants to listen can be comforting.

KELLER: It's certainly worth a try.

WALTERS: Sam, if you think it would be helpful to have Bioethics consult on your case, let us know.

We haven't explicitly addressed the futility issue, which is lurking at the edges of these cases. Other states accord families more authority to make treatment decisions for their dying relatives, which makes a significant difference in how these situations are handled.

LEVIN: That's a great segue into something that I hope will be useful in our discussion. Because states differ, sometimes significantly, in how they deal with end-of-life issues, I thought it might be worth looking at how forgoing life-sustaining treatment is handled elsewhere. Keeping in mind that this is an ethics discussion, not a legal one, it seemed useful to look at policies in some other states to enrich our thinking about the ethical issues involved. We've said many times here that we don't want policy to drive the ethical analysis, but reflection on how other institutions deal with these issues might reveal ways of thinking about end-of-life issues that could benefit us.

In that spirit, I asked four committee members to do a little research and give us a brief sketch of what happens in four states: California, New York, Oregon, and Texas. To keep the discussion moving and prevent us from getting bogged down, I've asked that these summaries focus just on the key issues that have the greatest relevance to our policy discussion, with the understanding that the statutes and the policies reviewed are much more detailed. So, Abby, please start us off with a picture of what happens in Texas.

PRINCE: I reviewed the relevant Texas statute and one hospital's policy on forgoing life-sustaining treatment. They both clearly lay out the decision-making process and the underlying philosophy, beginning with an acknowledgment of the right of patients to consent to or refuse any treatment, and the recognition that, under certain circumstances, life-sustaining treatment may impose more burden than benefit.

The Texas structure authorizes health care decision making under a wide range of circumstances. Decisions, including the withholding or withdrawing of life-sustaining treatment, may be made in any of the following ways:

- by a competent adult after consultation with a physician
- by a written or verbal advance directive, previously executed by a competent patient
- by a spokesperson designated by the competent patient in an advance directive
- by the attending physician and either the patient's legal guardian or agent under a medical power of attorney, the latter previously designated by the competent patient
- in the absence of patient competence or ability to communicate, advance

directive or appointed medical power of attorney, by a spokesperson selected
from the following in order of priority:

- the patient's spouse
- the patient's reasonably available adult children
- the patient's parents; or
- the patient's nearest living relative

MARTINEZ: What about the patient who is incompetent, has not left an advance
directive, and has no family or friends to act as decision maker?

PRINCE: In that case, a treatment decision can be made by the responsible physician as
long as it is concurred in by another physician who has not been involved in the
patient's care.

SEEGER: Well, that pretty much covers all the possibilities in a clear and orderly manner.

PRINCE: Let me tell you a few other noteworthy features of this policy.

- It focuses attention on two categories of patients especially likely to need
decisions made about life-sustaining treatment: those in terminal conditions
and those in irreversible conditions.
- The policy makes a point of addressing the broader issues of deciding about any
and all life-sustaining treatment, rather than specific interventions.
- Physicians are strongly and repeatedly encouraged to initiate timely discussions
with patients about advance care planning, including life-sustaining treatment.
- Decisions on behalf of an incapacitated patient are to be based on the patient's
wishes, if known, or on an assessment of the patient's best interest.
- The institutional ethics committee is either encouraged or required to be
involved in several parts of the process, especially when conflict exists.
- Decisions about life-sustaining treatment for children have additional
safeguards, but I imagine that's pretty standard in all states.

WALTERS: Does the policy address futility?

PRINCE: Not directly, but the law and the policy have one really interesting and detailed section dealing with decisions that physicians consider inappropriate.
These are decisions by or for patients that either request or refuse life-sustaining
treatment. When the patient or surrogate refuses treatment the doctor considers
medically indicated, the policy lays out a process for review, discussion, and, if
consensus is not possible, transfer of the patient's care to another provider. When
the patient or surrogate insists on life-sustaining treatment that the doctors consider not medically indicated, the policy sets up an even more elaborate eight-
step process, including medical review, mediation, efforts to transfer the patient,
and extensive ethics committee review.

All told, the Texas law, reflected in this policy, seems to provide consistent and
helpful guidance for clinicians dealing with a set of difficult issues.

LAWRENCE: It certainly provides a useful model, assuming it would be consistent with law in this state.

LEVIN: Next up, let's look at California. Eric, did you research that?

POWELL: Yes. California has a specific Health Care Decisions Law, which includes several of the same features that Abby just described. The statute also begins by affirming the patient's right to refuse treatment, the inappropriateness of prolonging the dying process when treatment will not benefit the patient, and the importance of keeping health care decision making out of the courts when there is no controversy.

Similar to Texas, the California law lists several ways in which health care decisions, including the withholding or withdrawing of life-sustaining treatment, may be made, including:

- by a competent adult
- by an individual health care instruction, previously written by a competent adult
- by an agent authorized by a power of attorney for health care, previously designated by a competent adult
- by a surrogate designated by a competent patient only for the duration of current treatment, illness, or stay in the health care institution, or sixty days
- by a court-appointed conservator with the authority to make health care decisions

KELLER: Except for decisions by the competent patient, all of these require advance authorization, usually by the patient when competent. What happens if that hasn't been done? Is there a default priority list that includes family, as in Texas?

POWELL: I found that curious, too. Neither the statute nor the policy I reviewed specifically mentions family. Yet the statute does say that a domestic partner can make decisions with the same authority as a spouse, although the authority of spouses is not described. Fact sheets about the decision-making law, however, explain that, when a patient lacks capacity and has not delegated decision-making authority, care professionals do what they do in most of these situations—turn to close family or friends who are most likely to know the patient's wishes and values. This informal appointment of a decision maker has apparently been customary in California for years, even though it does not appear in the statute.

NORMAN: What are the criteria for decision making on behalf of incapacitated patients?

POWELL: Similar to Texas, the agent or surrogate bases decisions on the patient's instructions or wishes, if known, or on an assessment of the patient's best interests, considering personal values.

LEVIN: Any other questions about California? Thanks, Eric. Sam, what can you tell us about Oregon?

KELLER: You might expect that a state that has worked through an assisted suicide law has given a lot of thought to end-of-life issues, and it shows in the legislation and the policy that I reviewed. As in Texas and California, Oregon provides several ways that treatment decisions, including those about life-sustaining treatment, can be made, including:

- by a competent adult
- by a written health care instruction
- by a health care representative, who can be one of the following:
  - an attorney-in-fact for health care, designated by a previously competent adult
  - a person who has authority to make health care decisions for the patient, selected from a priority list when the patient is in specified clinical conditions
  - a guardian or other person appointed by a court to make health care decisions for a patient

As in Texas and California, when a patient lacks capacity, the health care representative must base decisions on the patient's wishes, if known, or an assessment of the patient's best interest. But Oregon goes further and builds in additional safeguards. For example, the health care representative may only make decisions about life support or tube feeding in the following circumstances:

- the capable patient had expressly initialed the relevant permission sections in the directive, or
- the patient has been medically confirmed to be in one of the following conditions:
  —a terminal condition
  —permanent unconsciousness
  —a condition in which life-sustaining treatment would not benefit the patient and would cause severe and permanent pain
  —the advanced stages of a progressive, debilitating illness that will be fatal, prevents the patient from swallowing nourishment or water safely or recognizing family, and it is extremely unlikely that this condition will improve

An additional list of safeguards covers the withholding or withdrawing of artificial nutrition and hydration, which can only be done by a statement of the capable patient, an authorized health care representative, or the confirmation that the patient is in one of the specified conditions that I just listed.

The instructions section of the advance directive described in the statute is very specific in explaining conditions under which decisions about life support can be made. These conditions include close to death, permanently unconscious, advanced progressive illness, and extraordinary suffering, all of which are defined. The instructions even explain the phrase "as my physician recommends" to mean that the patient wants the physician to try life-sustaining treatment as long as the physician believes it will be beneficial, after which it should be discontinued. This level of explanation would seem to address concerns about people consenting to things in advance directives without knowing what they mean and care professionals misinterpreting what directives intend. I know I would find clear definitions like this helpful, as I indicated earlier in the discussion about our policy.

NORMAN: You mentioned a priority list for selecting a health care representative. Is that similar to the ones in Texas and California?

KELLER: Yes, thanks for reminding me. If the patient has been confirmed to be in one of the four specified conditions and has not appointed a health care representative or left an advance directive, a representative is named in order from the following list:

- a guardian authorized to make health care decisions
- the patient's spouse
- an adult designated and agreed to by the other people on the list
- a majority of the patient's adult children
- either parent of the patient
- the patient's adult siblings
- an adult relative or friend

And, if none of those people is available, life-sustaining treatment can still be withheld or withdrawn under the direction of the attending after consultation with appropriate people, such as the patient advocate or another physician who is not involved in the patient's care.

The bottom line seems to be that, in Oregon, decisions to forgo life-sustaining treatment can be made in most circumstances, but specified conditions and safeguards have to be met.

LEVIN: Thanks, Sam. Any other questions about Oregon? Ellen, I think you looked at New York.

SILVER: New York's situation is more similar to what we have in this state. Because no decision-making law governs these issues, there is no clear statutory structure for making health care decisions, including those regarding life-sustaining treatment, on behalf of patients without capacity. The legislature has provided some targeted regulation and laws, including a statute authorizing the appointment of health care proxy agents and a statute creating a hierarchy of surrogates who may consent to do-not-resuscitate orders for incapacitated patients. The legislature has also authorized surrogate health care decision making on behalf of specific vulnerable patient populations, including incompetent adults who may have court-appointed guardians, the mentally ill and developmentally retarded, residents of mental hygiene facilities, and minors.

The lack of a surrogate decision-making statute in New York means that health care decision making is governed almost entirely by case law. A line of New York cases has held that, when a patient lacks capacity, a decision to withhold or withdraw life-sustaining treatment requires "clear and convincing evidence" that the patient would have chosen to forgo the treatment in question in the patient's current circumstances. Missouri also requires this rigorous evidentiary standard in the clinical setting. Because the clear and convincing standard is very demanding, it is often very difficult for families to provide the level of evidence necessary when patients may not have explicitly articulated their wishes about life-sustaining treatment. A statement of patient wishes, such as a written living will or oral instructions, is considered to meet the clear and convincing standard.

The fact is that most patients without capacity are not part of specified vulnerable populations, have not appointed health care agents, and may not have articulated their wishes orally or in writing. They are vulnerable just because they need decisions made for them. As Eric pointed out, common practice is for care professionals to turn to family or close friends to make decisions for incapacitated patients. Unlike most states, however, there is no clear surrogate authority in New York for those who can provide insight into their wishes and values. As a result, the customary but informal practice in New York is for family members to consent to treatment but, unless they have clear and convincing evidence of a patient's wishes about life-sustaining treatment, they are unable to make decisions about withholding or withdrawing these measures. The legislature is considering a family health care decision-making bill, which would create a hierarchy of surrogates, similar to the ones in Texas and Oregon.

MARTINEZ: So what happens now in most cases when the patient lacks capacity and has not appointed a proxy agent or left clear instructions? How do policies deal with that?

SILVER: The policy I reviewed focused on the right to reject unwanted treatment, authority of appointed surrogates, the importance of initiating early discussions with patients and families about care wishes, and the process for eliciting and documenting clear and convincing evidence of the patient's wishes. It is my understanding that most institutions have mechanisms for addressing cases that don't meet these criteria, including exhaustive review by the clinical team, medical director, legal office, and bioethics.

LEVIN: Thanks to all of you for researching and presenting this material. Let's return to discussing our own policy.

LAWRENCE: We have another important resource that we haven't mentioned. The integration of palliative care is an important fact for bioethics, critical care, geriatrics, pediatrics—clinical care in general. So if we have questions about whether a patient is dying, we have this other valuable resource—a team of people who are experts in determining when a patient is dying and how best to arrive at the most appropriate plan of care. In these situations, we should routinely bring in those experts and try to get some kind of consensus that we're dealing with a patient in the process of dying, a patient who would be appropriate for palliative or hospice care.

WALTERS: Excellent point. If a patient moves from curative treatment to hospice care, my argument is that we're not withdrawing or withholding care from the patient. Although we are withholding what may be life-sustaining care, we're providing appropriate aggressive palliative care for a patient who is dying.

LEVIN: I think part of the problem with the policy is that it defines life-sustaining treatment in terms of specific interventions, rather than the broader context that we heard about in other policies. Specific interventions in some cases may indeed be life-sustaining, but in your example, the very same intervention would not be life-sustaining. So I wonder if there is a way to address the fact that we're not just focusing on the intervention in isolation from the patient's overall prognosis, but that it has to be looked at in context.

LAWRENCE: What would that mean? How would you frame it?

LEVIN: Well, we would have to frame it without actually getting into the slippery slope problem. Without talking about the dying patient, how do we define that category? How do you do it clinically? I don't know.

POWELL: Something like an APACHE or an Apgar score, something that gives specific and clear criteria?

MARTINEZ: I think that might be too specific. But can we leave it nonspecific and yet have something that's meaningful? I'm sorry, I interrupted you.

LAWRENCE: No, just one possible thought. As I was looking at these procedures, the palliative care medicine consult seemed helpful. It seemed to me in some cases, there should be a presumption when you're considering forgoing life-sustaining treatment that a palliative care consult would automatically be part of the plan. Maybe that would help to convince families that you're not abandoning the patient. It's just a different kind of care. I don't know if that's practical.

KELLER: Can I just point out on page 4, that C2 already acknowledges the point that we're making about the importance of palliative care? But somehow that gets lost when we focus on specific interventions.

[TECHNICAL DISCUSSION OF HOW AND WHEN VARIOUS INTERVENTIONS ARE LIMITED OR WITHDRAWN]

LAWRENCE: Clinically also in terms of palliative care, it's not a yes/no thing. I mean, it's often a time line where we say, "Let's try one course of antibiotics," thinking of your patient at home. We'll do that once or twice. Then after twice we'll stop because we'll know we're in the territory where nothing is working. It's a process, not an event.

WALTERS: Just let me make one comment and then Michael, you've been very patient again. One of the things we do in bioethics when we negotiate plans is time-limited trials, similar to what Sophia is describing. We say, "For the next thirty-six or forty-eight hours, we're going to do X. Then we'll come back and reevaluate whether X is right, or X plus 1 or X minus 1." I like the idea of having a policy that reflects a process, rather than specifics. Maybe that would help. Michael?

SEEGER: That's actually a very interesting concept. Then it puts in something that could be defined in the documentation—that we have a process of testing a therapy and determining whether it was effective, promising, or futile. We set a parameter and define by these criteria, and at the end of X we will evaluate it accordingly. Thus, we can determine that it's futile.

MARTINEZ: Isn't that similar to the section of the Oregon statute that Sam mentioned? Something about the advance directive providing for the attending physician to try life support as long as it was beneficial and then, when it was no longer helping the patient, being able to discontinue it. That sounds like the policy is able to build in the idea of trials.

WALTERS: This is what people argue in the ethics literature. You try something and see if it works. If it doesn't work, you are justified in stopping it.

RICE: While I agree with what you said about people, families, and the world thinking, "Oh, life will go on forever," I think that in the hospital, it's more a sense of, "You're going to abandon me because I'm dying." Patients and families fear that. So this approach, this process really mitigates that fear. It says, "No, you're involved with me. You're dying, but we're in this together."

CARRELTON: I think you're on to something. There are a lot of problems coming to terms with clinical reality. But I do find that often what's necessary is helping people realize that they're still part of the process.

KELLER: I want to go back to your palliation concept. When you have an engaged family with an active dialogue and an understanding of the situation, you don't even need to go through the palliative care consult. They're already on board. They get it.

The problem with palliation as required policy for this is that it's most useful for the families that are either not understanding the clinical situation or not dealing with it in a way we view as rational. We say, "Difficult family, difficult doctor." Palliative care is for dying patients whom we are not able to treat adequately within the limits of what society allows. If you want to go to hospice, you have to specifically say, "I accept the following limits on the kinds of treatments that will be available to me."

PRINCE: Not any longer. Under new hospice interpretations, patients can continue to receive some kinds of care that used to be considered strictly curative and not appropriate for hospice. You don't have to make the same kinds of stark decisions about treatment.

LEVIN: Could I bring us back to a suggestion on the policy? I find an inconsistency in it. There are all these really good things here, like principle 1, the very first bullet on page 2. "Physicians and other providers have no medical, legal, or ethical obligation to offer or provide treatment(s) that are not medically indicated." Then there is that other statement, C2 on page 4, which repeats the same thing. That, I think, is all fine and should remain.

WALTERS: Yes, I understand what you're saying. When I sat down to read this policy for the first time in a long time, I thought, "What a lot of words!" By the time you get through it, you don't know where you've been. The first thing I'd like to see is a two-page policy. You've got to get it in two pages or it's not helpful in the trenches.

Second, I think it should have a different starting point. I love this discussion we've been having. It's been very clarifying. When patients are actively dying, the focus should be on their physical, emotional, and spiritual comfort, and the comfort of their families. When a patient is not clearly dying—when there is potential for clinical improvement—we have a different discussion and different decisions. But, in the presence of active dying, we want to focus on what will benefit this patient most at this time. Then we need a process that gets us to that decision and a policy that speaks to that goal.

LEVIN: I would argue ethically and legally that we need a policy that helps caregivers figure out what they're supposed to do.

Unfortunately, we are just about out of time. We knew when we began this discussion that we couldn't hope to resolve these difficult issues in one session. But we've made a start and I know that this matter will come back to this committee again. Sophia, as the point person on this policy, you had the first word and now you get the last.

LAWRENCE: Someone asked before what the purpose of the policy is. My understanding is that hospital policies are intended to provide structure, information, and guidance to help clinicians and administrators through a set of consistent processes. This is an especially difficult policy because it deals with hard issues, which are made harder by the constraints of state law.

My goal—and this discussion has been enormously helpful—is to develop a policy that reflects the clinical realities of end-of-life care, the professional and ethical obligations we have to dying patients, and the legal realities that shape to some extent what we do. I will take my notes of this meeting and try to do a first draft of a revised and simplified policy that captures what has been said here. Again, thank you so much for your thoughtful comments and suggestions.

INDEX

ABOUT THE AUTHORS

LINDA FARBER POST is a bioethicist and clinical ethics consultant. She received her B.S.N. from Skidmore College, her M.A. in psychiatric nursing and education from New York University, and her J.D. from the Benjamin N. Cardozo School of Law. For almost nine years, she was a full-time member of the Division of Bioethics at Montefiore Medical Center and an assistant professor of bioethics at Albert Einstein College of Medicine. In those capacities, she conducted clinical ethics consultations and case conferences for clinical staff, presented bioethics teaching sessions and grand rounds for medical students and residents, advised on the development of institutional policies and procedures, and developed and conducted research on bioethical issues. She also coordinated and was a core faculty member in the postgraduate Certificate Program in Bioethics and Medical Humanities. Ms. Post lectures and publishes articles and chapters on bioethical issues, including advance health care planning, ethics in long-term care, decisions about care at the end of life, ethics in palliative care, maternal-fetal issues, and organizational ethics in health care. With colleagues, Jeffrey Blustein and Nancy Neveloff Dubler, she co-authored *Ethics for Health Care Organizations: Theory, Case Studies, and Tools* (United Hospital Fund, 2002). She teaches bioethics in residency training programs, sits on ethics committees, and consults on clinical cases in acute care hospitals, long-term care facilities, home health agencies, and hospice facilities.

JEFFREY BLUSTEIN received his Ph.D. in philosophy from Harvard University under John Rawls and Robert Nozick. He is professor of bioethics at Albert Einstein College of Medicine and clinical ethicist at both the Einstein and Moses Divisions of Montefiore Medical Center. At Montefiore, he conducts bioethics consultations, regular clinical case conferences with various departments and services of the medical center, and grand rounds. Dr. Blustein is a frequent speaker on topics in bioethics to professional and university groups and health care-related organizations and agencies regionally and nationally. He annually teaches an undergraduate philosophy course at Barnard College on ethics and medicine and is a core faculty member of the Certificate Program in Bioethics and Medical Humanities, conducted jointly by Montefiore Medical Center/Albert Einstein College of Medicine and Benjamin N.

Cardozo Law School of Yeshiva University. He is the author of *Parents and Children: The Ethics of the Family* (Oxford University Press, 1982) and *Care and Commitment: Taking the Personal Point of View* (Oxford University Press, 1991). With Carol Levine and Nancy Dubler, he co-edited *The Adolescent Alone* (Cambridge University Press, 1999), and with Linda Farber Post and Nancy Dubler co-authored *Ethics for Health Care Organizations: Theory, Case Studies, and Tools* (United Hospital Fund, 2002). Blustein has published numerous articles and reviews in such journals as *Southern Journal of Philosophy, Journal of Medical Ethics, Theoretical Medicine and Bioethics, Bioethics, Hastings Center Report, Metaphilosophy, Journal of Social Philosophy,* and *Dialogue.* He is currently at work on his third monograph, *Memory and Responsibility: Reflections on Our Relations with the Past.*

NANCY NEVELOFF DUBLER is the director of the Division of Bioethics, Department of Epidemiology and Population Health, Montefiore Medical Center, and professor of epidemiology and population health at the Albert Einstein College of Medicine. She received her B.A. from Barnard College and her LL.B. from the Harvard Law School. Ms. Dubler directs the Bioethics Consultation Service at Montefiore Medical Center (founded in 1978) as a support for analysis of difficult clinical cases presenting ethical issues in the health care setting; this service uses mediation as its process. She lectures extensively and is the author of numerous articles and books on termination of care, home care and long-term care, geriatrics, prison and jail health care, and AIDS. She is co-director of the Certificate Program in Bioethics and the Medical Humanities, conducted jointly by Montefiore Medical Center/Albert Einstein College of Medicine and Benjamin N. Cardozo Law School of Yeshiva University. Her most recent books are *The Ethics and Regulation of Research with Human Subjects,* Coleman, Menikoff, Goldner and Dubler (LexisNexis, 2005); *Bioethics Mediation: A Guide to Shaping Shared Solutions,* co-author, Carol Liebman (United Hospital Fund, 2004); *Ethics On Call: Taking Charge of Life-and-Death Choices in Today's Health Care System,* with David Nimmons (Harmony Books, 1993); and *Ethics for Health Care Organizations: Theory, Case Studies, and Tools,* with Jeffrey Blustein and Linda Farber Post (United Hospital Fund, 2002). She consults often with federal agencies, national working groups, and bioethics centers.